TOWARDS
Outstanding

A Guide to Excellence in Health and Social Care

Towards Outstanding

A guide to excellence in health and social care

© Pavilion Publishing & Media

The author has asserted her rights in accordance with the Copyright, Designs and Patents Act (1988) to be identified as the author of this work.

Published by:
Pavilion Publishing and Media Ltd
Blue Sky Offices, 25 Cecil Pashley Way
Shoreham by Sea, West Sussex
BN43 5FF

Tel: 01273 434 943
Email: info@pavpub.com
Web: www.pavpub.com

Published 2021

A catalogue record for this book is available from the British Library.

ISBN: 978-1-913414-69-6

Pavilion Publishing and Media is a leading publisher of books, training materials and digital content in mental health, social care and allied fields. Pavilion and its imprints offer must-have knowledge and innovative learning solutions underpinned by sound research and professional values.

Author: Terri Salt
Production editor: Mike Benge, Pavilion Publishing and Media Ltd.
Cover design: Emma Dawe, Pavilion Publishing and Media Ltd
Page layout and typesetting: Emma Dawe, Pavilion Publishing and Media Ltd
Printing: CMP Digital Print Solutions

Contents

For all those working in health and social care who have provided the inspiration for this book, and who continue to provide world class care and treatment in the most challenging of circumstances.

"If you think you are too small to make a difference, try sleeping with a mosquito."

Dalai Lama

For Toby Henshaw, who I failed by booking a holiday where the pool had no lines on the bottom – it really is all about what is important to people using services.

For my children and foster children, all genuinely good young adults, who have taught me that if you put in the effort you enjoy it far more and improve outcomes, almost as a side-effect.

For my long-suffering husband, Toby, who has taught me more than he will ever know; who questions bravely and makes me think.

Foreword

This innovative book has been written by someone who has been actively involved with health and social care regulation for many years. Terri Salt has a nursing background and, although all individuals involved in all aspects of health and social care will find this publication extremely useful, nurses especially will profit from an exploration of this text.

This is not a traditional textbook where one can commence reading any individual chapter; rather it takes readers through the various components of the current regulatory framework and where the whole is greater than the sum of the parts. Given the COVID-19 pandemic it is difficult to predict the format of future health and social care inspections, but the five regulatory domains of Safe, Effective, Caring, Responsive and Well-Led and the corresponding key lines of enquiry are likely to endure for the foreseeable future.

Terri Salt does give a caveat at the beginning of this text that simply reading it won't get the reader an improved rating at an inspection; whilst everyone would like to achieve an outstanding grade for the care they deliver, this is not always possible. However, reading this book will illuminate what is and what is not outstanding practice. The style reminds me very much of Florence Nightingale's *Notes on Nursing: What it is and What it is Not* published in 1859. In this, perhaps the very first nursing textbook, Miss Nightingale stresses that her book is not meant as a comprehensive guide from which to teach oneself to be a nurse but to help in the practice of treating others. In a similar way, through narrative dialogue and helpful real-life vignettes, Terri explores her vision of what outstanding practice looks like.

Towards Outstanding is easy to read and, while its caveat is a wise one, it does help clarify what CQC inspectors look for and triangulate when weighing up the factual objective evidence provided by the institution with that of more subjective evidence they solicit through observation and interview with service users and individual staff members. For the uninitiated the complexities of a CQC inspection may appear daunting, and for some quite stressful. *Towards Outstanding* simplifies the processes involved and makes it absolutely clear what they seek to elucidate. I whole heartedly recommend this publication.

Dr Alan Glasper
Emeritus professor of Nursing Studies
The University of Southampton.
Formerly a CQC specialist advisor

About the author

Terri Salt is an Inspection Manager for the Care Quality Commission (CQC), and has previously been Head of Hospital Inspection for North London. She has previously been a team leader for inspectors working in adult social care and primary medical services and is among the most experienced regulators of health and social care in England. A registered adult and sick children's nurse and coach with postgraduate qualifications in public sector leadership, adult education, and healthcare, Terri is a regular contributor to *The British Journal of Nursing*. She is the Founder and Director of Towards Outstanding, which offers education and support to health and social care providers and staff wanting to use reflective practice to improve the care and treatment people receive.

Towards Outstanding is built upon the principle that all services can, and should, provide excellent care. It's about learning through reflection and sharing outstanding practice.

The company is affiliated to Salt of The Earth Consulting Limited, which provides executive coaching, keynotes, board development and organisational assessment for providers of health, social care, and education leadership. From February, the Centre for Reflective Practice Education will offer assessed courses for providers who want to support staff in developing their use of reflection, to improve outcomes for all. We are also able to offer bespoke training packages for specialist services and providers outside of the English health and social care regulatory system.

The Towards Outstanding Limited website will go live in February 2021 and will offer further support to providers and staff wanting to use reflective practice to improve the care and treatment people receive.

To discuss how Towards Outstanding could support your organisation, or for any other enquiries, please contact terri@saltoftheeartconsulting.com.

Part 1 – Introduction

Disclaimer

In writing this book, some names and identifying details have been changed to protect the privacy of individuals. Their inclusion is because they have demonstrated good practice and it would be nice to acknowledge those mentioned in the case studies, but I have not always been able to ask them and so feel I cannot name them. Hopefully, they may recognise themselves and their stories and feel justifiably proud.

I have written this book based on far too many years' experience of health and social care and regulation. A number of my examples pre-date the establishment of the current regulator for England, the Care Quality Commission, but I hope the messages to be drawn from reflecting on them may prove useful in considering how to improve the experience of the people that you care for. Good care hasn't changed much over the years; it has evolved and become more accountable, but the underpinning foundations of compassion, kindness, team working, attention to detail and personal preferences remain as true today, as ever.

The book is my work and has not been endorsed by the Commission. I rather hope that there is nothing contained within that would be at odds with the views of others who work in health or social care or in regulation, and that the key messages allow reflection on how well a service meets the expectations of the legislative framework, but I am not going to tell you, in detail, how to run your service nor can I give you an unearned advantage in the inspection process.

Simply reading this book isn't going to get you an improved rating. I have no influence over that process, there is a strict quality assurance and benchmarking process, whereby inspection ratings are agreed. I hope you do get improved ratings. If you are reading this book, the chances are we are on the same side and we both want people to experience high quality care.

The premise of the book is that providers and staff will reflect with honesty on how they deliver care and treatment and then use those reflections to drive improvements. There are no guarantees: you and your staff have to put the effort into understanding your own service, being honest about shortcomings and recognising the strengths that you can build on. The book will hopefully guide you towards an understanding of where you need to travel but it is not a free ticket. There is no easy ride to excellence. Indeed, putting the work in and harvesting the fruits of your labours is part of the joy that comes with improved outcomes. It offers a way of thinking, not a replacement for thinking.

Information produced by public bodies in the UK, such as the Care Quality Commission, NHS England and the Department of Health and Social Care is included and used in accordance with the Open Government Licence v3.0.

The licencing conditions can be found at http://www.nationalarchives.gov.uk/doc/open-government-licence/version/3/

Information produced by the Care Quality Commission can be found at https://cqc.org.uk/

The context

The Towards Outstanding series of books and training materials is intended to support services in England that are registered with the Care Quality Commission to provide regulated activities. They should have applicability to all sectors, and materials can be adapted to make them more relevant to specific organisations. They are not so closely aligned to the inspection methodologies that they will become less useable as the way inspections are carried out changes – this will inevitably happen over time, but the basis of good care is timeless. The global impact of the Coronavirus pandemic has impacted on the way services are provided and the way they are regulated. There is likely to be a move towards more remote monitoring through the use of data and intelligence, which is why it is so important to have clear evidence of what you are doing well and to share this through engagement with the regulator.

The book series does focus on the legislative framework for England, but with very little work can be adapted to be relevant in other countries that embrace health and social care regulation as a force for bringing about improvements, particularly where ratings are given.

The Welsh regulations for providers of adult social care, for example, have significant overlap and include many of the same requirements as the regulations that providers of adult social care in England must adhere to. The Regulation and Inspection of Social Care (Wales) Act 2016 makes many similar requirements to the Health and Social Care Act 2008 (Regulated Activities) Regulations 2014. Scotland's Health and Social Care Standards are worded differently but impose very similar requirements on providers. The Regulation and Quality Improvement Authority (RQIA) operates in Northern Ireland, and while its standards are, perhaps, more explicit, they set the same requirements. The framework for the Health Information and Quality Authority for Ireland has more in common with the English framework than is different. While Canada has different guidance and standards for each province, the content is remarkably similar.

My experience and the case studies in the main text are predominantly from England. The messages are international and have relevance to most countries where health and social care is delivered with similar national or provincial standards. The list of English-speaking countries with aligned regulation frameworks is long and includes, but is not limited to (in no particular order):

- Canada
- Ireland
- Scotland
- Wales
- Northern Ireland
- Bahamas
- Malta and Gozo
- United Arab Emirates
- Mauritius
- South Africa
- Singapore
- Hong Kong
- Jamaica
- Australia
- USA
- India

Many non-English speaking countries also have aligned regulation of health and social care settings, too, particularly across Europe.

Good care is good care regardless of where it is provided. There is a commonality of understanding among health and social care professionals the world over about what excellence looks like. Achieving it can be a little harder.

Excellence in health and social care has changed very little since I started training; it has always been about providing personalised care that meets the needs and preferences of individuals. The legal framework has changed, the level of accountability has changed, the way services are regulated has changed a little (but not as much as might be imagined) and the expectations of society have changed, but if one reads the works of long ago one can see the essence of care has remained the same: Florence Nightingale wrote, "The symptoms or the sufferings generally considered to be inevitable and incident to the disease are very often not symptoms of the disease at all, but of something quite different – of the want of fresh air, or of light, or of warmth, or of quiet, or of cleanliness, or of punctuality and care in the administration of diet, of each or of all of these." If slightly more modern words were used, the statement could easily have been written by any Director of Nursing of an acute or mental health trust or any care home manager today.

From a medical perspective, Hippocrates himself said, "It's far more important to know what sort of person has a disease than what disease the person has". The modern version of the Hippocratic oath says, "I will remember that I do not treat a fever chart, a cancerous growth, but a sick human being, whose illness may affect the person's family and economic stability. My responsibility includes these related problems, if I am to care adequately for the sick."

The basic underpinning tenets of outstanding care really have changed very little. We just need to remember them, and that can be challenging in our fast-paced and ever-changing world.

Introduction

"Outstanding does not mean perfect"

Professor Sir Mike Richards (CQC Chief Inspector of Hospitals 2013-2017)

If you are looking for a book that provides a set of checklists and tools to complete, then this probably isn't the right book for you. I aim to set you on the path towards excellence by suggesting ways of thinking, ways of growing yourself and your organisation and by sharing stories of excellence in health and social care. The journey towards an 'Outstanding' rating is about being a learning organisation; about reflecting on what you do well and building on that by creating a compassionate and person-centred model of care. If your focus is on receiving an 'Outstanding' rating from the regulator, I would venture that you have a long way to go. The best organisations are delighted to receive their rating but that isn't the key driver. The only effective reasons for aiming towards an 'Outstanding' rating is to improve the care and treatment of the people using your service and to improve the working lives of your staff.

Some of the content may come across as autobiographical, indeed some of it is. That is not because I want to be the subject of the book, on the whole I dislike being centre stage, but rather to demonstrate how our own experiences impact on how we react to the world. Without understanding *why* we hold certain views, how our own opinions were formed, it is difficult to be truly objective. Self-awareness is necessary before we understand others.

Our own reflection should enable us to see others through kinder spectacles and to understand why they think and act as they do. I grew up in a fairly feral household, unfettered by many restrictions at all. I can see why my husband, who grew up in a much more risk averse family, worries more than I do and how this leads to the children getting cross when he is perceived as being overly protective and overly helpful, now that they are adults.

It is clear to those who have worked across several sectors that the highest performing organisations have much in common, regardless of the services they provide or their size and complexity. This book offers insights across various provider types but has more about the services I know very well. There is much about acute healthcare providers, as that is where I have worked most recently. There is a lot about residential and nursing care homes too, as there are far more of these and they vary so much in what they provide and the quality of how they provide it. The setting probably doesn't matter much. The messages are often universal and can be transferred between settings. Listening to staff is important whether you are a GP, a sexual health clinic, an ambulance service or a small home for people with learning disabilities.

People want and expect to receive high-quality safe care that is close to home and at the right time – without undue waits or time lapses that allow for a deterioration in their condition. I have yet to meet many staff who didn't enter the caring professions to deliver the best health and social care; most staff genuinely want to provide good care. Despite this, we know that the quality of care is variable – between organisations, different conditions, and different patient groups.

So why aren't all health and social care services rated as 'Outstanding' by the Care Quality Commission? What differentiates one service from another, similar service? Is the rating indicative of the quality of care or is it down to idiosyncratic judgments by the inspection team?

This is probably a good point at which to make it clear that this book represents my own experience, knowledge and opinion and does not carry an endorsement from the Commission, although I hope few in the Commission would disagree with what I have written. There is no guarantee that by using the ideas within the book an 'Outstanding' rating will automatically follow. Any rating must remain unbiased and a judgement about the care and treatment people are receiving; it cannot be about having used a particular model of care or reading a particular book.

Interestingly, the proportion of services who achieve the top 'Outstanding' rating is fairly evenly spread, both geographically and across different types of services. In 2019, just 4% of adult social care providers were given the highest rating, with a further 80% rated good. Primary Medical Service inspection teams rated just 4% of GPs as 'Outstanding' and about the same figure for NHS Trusts.

Hospices fare the best with 25% rated as 'Outstanding' and a further 75% as good. Eight percent of independent hospitals achieved an 'Outstanding' rating and a further 62% were rated as good.

There has been some slight improvement in the overall figures over time across services, but no dramatic change. The race to the top is made ever more difficult as the benchmark goes up and societal expectations change. For example, more NHS patients are now operated on in independent hospitals through Clinical Commissioning Groups contracted services; it becomes more usual to have better hotel type services – single en suite rooms, a better menu and easier appointment-booking system. There is a risk that people become less content with the more common NHS bays and tiny pull down, pay-as-you-go television consoles.

Hospices generally provide an exceptional service (so the bar for them to reach 'Outstanding' is, perhaps, set a little higher – we all need something to challenge us). It would be hard for an NHS hospital to compete directly in terms of facilities, volunteer support services, personalised care and symptom control. A few do but they really are the exception. Independent hospitals are not usually set up, staffed or resourced to provide exemplary end of life care and there is something to be said for providers knowing where their strengths lie. A small independent hospital is not going to hold its own in the quality of provision for end of life care when compared to a hospice with a multi-faith chaplaincy, round the clock specialist palliative medicine support and an entire education faculty geared towards ensuring their staff have real expertise in end of life care. The hospices are leading the way with true virtuosity and perhaps that is right and proper. If we can't get it right as someone approaches life's end, when can we?

> The Care Quality Commission (CQC) is the independent regulator of health and social care in England.
>
> Their role is to make sure health and social care services provide people with safe, effective, compassionate, high-quality care and they encourage care to improve.

The current inspection ratings are widely reported; there is a legal obligation for these to be displayed on the provider's website and in the service. People are promoted and receive tangible rewards for high ratings, but inspection teams are also very aware that, sadly, some people lose their jobs in response to an 'inadequate' rating. Staff agreeing the ratings do so with full consideration of the impact for individuals and the wider health and social care economy, but patient safety and the quality of care must remain the primary consideration. Ratings are given not as a marketing tool but rather because it is important that people who use services see them. The aim of the regulation is to increase transparency about quality of health and care services, encourage improvement and help people who use services to make choices about their care.

The bonus for providers of 'Good' or 'Outstanding' services is that they can use the rating as a route to support recruitment of high-calibre staff, to secure contracts tendered by local commissioners, to encourage people to choose their service and to reduce the burden and frequency of regulation.

Current inspection frequency rules mean that services rated 'Good' or 'Outstanding' get inspected less frequently. Inspections are more frequent where it is believed there is a risk to the safety or well-being of people who receive the service or there has been a significant deterioration in the quality of that service. If there is no intelligence to inform the inspection of the service, then frequency rules apply. If your adult social care service is rated 'Outstanding' then the next inspection takes place within 30 months; if it has been rated inadequate for any of the key questions or for the overall rating, then the time between inspections is reduced to six months.

The Health and Social Care Act 2008 (Regulated Activities) Regulations 2014: Regulation 20A says that providers must ensure that their rating(s) are displayed conspicuously and legibly at each location delivering a regulated service, and on their website (if they have one).

CQC can prosecute for a breach of this regulation or a breach of part of the regulation and can and do move directly to prosecution without first serving a warning notice.

As data quality improves and as resources become ever more straitened, the Commission is moving towards a much more risk-based inspection programme and is considering changes to the publicised frequency rules. This will mean that where services are identified as higher risk, they will be more likely to be targeted for inspection; it will no longer be possible to estimate when you are likely to be inspected simply by knowing the rules. Acute hospitals have realised for some time that the Commission cannot sustain an inspection programme that meets the published frequency intervals for all core services. This will inevitably make it harder to move to 'Outstanding' through one inspection; the things that make a provider 'Outstanding' will have to be sustained and more widely spread across the services. That must be a real benefit for patients and people using services as providers simply have to try harder and sustain best practice. The genuinely 'outstanding' services understand this and will continue to work towards improved ratings through improved care quality.

The Primary Medical Services Directorate, which includes GPs, dentists, private doctors, and telemedicine services, have started a new approach to monitoring, inspecting and rating services that are rated 'Good' or 'Outstanding' by implementing the Annual Regulatory Review (ARR) and focused inspections to re-rate. The ARR will be the main vehicle for monitoring the activity of general practice services for locations rated 'Good' or 'Outstanding'. Services with any other rating will be inspected. This process is intended to streamline the monitoring activity and bring more consistency to the Commission's decision-making. If change in quality is suspected because of data or other intelligence, then the service will be inspected. Clearly for Primary Medical Services (PMS), this means there is a real benefit from providing a level of service that meets the threshold for a solid 'good' or 'outstanding'. The better you are the less you are inspected.

The Adult Social Care Directorate is also working towards more efficient and effective ways of working. Providers and services will be inspected in response to risk and at frequencies determined by their rating and type of service. A clear message that the monitoring of services will increase but that the inspection frequency will be determined, in part, by the existing rating.

Where pertinent, I will explain a little about the inspection frameworks, the regulations and the quality assurance processes in later chapters, but this book is essentially about the quality of care and how providing high-quality care benefits both the provider and the people using services. It's a win/win situation.

Hospitals Business Plan 2019/2020

During 2019/2020, the Hospitals Directorate planned to make ambitious changes to the model of inspection to make significant progress in delivering intelligence-driven regulation of the sector. The aim is to move to a more flexible approach with greater emphasis on monitoring service quality, enabling a programme of inspection that responds to the risk to service users as opposed to being driven by a strict and inflexible reinspection cycle. This change in approach will improve the experience of regulated organisations with a reduction in the burden of inspection activity.

Primary Medical Services Business Plan 2019/2020

Primary Medical Services and integrated care is at the heart of widespread and rapid changes to the health and social care landscape. The way we approach our work mirrors the landscape in which we regulate. We are focused on encouraging improvement and innovation across the providers we regulate. We will continue to engage with stakeholders and work closely with providers to ensure that our approach meets our purpose of ensuring that safe and effective care is provided; we reduce the burden on providers and we use intelligence to direct our resources in the most meaningful way possible.

Adult Social Care Business Plan 2019/2020

Across Adult Social Care (ASC), efficiencies are required to support leaner ways of working. We remain entirely focused on the quality of care and encouraging improvement and will continue to be risk based and responsive to changes in risk. Our plan therefore needs to enable us to respond to risk and keep people safe but also flexible enough to enable us to properly resource and lead improvements to how we work.

What is sometimes missing in the regulatory cycle is the provider demonstrating and providing evidence of the particularly good work they are doing. As an inspectorate, the default assumption is that the service will be sitting within the range that is 'good' for each key question on the report. My experience tells me that it is easy for inspection teams to find the evidence that drops this to a 'Requires improvement' or even 'Inadequate', but much harder to see the excellent practice that tips it into 'outstanding'. The provider needs to ensure that they show the inspection team the evidence; just saying, "We have a lovely team who are kind" simply isn't evidence – it's an opinion. We will look at the difference between evidence and opinion later.

> Evidence is the available body of facts or information indicating whether a belief or proposition is true or valid. If you are telling an inspection team the greatest thing about your service is the team, then you need to provide evidence to support this opinion.

It might surprise some to learn that inspection teams are human too. While every effort is made to ensure that ratings are awarded objectively and entirely based on evidence, there is always going to be a degree of subjectivity and personal values that impact on the final report. Providers and inspectors need to be aware of those human factors and work to ensure that they are used for the good of the people using services. Self-awareness is, in my opinion, key to raising standards. That self-awareness includes starting with consideration of how people have been formed into who they are today, how their values and beliefs have been formed and who have been key influencers. It radiates up as the experience of the individual impacts on how they perform their work and how they interact with their colleagues. This will without doubt affect team performance, norms and values. Peer pressure is powerful and needs harnessing to be advantageous to all.

Team performance impacts on the care delivery and the management response. It also impacts on how the inspection teams perceive the provider – as I said, we are but human. Part of the role of the 'Outstanding' provider is to lead these individuals towards self-awareness and a desire to achieve excellence; to do that they need to understand the people they employ, and work with them to develop a shared value, a shared understanding of what constitutes good practice and a commitment to the team. Not only do individual staff need to be self-aware, but so do teams and leaders. Really honest reflection is essential as a tool for driving improvements. My favourite mantra is that, "A tick box chart is never going to cut the mustard". All the lists in the world won't ensure you are given an 'Outstanding' rating; it has to come from leaders who value and support their team to deliver excellence because it is the right thing to do.

> A Key Performance Indicator (KPI) is a measurable value that demonstrates how effectively a company is achieving key business objectives. Organisations use KPIs at multiple levels to evaluate their success at reaching targets. High-level KPIs may focus on the overall performance of the service, while low-level KPIs may focus on processes in departments or the work of individual team members.

Ensuring a team meets their Key Performance Indicators may get you a 'Good' rating but is less likely to get you to 'Outstanding' – that needs a sustained positive culture that is inclusive and listening.

So, now to think about how I came to my understanding of 'outstanding', or 'excellence', and what is the trigger that makes me feel a service is 'outstanding'. I do mean *feel* – all the data in the world won't necessarily tip it over into the top rating. It must be about the patients' or service users' experience and how standardised good care is personalised to make it excellent care.

As I began to write this book I thought back to my younger years and remembered with pleasure some of the lightbulb moments that have helped me understand excellence in health and social care, so here are a couple of personal stories.

Emma

As a teenager I volunteered at British Red Cross summer camps for physically disabled children. Each volunteer was paired with a guest and was required to support them by providing all their care and entertainment. We became their best friends and carers for two weeks. There was a registered nurse on site and a team of adults supervising the cooking and activities, but we were given huge responsibility for 14-year-olds. We'd never heard of risk assessments and were fairly uninformed about the limitations that some disabilities brought.

Emma was an 11-year-old girl who had a degenerative neuromuscular disease. She was entirely dependent on a wheelchair and attendant to move around. This was well before electric wheelchairs became mainstream. She couldn't sit unsupported and life was generally quite limited.

I don't know if many will remember the summer of 1976, but it was hot – ridiculously hot – and sitting in a plastic wheelchair surrounded by support cushions was even hotter. On site was a fabulous outdoor pool. Emma really wanted to swim like most of the other children on the camp. She had never been in a pool before. For the first couple of days we sat at the top of the steep steps watching others who were more mobile splashing around. Then we decided this was so unfair; Emma wanted to swim, and she should be able to do so. I can't say the carrying down the steps was particularly elegant, but she was well covered in towels and squealed as the chair rocked and rolled in the hands of four big, teenage lads. Then without any great dignity (but, at the same time, with the utmost dignity, kindness and respect) she was lifted by the same four lads grabbing various parts of her body and lowered into the water. She had a Heath Robinson safety harness in the form of a sheet held by two other lads. I was already in the water to 'catch' Emma.

My goodness, it was a loud scream when she realised the water was unheated. I still have the photograph that one of the adults took and it remains one of my favourite pictures ever. The sheer joy, the absolute trust, the experience of weightlessness for a child who was pretty heavy and whose limbs felt like lead most of the time.

I won't describe the method of getting her into an unadapted rowing boat in the park where we picnicked, but it was great fun and another entirely new experience. Lifting her out of the window for midnight feasts on a 'secret' lawn was also great fun, now I think about it.

How does this impact now? Clearly expectations around risk assessment and the balancing of personal choice against the degree of risk have changed, but that's not really the most important message. What it really taught me – more latterly, when I reflect, than at the time – is that it is difficult to provide truly personal care that meets the needs and preferences of the individual if we don't take some risks. I've seen good examples of this in regulated settings and will expand upon this in other chapters. It also taught me that most things can be achieved with good team working and a shared sense of purpose; again, more later.

A reminder at this point that times and expectations around risk assessment and child volunteering have changed since the 1970s. I am not suggesting you take people using services to a swimming pool and throw them in, nor am I suggesting that you can use unsupervised child volunteers to deliver care.

Lexie

This little girl taught me one of the most valuable and enduring lessons of my professional life. Lexie was a tiny seven-year-old child who was significantly disabled by cerebral palsy with an associated learning disability. I met her when she was admitted to the respiratory unit at what was then the Hospital for Sick Children, London, but which is now Great Ormond Street Hospital. Lexie was a regular visitor with frequent episodes of pneumonia. She usually lit the ward in a warm glow, a raspberry blown on her foot or tummy resulted in loud, contagious giggles. On this occasion she was admitted to the ward having had orthopaedic surgery to manage contractures. She needed to be in long leg plaster casts for a few weeks. She came to us because we knew her well and she was more familiar with the staff and surroundings.

I was a newly qualified staff nurse with a lovely, bright red, petersham belt and shiny silver buckle. I wore a ridiculous frilly hat atop my head and a crisply starched white apron: I really thought I was the bee's knees. The ward sister was having a long weekend off to go to Wimbledon and I was left in charge. I was confident that I could do it and do it well. Everything went smoothly, linen cupboards were tidy, the medicines had been restocked, new consumables ordered, the staffing rota for the next month done. I was flying!

The ward sister, a wonderful mentor and guide, returned for her handover. She was very thorough, very well informed but also exceedingly kind and supportive. She walked around the ward checking I had completed all the essential tasks and giving positive feedback. We stopped by each bed while she spoke with the children and any parents that were there. She looked at each child's charts. I knew they were all perfectly completed, so was beginning to feel a bit smug.

We reached Lexie, who was still a bit miserable and whiny. She'd been 'off colour' all weekend and I explained this in my handover. I said I thought it was a combination of the heat and being fed up with being in the cast. No response from Sister. She just looked at the charts and tickled Lexie gently. We completed the handover round and went back to her office. I was expecting a pat on the back and to be allowed off a few minutes early. The sister simply looked at me and said, "Before you finish, please could you go and give Lexie some analgesia and then look at her again in an hour and if she is still uncomfortable, perhaps you could ask the doctor to review her medicines? Then perhaps you could ring her mother and apologise."

What a powerful lesson. I have never made assumptions about behaviours since and have always ensured that anyone in my care – or in services I am inspecting – have adequate pain management. I cried myself to sleep that night, knowing I had been too pleased with myself to see what was before me and as a result a small child, who was unable to tell us what they were feeling using the spoken word, was left in pain.

As importantly, and without realising it until many years later, I also learned that the best way to address staff shortcomings was not to shout at them in public, not to humiliate them, not to apportion blame but to allow the member of staff to think through their failing and to try and put it right.

These two personal stories are intended to demonstrate that our earlier and ongoing experiences impact on how we interact, our values as we go through life and our perception of what 'good' or 'outstanding' care looks like. By reflecting on our individual and collective experiences we can identify organisational and personal strengths and build on those. A focus on understanding why something is good and how best practice can be disseminated leads services towards that cherished 'Outstanding' rating.

That is not to say that we don't address shortcomings but rather that by focusing on areas of good practice, the 'less good' becomes more evident to the staff themselves. An 'outstanding' provider usually knows that the staff have the answer to making improvements and supports them to do so.

"Knowledge of the self is the mother of all knowledge. So, it is incumbent on me to know myself, to know it completely."
Kahlil Gibran

This book is not going to show you any magic tricks. It isn't going to provide you with a script. If you want to be part of the exclusive '5% club' you must work at it. You need ambition and must want to improve and to be the best. There is no quick way, no tricks, no easy path; excellence is what you need to aim for, with a focus on delivering care and treatment that meets people's individual needs and preferences. It's an attitude rather than a task-focused checklist.

If you are a leader, you must persuade your staff that this is what they want to do. You have to support them and listen to them. You must set the direction of travel and show them the aspiration, but they will be the ones who deliver.

That working together to journey, as a team, to a distant point where excellence is sustained (but continually adapting) should be fun and rewarding. We must never lose sight of what draws people to provide health or social care.

As the modern Hippocratic Oath says:

May I always act so as to preserve the finest traditions of my calling and may I long experience the joy of healing those who seek my help.

Part 2 – What is outstanding?

What inspectors think outstanding means?

There are two definitions of 'outstanding'. The first is obvious – it means something is clearly much better than the usual. The second is perhaps more pertinent and is the definition you need to use if you want to provide a truly outstanding service. It means not yet paid, solved, or done: in the context of health and social care services, an outstanding provider will understand there is always more to do, there are always improvements that can be made. Outstanding services do not stand still and think they are good enough. There should never be complacency.

Even if you purchase a commercially produced package that ensures you tick the boxes and have all the right policies in place, all the equipment checks and audits completed, all the staff files up to date, you won't necessarily become outstanding. I would go as far as to suggest that if you expect to become outstanding because you have purchased a package, and found a file to put the newly created policies in, then you are unlikely to receive an 'Outstanding' rating without a significant change in attitude.

To be outstanding takes skilled leadership, engaged staff, determination and sustained effort. It requires you to truly know your service and to want to provide excellent care rather than to simply want an improved rating. There is no easy way.

You cannot usually take what works for one provider or in one location and just transfer the fairy dust across. Each location, each type of service, each leader, each staff group has a unique identity. The provider aiming for an 'Outstanding' rating needs to work with that uniqueness and develop the service towards excellence, building on the strengths of that particular location. That is not to say that there shouldn't be strong corporate governance or standard operating procedures, but that these things alone will never be enough. Going further, to be truly outstanding, the service offered needs to be a bit quirky, it needs to accept and work with the individuality of staff members and people who use the service. It needs to be brave enough to take risks; considered risks perhaps, but risk, nevertheless. It is the uniqueness that makes places and people unforgettable – hopefully in a good way.

A lampshade from a well-known Swedish flat-pack furniture company is never going to hold its own against a Murano glass chandelier. The lampshade isn't bad, it serves its purpose, but it is never really going to stand out. Yes, the Murano is more expensive to buy, but it will probably still be in use after several generations and may well have increased in value since it was made in the 18th century; it could be considered an investment rather than an expense. Expenditure on good care is much the same. Used wisely, investment in care can save money over time; asset stripping or using the cheapest option without consideration of quality rarely results in better outcomes.

I am not suggesting that you cannot learn from others and adapt initiatives or practice to suit your environment; what I am saying is that you can't take an initiative and impose it on the staff and service users without thinking about whether it is appropriate or is wanted. What works in one setting is by no means going to be appropriate in another. Some settings don't need to offer activities – although if you really think outside the box, many types of service could benefit from greater consideration of the importance of activity and distraction. A student bedsit would not suit a Murano Chandelier, after all.

Pendean

I recall a good few years ago visiting a residential home near Midhurst in Sussex, called Pendean (and it did feel like a visit, not an inspection). It was a beautiful country house decorated in a very traditional way with glass doors opening onto a wide terrace from the morning room. They offered a French club, bridge afternoons, a book club, chamber orchestral performances and had several mobility scooters for guests to use to visit the local shops. People said they really enjoyed living there and felt well cared for and fulfilled. My visit was long before ratings were introduced, long before the Care Quality Commission was even established, but I remember it still as being quite exceptional.

What it is important to understand is that the model of care offered by Pendean is not going to work everywhere; many people would feel uncomfortable among the grandeur and activities that the home offered. Some would much prefer fish and chips on the seafront watching the sunset or enjoying the FA cup final on a huge television with a cold beer and a curry. In some places you simply couldn't offer that sort of activity because people are too poorly or do not have the cognition to engage with that level of activity – but you can ask yourself, your staff and your service users, what is appropriate in your setting and what would people enjoy? I know of one GP practice that offers afternoon tea to their very elderly patients.

When I was reflecting on what 'Outstanding' services meant, I asked some current CQC inspection staff from across directorates and of differing grades, what 'Outstanding' meant to them and was surprised that, although they came back with different answers, there was a common thread running through them. I should perhaps point out here that there is a strict quality assurance process and ratings are not determined by inspectors. I use these examples more to share how the inspectors experiences of services have enabled them to understand the commonalities shared by particularly good services.

This is what they said:

"As an inspector who has managed healthcare services in the past, I tell my new colleagues two things about outstanding practice: firstly, it can be quite hard to distinguish between consistently good practice and outstanding practice. Secondly, the best definition of outstanding practice is something the provider is doing that would make managers of similar services want to drive over and see it for themselves. What I have learned is that while outstanding practice may be harder to define, you know it as soon as you see it during your inspection."

Matthew Preston

"I know a service is outstanding when I see hardworking staff empowered and supported by their managers to deliver a programme of constant improvement to exceed their patient's expectation. An outstanding service is an organisation that is in touch and responsive to their workforce, where managers are mindful of getting the basics right consistently with energy and flair."

Sue Johnson

"A service is outstanding if it can palpably demonstrate a positive impact in the services it delivers for patients."

Claire Martin

"I know a service is outstanding when staff at all levels speak with passion and enthusiasm about their role and services. They talk about challenges in a positive way, the culture is open and inclusive, with a common goal to provide the best possible care for people who use services."

Lou Thatcher

"I know a service is outstanding when the leadership, and the culture driven by the leaders at all levels, can demonstrably be shown to improve patient safety and patient outcomes."

Russell Brown

"People were truly placed at the centre of the service and were involved in decisions about their care to an extent that they achieved outstanding and transformative outcomes in their lives. The registered manager and staff have an excellent understanding of people's needs and where staff find ways to improve people's lives by introducing creative activities that opened up new possibilities for them. Both services were services for people living with learning disability."

Zdzislaw (Zee) Matusiewicz

"'Outstanding' to me is not always something you easily put into words in a report or verbalise in a quality assurance meeting; it's a feeling you get when you talk to service users and staff and you just know."

Jacquie Nye

"I know when a service is 'Outstanding' when many patients and their carers can give accounts of when staff went above and beyond to provide care that had a positive effect and a lasting impression on that patient and/or their carers."

Emma Carroll

Those common threads are the things that are sometimes hard to measure, but are the very things that are important if a service is going to grow and develop. One inspection manager, Shaun Marten, gave a clear picture of what he expected of an 'Outstanding' service:

"I know a service is 'Outstanding' when:

- staff have an absolute focus on the patient and their loved ones, can describe all individual needs and care preferences, and patient feedback is overwhelmingly positive

- staff demonstrate in-depth clinical knowledge and technical prowess, and anticipate patient's needs

- patients are obviously well cared for and engaged with what is happening to, and around, them

- staff use data and audit to judge their performance and identify risks to quality and safety; outcomes data is consistently positive and exceeds benchmarks and standards

- when everyone is empowered to challenge and change the ways things are done for the better, talk openly about their failures and the learning and actions that have resulted from this

- patients and staff are encouraged to take risks, but those, and all other, risks are considered and managed

- patients can access the service promptly and easily when they need it

- managers "know their business", know how well they are doing and what they need to do in the short, medium and long-term to deliver an ever-improving service."

For each directorate (Hospitals, Primary Medical Services, Adult Social Care and some specific service types such as hospices) the commission publishes Characteristics of each rating level. They are all based on a four-point scale from Inadequate through Requires Improvement and Good to Outstanding. The default rating is Good with inspection teams needing to provide evidence and justify another rating. It is very easy for inspection teams to find evidence that lowers the rating from Good, but it is much harder to see Outstanding because it is far less tangible.

The characteristics are not a checklist and are not exhaustive but are written to give a picture of a service in respect of the five key questions. Inspection staff make a professional judgement, based on the history of the service and the evidence gathered. Some of the characteristics may not always be appropriate for all different types of services. A service does not have to meet every area covered in the characteristics to fit in that rating section.

Do the reports issued reflect the inspector's definitions about what outstanding means? I think they do. What takes providers over the threshold into 'Outstanding' is the focus on personalised care and the culture they have built with their staff.

I think anyone reading these two paragraphs below, published in a CQC report in 2014, would certainly feel it was deserving of its 'Outstanding' rating. It was the first core service 'Outstanding' rating that was declared nationally within the hospitals directorate and set the bar quite high. This wasn't about fridge temperatures or neat staff records; this was about the impact of staff behaviour and attitudes on patients and those close to them. It was about seeing and feeling, that sense of this being something special.

Frimley Park Hospital

"A porter told us that all his team treated the people who had recently passed away on the wards as if they were, 'Our own nan or mum'. We make sure we look after their dignity and that they are comfortable. Most of us talk to them about where they are going and explain what the mortuary will be like and that their fridge will be cold. It makes our job better if we do it properly and kindly."

"We sat with one elderly person who was being cared for in bed, in a single room, as they were expected to die shortly. This person slid their hand out of the covers to hold our hand and said they weren't really frightened as everyone was so kind to them. They said their grandchildren had visited and bought them lovely presents that were displayed around the room. Then they showed us the bright nail polish that they said one of the night nurses had used when they gave them a manicure. They said, 'I used to like dancing and parties and my nails make me smile and remember those days'."

And from other sectors, the message is equally clear. What makes a truly outstanding service are often the intangibles. Time and again inspectors, managers and specialist advisors say they 'just know'. It cannot and should not be reduced to a simple checkbox exercise; that would be unfair on all those staff who genuinely go the extra mile. For a service to shine out as a beacon of good care it must focus not on gaining an 'Outstanding' rating but on each and every staff member buying into a vision, a strategy, and embedded, everyday practice that truly considers the needs of individuals. The excerpts below from published reports show a variety of ways providers have really considered the needs of the people they care for and given a sense of 'Outstanding' care that goes well beyond the definition of 'good'.

Mountfitchet House

"Throughout the home were 'themed' areas reflecting resident's interests and promoting reminiscence. For example, a library corner, Hollywood wall, dressing table with jewellery, a safe ironing station and rummage boxes."

Birmingham Children's Hospital NHS Foundation Trust

"A young person's advisory group was involved in the development, design and delivery of services for children and young people. They also played a part in the recruitment of senior staff and joined interview panels."

Getta Life Limited, Coventry

"Staff showed inspectors how their care plans were invaluable for personalised care – they could help people to maintain their preferred routines and make life choices in a meaningful way. Two people who used the service had formed a relationship and now lived together as a couple – staff and family had supported them in this, including a celebration of their relationship at their local church. The couple showed inspectors pictures of their ceremony with pride and happiness."

Beverley Parklands Care Home

"A 'Make a Wish' project had been introduced to offer people the opportunity to carry out aspirations they had. We saw one person had always wanted to do a sky dive and had achieved this using a virtual reality headset system. We saw the person who said, 'I felt free and I cannot wait to tell my family I have done a sky dive. They won't believe me.' Other people had been on safari and walked the Great Wall of China using this technology."

Waterloo GP Surgery, Millom

"A member of staff from the practice was delivering training to the local population in a bid to make Millom a 'dementia friendly' town. The practice had also purchased software which aided communication between patients with dementia and their relatives and carers."

Nuffield Health Cambridge Hospital

"There were also courses specifically designed for family members, which included 'Kid's days', which offered the chance for young people whose parents had cancer to find support and answers, and a six-week friends and family course for anyone caring for a person who had cancer. For example, one patient stated, 'The nurse helped me enormously by bringing my children to the unit and explaining to them why I have to have chemotherapy and how it is given which took out all of the mystery for them.'

Northumbria Healthcare NHS Foundation Trust

(A specialist community mental health service for children and young people)

"During a visit to four locations, inspectors heard from young people who used services and carers, as well as managers and staff members. Young people and their parents and carers spoke very positively about their experience of the service – they felt involved in the planning of their care and spoke highly of the staff. Everyone said that staff were respectful and caring."

"Staff were passionate and motivated to improve the health and well-being of young people accessing a service which actively encouraged feedback. There was also an analysis of the comments from parents and young people about their views of the service, with 84% of parents and 75% of young people stating that the service was good, and nothing needed to change."

Woodbury GP Surgery, Exeter

"The practice had an established triage system, with GPs telephoning the patient or carer in advance, within 30 minutes of contacting the practice, to gather information to allow for an informed decision to be made on prioritisation according to clinical need. In cases where the urgency of need was so great that it would be inappropriate for the patient to wait for a GP home visit, alternative emergency care arrangements were made."

Northumberland, Tyne and Wear NHS Foundation Trust

(A mental health and disability trust)

"Staff used flexible methods to ensure that patients and those close to them were involved as partners in their care and treatment. Where patients had complex needs, staff had used equipment to facilitate patient involvement. They recorded patient voices expressing their views and questions to be played in multi-disciplinary meetings they could not attend."

First Community Health and Care CIC

"We saw several notable examples of where the senior managers had flexed to ensure that the staff needs were met. Staff knew their executive team well and there was a genuinely open-door policy. Many staff worked from the office where the executive team were based, which coupled with the small size of the organisation, led not only to personalised care for patients but also to personalised care of the workforce."

"There was a unanimous feeling that every individual member of staff counted and was valued, regardless of their role or position. Staff felt they could genuinely effect change and have a positive impact on the service delivered and the teams they worked in."

"'Outstanding' is when we find patients are genuinely valued and involved in strategy and service development. It is also discovering a healthy culture where staff feel empowered, valued and wilfully display their commitment and happiness."

"I know I've found 'Outstanding' when I walk away feeling this is somewhere I and my loved ones would be well cared for, and I have to fight the desire to put my nursing uniform on and work there."

Geraldine Wilkinson

First impressions
and lavatories

"In the same way that I tend to make up my mind about people within thirty seconds of meeting them, I also make up my mind about whether a business proposal excites me within about thirty seconds of looking at it. I rely far more on gut instinct than researching huge amounts of statistics."

Richard Branson (*Losing My Virginity: How I've Survived, Had Fun, and Made a Fortune Doing Business My Way*, 1999).

As regulators, Commission staff try to be objective and base judgments on evidence alone. The very best inspection staff always use all their senses to understand the quality of care being provided – and that starts, unsurprisingly, before they turn into the driveway, before they see the establishment as they walk from the station or before they enter reception. This won't tell them whether the provider is meeting the Referral to Treatment target for surgery, what the staff survey says or how the provider manages the care of people with learning disabilities, but it will send them a whole host of conscious and subliminal messages. Some of the messages are probably valid (who wants a care home to smell of stale urine?) and some probably less so.

What it is important to understand is that, regardless of how objective someone strives to be, how clear the framework is, how much one tries to lay aside the first impressions, they cannot be unseen, unheard or unsmelled. First impressions cannot be readily archived to a shelf in our brains that doesn't impact on our perception.

The Commission website talks about what happens at the start of the inspection and says, "The inspector or inspection team usually meet senior staff. At this meeting, we will explain:

■ Who the inspection team are.
■ The scope and purpose of the inspection.
■ How we will communicate our findings."

Inspections of acute hospitals, GP practices and GP out-of-hours services often begin with a presentation by the care provider, in which they can give their own view of their performance".

It is human nature to form opinions and to be affected by first impressions. They are important not only for inspections but for how your service users, patients, clients, visiting professionals, neighbours and staff feel. It would be difficult to persuade anyone you were outstanding if you had not given much thought to first impressions and how your service presents itself to the wider world.

First impressions of what, perhaps you ask? I think a wise provider or leader would want to consider the first impressions given by the approach and outside of the premises, the reception area and most importantly the staff and leadership team. Within large organisations and services, the staff teams might want to consider how their part of a service presents itself. This might be a directorate within an acute or mental health trust – what do you sense when you walk onto the stroke ward or long-stay ward? It might be a small community hospital or child development centre. It might be the nursing floor of a large care home. It might be the reception team at a GP surgery or a large dental practice.

The Newcastle upon Tyne Hospitals NHS Foundation Trust

From their CQC emergency department report, the Newcastle upon Tyne Hospitals NHS Foundation Trust stated, "We observed staff smiling and making eye contact with patients during our inspection. Patients and relatives who had visited the department previously told us staff always smiled and made eye contact".

It seems so simple; have your staff make eye contact and smile. It makes a huge difference to their colleagues, their patients or residents and to themselves. Smiling makes people feel better; people who report more positive emotions live longer and healthier lives (Danner et al, 2001). Both smiling and laughter have been found to boost your mood (Neuhoff & Schaefer, 2002).

Unfortunately, people visiting emergency departments aren't always greeted with eye contact and smiles. In stark comparison to Newcastle, the emergency department report for another trust said, "We observed the reception area for a short period of time and saw parents arrive genuinely concerned about their three-week-old baby. We saw the receptionist did not make eye contact or smile. Reception staff did not advise the parents on the current waiting times or who would see their child. The parents' first language did not appear to be English, but there was no offer of a translator." Unsurprisingly, this trust was rated as Inadequate.

Sometimes we cannot see what others see, hear or smell because we have looked too often, and it has become the norm; we ignore the yellow waste skips in the car park, the out-of-date, peeling laminated signs barking orders at people on the front door. We no longer smell the overwhelming odour of stale urine covered up with cheap air freshener or notice the incessant call bells ringing. We accept being ignored by the receptionist and just walk past without expecting interaction. I notice these things each and every time I go somewhere that I haven't been for a while. My children used to play 'Be an inspector' whenever they had GP or hospital appointments – spotting things that were out of place or inappropriate for a patient facing area; it passed the time and heightened their observation skills. If a child notices, then sure as figs are figs, visitors and CQC staff inspecting the service will notice.

It takes a tenth of a second to form an impression of a stranger from their face, and longer exposures don't significantly alter those impressions, although they might boost your confidence in your judgments (Willis & Todorov, 2006).

Those first impressions really do stick – even when we learn new information that should cause us to question that impression. For example, in one set of studies, participants formed impressions of two groups based on a story in which one group coldly massacred the other. The participants formed implicit and explicit evaluations consistent with what they learned (Gregg *et al*, 2006). Subsequently, they were told that the groups had been labelled incorrectly due to experimenter error and should be reversed. Did participants change their perception of which group was 'good' and which was 'bad'? No. Not at all. They continued to respond more positively to the first group despite knowing they had been the murderers. This rather suggests that our first impressions may continue to influence and guide us, even after we have explicitly rejected them.

Considering that implicit reactions predict behaviour in unique and important ways, this suggests that our first impressions may continue to influence and guide us, even after we have explicitly rejected them.

We are all told throughout our lives not to 'judge a book by its cover' and inspection teams try their very best to be objective and form judgements based on evidence, but I would suggest that the 'Outstanding' providers understand that those first impressions set the tone and are hard to overcome if they are not positive.

So, let's talk a bit about the entrance to your property. I think the easiest way to do this is to describe a service I have known since it was a piece of woodland, close to a dual carriageway.

Chestnut Tree House

Chestnut Tree House is a children's hospice in West Sussex. If you don't know much about children's hospices you might imagine places that are shut away from the rest of society, with drawn curtains, muted colours and a mist of misery. Nothing could be further from the truth; while there is inevitably huge sadness and even despair sometimes, they are generally light-filled, joyous places, which are more likely to be filled with laughter than tears.

Most of the children's hospices that I have known are very conscious of their first impressions. Parents and children need to feel reassured and welcomed when they arrive; they need to have their fears dissipated. They want to feel that they are entering a special place that may be where they say their final goodbye to their child, at some point in the future. If the parents are bringing their child who has already passed away, to rest peacefully until the funeral, then the first impression is even more important. You only have one chance to get a first impression right.

You turn off the dual carriageway into a lightly wooded lane. A few yards along the lane are traditional wooden fences with a gateway that leads to what looks like a large country house. The scale is big but not institutional. The grounds are immaculate with neat lawns, manicured flower borders, gravel pathways and plenty of parking. As you drive in you see the bronze statues of three children playing in the gardens. These are happy children, at home in the environment and enjoying life. A good image to portray to people who are perhaps scared, worried about what is through the entrance and what may lie ahead.

There used to be (in my opinion) the most beautiful and tactile giant bronze chestnut half out of its spiky casing that I could never resist touching, but in response to people who felt it looked a bit too much like a baby's bottom, it was moved to a less prominent position. This is a provider that is aware of the impact of the environment on people using the service and who responds to comments and concerns.

The front door has a glass panel that you can peep through – it is much like any front door you might expect to find on a small country house. It is simply a normal door. Nothing scary, no huge signs, nothing to suggest this place is anything but a pretty place to visit. You catch glimpses of bright colours through the huge arched windows that reach from floor to ceiling in the communal areas of the house. The doorbell is answered almost immediately by a smiling volunteer who is tasked with staffing the front reception. You enter and find a large, airy and bright space that has doors through to the main house, where we can see children and staff playing happily while a parent watches and drinks coffee. The receptionist is charming, smiles all the time and asks whether we'd mind signing the visitor's book. There are comfortable, colourful sofas to sit on while the receptionist goes off to find the person in charge. A newsletter and some additional information are provided to look at while waiting. It all feels very calm and relaxed. Just as it should be.

The other part of the hospice where first impressions are paramount is the direct entrance to the Stars suite. This is an area where you arrive through private gardens with a pretty pond and a door directly into the bereaved family's accommodation. I've seen inspectors unfamiliar with children's hospices hold their breath and pale at the thought of entering this area, fearing they might be unable to cope. Imagine then how vital it is that the first impression for parents isn't fearful or overwhelming. Those same inspectors, having crossed the threshold, invariably exhale, look around and smile. Usually they comment on how lovely the space is. The child's bedroom is a wonderfully comfortable, light-filled and personalised room that has been made ready to receive the child. While the bed is designed to keep the child very cool, that isn't obvious; it just looks like a child's bed or cot. Lighting is gentle and a warm white. A small sitting room provides a space for families to sit, cry without being watched, have a drink, eat in privacy. A safe and protective space for the family to spend their time together until the funeral. It is simple but very welcoming.

Ward F6 Queen Alexandra Hospital, Portsmouth

QA is not a hospital that is rated 'Outstanding' at the time of writing, it's rated as 'Requires Improvement' for all five key questions. First impressions (unless there is something indicative of a breach of regulation or that is amazing) aren't going to necessarily impact on your rating directly – they are going to impact on how people perceive your service. Services that are rated as Requires Improvement or even Inadequate can have pockets of particularly good care and some areas may provide an exceptional patient experience within a service where there are challenges. A provider and their managers should know where the good is and build on it.

Ward F6 is an acute stroke unit with some seriously unwell patients, many elderly, frail people and some very confused people. It is busy, and patients have high levels of need. Relatives arrive worried about their family member, possibly having read about failing elderly care in the NHS or with other preconceptions that mean they are not feeling terribly positive when they pull up in the hospital car park.

The corridor from the lift to the ward is reassuring, it's just a corridor but there are doors marked with the names and job roles of specialist stroke staff. It's good to see that there are so many experts involved in caring for patients with strokes and they all work close to the ward. There are some neat information posters that give information about strokes too; not tatty, peeling or out-of-date pieces of paper about assorted random things that have been stuck up without thought, but genuinely useful information. The number of posters is minimised for maximum impact.

The door to the ward is secured but staff answer the bell very quickly. The voice on the other end doesn't make me feel it is a chore to answer the bell – although

I rather suspect it is. The ward clerk stops what they are doing, looks up and asks whether they can help? The ward seems to have lots of staff, all actively engaged with the patients or discussing patient treatment plans, but it's a calm kind of busy rather than chaotic rushing around. The ward sister offers to show you where the patient is being cared for.

No bells are ringing and there is a noticeable absence of people calling out. Given the cohort of patients they care for this is a little unusual and one wonders whether bells have been placed out of reach or disconnected. In the bay, it is clear why there are no call bells ringing but going unanswered. There are four members of staff working in a six-bedded bay. A registered nurse and a health care assistant are assigned to the bay for the shift. They are proactively asking patients whether they need anything, are offering assistance to drink and fetching fresh drinks of the patient's choice. As they bring drinks, they touch the patients reassuringly and hug those who appear to want a hug. They are chatting to each other and the patients and relatives as they work. One of them is singing intermittently – she has a lovely voice and the patients are clearly enjoying it. A quick look at the patients shows they all appear comfortable and well groomed. Nobody is calling out, although two are asking the same questions repeatedly; the response is kind and repeated as often as the questions are asked.

Despite having staff ever present in the bay, each patient seems to have a working call button close at hand.

There is also a speech and language therapist working their way around the patients, chatting to relatives and assessing how well they are managing to eat or drink. A physiotherapist is doing likewise but assessing people's mobility and encouraging them to move.

The first impression is of very well cared for patients and staff enjoying their work. That first impression must influence how relatives, visitors, other staff and external professionals perceive the quality of care. A nurse visiting from the emergency department to bring some clothing that had been left behind might well think this is a nice place to work – I might want to transfer here. A visiting relative might see the same and think that they would apply for a job as a health care assistant here. Families might relax and see their loved ones are being managed appropriately, so not fuss and make demands because they are fearful of poor care.

Most importantly, the patients might feel safe and cared for at a time that must be very frightening.

What can you do?

French novelist Marcel Proust wrote that, "The real voyage of discovery consists not in seeking new landscapes but in having new eyes".

NHS England provides resources for staff working in healthcare to assess and improve services. It was developed and published by the now closed NHS Institute for Innovation and Improvement. It came about because the mother of a young patient who needed frequent admissions said, "I can tell what kind of care my daughter is going to get within 15 steps of walking on to every new ward".

This idea can easily be adapted to suit all sorts of environments. It needn't just apply to hospitals. Practice your observation skills next time you stay at a hotel. The tourism and leisure industry should be the leaders in first impressions; if they don't get it right, they lose custom. As you pull up to the hotel for a conference or a city break, stop thinking about what to have for supper or what time the day will finish. Look with detachment at what the environment is telling you about this hotel. What is the drive like, is it well signposted, what does the style and state of repair of the entrance signage tell you? How well maintained is the exterior of the hotel. Does someone care about the less obvious places around the hotel – the bin store, the car park? How did the arrival leave you feeling?

All this is usually a subconscious assessment before you've even opened the front door. Once you've opened the front door (or someone has opened it for you) you should observe with all your senses – the term mindfulness comes to play here a little. Professor Mark Williams, former director of the Oxford Mindfulness Centre, says that mindfulness means knowing directly what is going on inside and outside ourselves, moment by moment. "It's easy to stop noticing the world around us. It's also easy to lose touch with the way our bodies are feeling and to end up living 'in our heads' – caught up in our thoughts without stopping to notice how those thoughts are driving our emotions and behaviour".

Professor Williams says, "Another important part of mindfulness is an awareness of our thoughts and feelings as they happen moment to moment. It's about allowing ourselves to see the present moment clearly. When we do that, it can positively change the way we see ourselves and our lives." While looking to see whether the front door is in good repair and foyer smells nice, we need to lay aside our own feelings about how we think we come across and be truly present and look anew at the reality. We need to see the service as others see it. Allowing yourself to be truly present as you enter your premises or area of control you will understand better how others perceive your service.

How do you do it in your service or your area of control?

"The only true voyage, the only bath in the Fountain of Youth, would be not to visit strange lands but to possess other eyes, to see the universe through the eyes of another, of a hundred others."
Marcel Proust, 'La Prisonnière' (1923)

Fresh eyes are really important when looking objectively at how your service, your home, your hospital, your GP practice, the sexual health clinic or the ward presents itself to others. There is no one right way, no shade of 'Farrow and Ball' that will do the trick. Each leadership team needs to reflect on how it wants to present itself. A sexual health clinic or termination of pregnancy clinic may want to present a more discreet entrance – or conversely, they may want to tell the world that sexual health is part of everyone's healthcare needs generally, to promote their service as entirely normal and free from shame. It is not for me to tell them which is right but for the leaders to decide and then look at whether the first impressions give the right messages. An independent hospital might want to project a feeling of luxury while a small care home for people with learning disabilities might want to appear as an integral part of the local community

Fresh eyes can help 'get it right'. Too often we become blinkered and fail to see what is in front of us. Fresh eyes can help overcome the obstacle of familiarity. This is true about more than the first impression of a service. The 'familiarity blindness' can impact on patient safety and many aspects of the quality of care. Just remembering to look afresh at someone can improve their care. Hospitals and care homes work with many, many very frail elderly people daily.

In 2019, there were 5.4 million people aged 75 and over:

- 1.6 million were aged 85+.
- Over 500,000 people were 90+ (579,776).
- 14,430 were centenarians.

Each Baby Counts is the Royal College of Obstetricians and Gynaecologists' national quality improvement programme to reduce the number of babies who die or are left severely disabled because of incidents occurring during term labour.

The Each Baby Counts (2015) report identified that out of the 556 babies for whom different care might have led to a different outcome, there were 409 babies for whom fetal monitoring was identified as a critical contributory factor by one or more reviewer. →

Two of the recommendations made were:
1. that maternity units should employ a 'fresh ears' approach to intermittent auscultation, whereby a second midwife confirms the fetal heart rate pattern every hour, to try and reduce interpretation errors.
2. A buddy system and a 'fresh eyes' approach to cardiotocography (CTG) interpretation should be used in all units interpreting continuous CTG as there is evidence this may reduce errors in CTG interpretation.

Are we guilty of seeing these people as just 'old folk' or do we see the people behind the age on their birth certificate, the person hiding within the dementia, the fun-loving person living with loneliness? Seeing each person and responding to their individual needs will go a long way to improving services. Hopefully, we're long past services that talk about 'the pneumonia in bed seven', but we're probably not as far along the journey to truly personalised care that comes from occasionally seeing the person anew.

An example of this 'seeing with fresh eyes' is the story about Hungarian statistician Abraham Wald, who worked with the UK Air Ministry during World War II. British planes were being shot down over Germany, and it was suggested by aircraft engineers that the planes should be reinforced with armour. The problem was that if you protect the entire plane with sheets of metal, it would be too heavy to fly. Wald was asked to perform a statistical study to answer the question, "Where should we place the armour?"

Records of planes returning from Germany showed where they had been hit, sometimes with large holes in the aircraft. So the Air Ministry wanted to put armour plates on all the areas that showed heavy damage. Wald pointed out that there was no data on bombers that didn't return from Germany. He looked at the exact opposite – those areas of the planes where holes were NEVER found. These were the areas that Wald said needed additional protection, because any plane hit in those areas must have been brought down and not made it back to England. Only after looking at the evidence with fresh eyes was it understood that what had previously seemed "obvious" was obviously wrong.

The Air Ministry staff were going down the wrong path because they saw what looked like a pattern and made an incorrect assumption. They were blind to the pattern that they couldn't see; the pattern of holes in all the planes that were shot down. That needed fresh eyes.

So back to your service. How can you look again at the first impression people get of your service with fresh eyes?

The most obvious way is to use someone who has genuinely fresh eyes. This needs to be someone who isn't necessarily aiming to please you or gain favour. It must be someone who will deliver a message that it may be hard to hear. Where do you find that someone? You might want to consider:

- Asking your local Healthwatch if they would like to visit.

- Asking someone from another part of the organisation. If you have three locations, then staff from one location could visit the other location. Ask the volunteers who do the flowers. Ask the chaplain.

- Asking someone loosely connected that you might meet at some local meetings or networks. If you are a child development centre, maybe ask a local headteacher. If you are a GP practice, ask someone from the deanery. If you are a care home, maybe ask someone from the Clinical Commissioning Group. Explain that you are trying to improve your service and most people will be keen to help.

- Use relatives and friends. Your spouse (if they don't work at your service) your adult children, your friend who is a magistrate or police officer.

- Use your imagination!

Don't simply say, "What do you think about our entrance". Walk the journey with them. Look properly yourself. Get staff engaged in looking too. Agree what message you want to give then ask the person with fresh eyes questions that draw that message out. Be specific about 'Kerb appeal'. Does the entrance look clean, in good repair, free from hazards and noxious smells? Are the signs readable or are there a series of laminated signs barking orders at visitors? How do people feel as they approach the premises? Does the bell work? Is it answered? Are the windows clean? Is waste secured and out of sight? The questions really aren't difficult to work out.

A random example: Wightlink Pierhead terminal

Nothing whatsoever about health or social care, but one example of staff making a difference to how their service is perceived comes from Ryde on the Isle of Wight. Wightlink run their Fastcat service into Ryde Pierhead. People coming off the train from London Waterloo can catch a ferry from the station to the island. Many commuters use it, and it's the gateway for the festivals and for lots of holiday makers and people on day trips. In fairness, it helped that it was a glorious sunny day, I'd been swimming already and was waiting for my daughter to arrive. What made this something to comment on? It was about the staff having pride in their environment, understanding who used the service and the impact of that first impression.

What we were greeted with when we arrived 40 minutes early, because we had been concerned about traffic that didn't materialise, was a cool haven on a blistering, hot day. The staff had put up colourful bunting, there was a red carpet over the concrete floor and good quality pictures about local attractions. It was clean, there was comfortable seating in sufficient quantities and the overarching impression was that we were on holiday. The staff were happy in their work; one chap was whistling cheerfully and helping a young family with too many bags and another staff member went and found a bowl and filled it with cold water for our dog. In the café the staff chatted and smiled as they made our iced drinks. What could have been a dreary, uncomfortable wait was turned into a positive experience because the staff had pride in the service they offered.

When people arrive, they are often visiting for the first time and confused about where to go. This is a ferry terminal on the end of a Victorian pier. The staff guide and help people where necessary, but the signage is clear and easy to follow – a few well-placed signs with large lettering giving clear instructions about where the trains go from and where the car park is.

The provider also celebrates success and drives interest in what would usually be considered a mundane, everyday boat service. Inside the terminal is a wall celebrating their annual review. It isn't scruffy, laminated signs or out-of-date information, it is a bright, succinct, relevant collage that draws you in to create a positive impression by humanising and adding scale and interest.

Who knew that there had been a marriage proposal or that the company had provided £800,000 worth of discounted fares to charities and to support island events?

They had also won a 'Loo of the Year award': their lavatories were spotless, airy, freshly painted and sufficiently private to accommodate everyone's needs.

Why lavatories? Quite simply, the state of your lavatories says an awful lot about your organisation and are often one of the first places inspection teams visit on arrival, having driven for two, or more, hours. If you want to make a good first impression, you could do worse than make sure that the loos are in good order.

King Edward VII's Hospital, London

King Edward VII's Hospital is an independent charitable hospital with a history of Royal patronage, located within London's Harley Street medical district. It is, understandably, very image conscious and they have a clear vision of how they want to be perceived.

The entrance is grand. A small grey sign shows that it is indeed the main entrance but that is the only signage to distract from the impressive art deco doors adorned with very tasteful and expensive looking Christmas wreaths. A doorman in morning suit, complete with a top hat, waits to assist people arriving or leaving. A flagpole stands proudly on the wrought iron balcony, above the doors.

Not every service would want a doorman or a marble column; it's about knowing what first impressions you want to give and then seeing anew whether that is what your service projects.

Having looked at the first impression your building creates, you may want to consider the first impressions your staff make.

It takes just one-tenth of a second for us to judge someone and make a first impression. Non-verbal behaviours are particularly important to forming impressions when meeting people in a professional setting. Specifically, components of social expressivity, such as smiling, eyebrow position, emotional expression, and eye contact are key to a good beginning. First impressions are more heavily influenced by non-verbal cues than verbal cues. In fact, non-verbal cues have over four times the impact on the impression you make than anything you say.

Christian Jarret (2014), in the *British Psychological Society Research Digest* summarises the society's research archives and surmised the following assumptions people made on first impressions or photographs – some may make people squirm but it's worth considering whether we hold the same perceptions and whether they are fair.

- People who make more eye contact are perceived as more intelligent. Other research has found that people who avoid eye contact are judged to be insincere and lacking in conscientiousness (this last result was found for women, but not men).
- Faster speakers are judged to be more competent.
- Dressing smartly communicates success.
- Smartness and the appearance of wealth brings influence.
- People make assumptions about others based on their choice of shoe. This is an interesting observation and one that I can relate to. More agreeable people tended to wear shoes that were practical and affordable (pointy toes, price and brand visibility were negatively correlated with agreeableness); that anxiously attached people tended to wear shoes that look brand new and in good repair (perhaps to make a good impression and avoid rejection).
- People who have multiple facial piercings are assumed to be less intelligent. As the number of piercings went up, the ratings of intelligence went down. What does your dress code say about piercings?
- Men with shaved heads are seen as more dominant.
- People who walk with a loose, expansive gait are seen as more adventurous.

Surrey and Sussex Healthcare NHS Trust

When we arrived at East Surrey Hospital for an announced inspection, we found the Chief Executive, the Chair, the Chief Nurse, the Chief Operating Officer and the Medical Director all waiting for us in the foyer. The CEO was chatting to the front desk receptionist but was keeping an eye out for our arrival. I don't think it's necessary to fawn all over inspection teams – that is likely to have the opposite effect to the one intended – but it felt nice that the senior team were so engaged and wanting to build a relationship with the team. It made us feel welcome.

The SASH staff began saying hello to individual inspection team members. I think the CEO shook every member of the team's hands and said, "Welcome", while smiling broadly. They then escorted us, chatting in small groups as we went, to the room allocated as our base room. The CEO and the Chief Nurse ensured we had everything we needed before suggesting they leave us for a short while to have a drink and settle in.

As the inspection progressed staff told us that the CEO was 'omnipresent', and we found that to be true. Everywhere we went he popped up to check we were being properly looked after. He lived up to his first impression of being someone that really cared about his organisation and staff, and who wanted us to understand why he felt so proud.

On an individual basis, there are things you can do about the first impression you present to people.

- Consider your attitude. People pick up your attitude (warmth, hostility) instantly. Before you turn to greet someone, or enter the interview room, or step onstage to make a presentation, think about the situation and make a conscious choice about the attitude you want to embody.
- Stand or sit up straight. Status and power are non-verbally conveyed by height and space. Standing or sitting tall, pulling your shoulders back, and holding your head straight are all signals of confidence and competence.
- Smile. You may be nervous, but a smile still does wonders. A smile is an invitation, a sign of welcome.
- Make eye contact. Looking at someone's eyes says you are listening, and you are engaged. (To improve your eye contact, make a practice of noticing the eye colour of everyone you meet.)
- Raise your eyebrows. Open your eyes slightly more than normal to simulate the "eyebrow flash" that is the universal signal of recognition and acknowledgement. Don't make it too obvious though.

- Shake hands. It takes an average of three hours of continuous interaction to develop the same level of rapport that you can get with a single handshake. The caveat is if you are in a situation where someone may be uncomfortable with a handshake or touch in general.

- Be respectful of the other person's space. That means, in most professional situations, staying about two feet away.

Is it enough for the leaders to be welcoming and smiley? The answer must be no. Leaders cannot usually meet everyone that crosses their threshold. They need to gain 'buy in' from their front of house staff. That first representative of your service is going to provide the enduring impression.

There is no one perfect type of staff member, no ideal way for staff to present themselves but there is scope for leaders to re-enter the premises and see what people visiting for the first time see and how they are greeted. Those fresh eyes and unknown people are useful here too. Generally, if a senior partner in a GP practice, the Chief Nurse or a care home owner, comes through the front door, they will (hopefully) receive a warm welcome. An elderly woman with a food stained shirt or a young man with learning disabilities might not have the same experience.

If you are using a fresh eyes approach to understand the reception that people get when they arrive, do use someone who understands the type of service and who can empathise with people using the service. Healthwatch might be willing to help you out here too – they want to work towards improving services just as much as you do. If your fresh eyed person turns up to a service for people who misuse drugs in a Saville Row suit, carrying an expensive briefcase and a clipboard they are likely to get a very different reception and may not see the service as service users see it. Think carefully who you ask.

Satisfaction surveys are another way of gauging opinions about the initial impression and experiences. My experience is that often surveys are done to ask the questions the provider wants the answer to (which is not necessarily the same as the most useful questions). It might be necessary to change the questions to ask specifically whether the reception staff were kind, helpful, attentive and patient. Sometimes the number of visitors to a service is low and a survey isn't enough to get truthful answers because people are worried, they may be identifiable. Positive results are nice – we all like to hear good things about ourselves – but criticism is more valuable if we genuinely want to improve. Surveys can only give you the answer to the questions you ask, and you might have included a degree of bias, either consciously or subconsciously.

Why would you want a survey to not tell the whole story? Imagine marketing your service with a headline that 98% of people felt the environment was pleasant as opposed to a headline saying 63% of people said they had waited more than five minutes for the receptionist to acknowledge their presence. Which do you think is the most useful? The marketing director would undoubtedly think the 98% result but if you think a bit harder, the less positive result is of greater use. In the short-term, I would be looking and monitoring the response of reception staff to understand why they took so long to acknowledge people and addressing that, but it is the longer-term actions that will help a service move towards 'Outstanding'. Understanding the service user's experience from the time they enter the building (or before) is important to improving how those same people respond to surveys and to any small lapses in service provision. If you were greeted with an eight-minute wait while the receptionist carried on working at her computer; if the receptionist just said, "Name? Date of Birth? First line of address?" and then pointed towards a vague area and said, "Area five", you are likely to perceive the entire service less favourably, aren't you?

The third, quite brave, way is to get the reception staff to critique themselves. The caveat is that this cannot be managed in a punitive or negative way; it cannot be public criticism of an individual. It must be the reception and front of house team looking at team practice and thinking how they could improve the experience they provide. The team could take it in turns to carry out an observation for about an hour. They could look at how long people wait to be acknowledged, whether conversations can be overheard and therefore some personal information is revealed, and they could count the number of times the reception staff smile when helping. The team could be guided to set up their own observational framework. The results will be far more powerful, and the lessons learned will be embedded far more deeply if the team are allowed to take ownership for the first impression they give.

Forty per cent of people say that having to talk through their symptoms with doctors' receptionists could put them off going to their GP (Moffat et al, 2016).

Dr Richard Roope, Cancer Research UK's GP expert, said: "This may mean more emphasis on training front desk staff including receptionists to deal more sensitively with patients".

How much more important does the first impression and approachability mean if you consider it might be a factor in delayed cancer diagnosis?

As a leader you might want to consider whether the staff appearance is supporting your ethos, creating a barrier or hindering your assertion that you are a particularly good, moving towards outstanding, provider. Here it is a case of little things matter. Inspection teams notice little things.

Research by Omri Gillath *et al* (2012) shows that you can tell a lot about someone's personality, politics, status, age and income just from looking at a photo of their shoes. How much more does the way your staff dress convey about your service?

I know that when we were sent away from Great Ormond Street to gain experience in the care of adults, in the 1980s, patients often asked for us. I suspect it was less about our skill set and more about our uniforms. We were 'Pinkies' in a very traditional, pink candy-striped dress with a crisply starched white apron, funny hats and thick black stockings. The hospital we were placed in used the new national uniform that was akin to dressing in a synthetic dishcloth. Much more comfortable and practical but much less impressive. We were hugely proud of our starched collars – despite a ring of blisters around our necks. Our uniform code was severe – no cardigans without a cape except at the nurse's desk on night duty which was to be removed before leaving the desk, no top buttons undone (ever), no crumpled or stained aprons. We spent a fortune on spray starch. The pale blue dresses with V-necks and a zip were so much easier to wear, so much cooler in hot weather, but it was long enough ago for many patients to want their nurses to look like Florence Nightingale, and we came close. We were more trusted and considered better nurses simply because we fitted the perception the patients had of what a 'proper nurse' should look like. My learning is that while dress codes and uniforms adapt with the changes in culture and expectations, what staff wear will impact on the perceptions of people using the services and, perhaps as importantly, on the way those staff perceive themselves and the pride in their work.

UBS Group AG is a Swiss multinational investment bank that made global news in 2010 by issuing a 44-page dress code. It wouldn't be for everyone, but it made very clear the company's expectations around the way their staff dressed. To many they may well seem excessive.

"Adopting impeccable behaviour extends to impeccable presentation."

"Jacket buttons should be closed. When seated, they must always be open."

"Piercings, besides earrings, and tattoos are prohibited. Tattoos, piercings or anklets are outdated and do not look professional."

"Your underwear must not be visible through your clothes or stand out."

"Ultra-trendy eyewear or too showy coloured glasses are not tolerated. Ultra-hip glasses or lenses in too gaudy colours are not allowed."

The level of detail isn't going to be appropriate for every sort of service, but you should consider what is and isn't acceptable wear for work. An explicit dress code or uniform policy does reduce conflict by making clear expectations. It may be made easier where there is a corporate dress code and you only need to ensure it is upheld locally; clothing for work may be supplied. Uniforms are definitely easier to ensure consistency. A dress code that says simply 'Business wear' as the only requirement, is open to discussion and debate.

Where do you stand as an organisation on make-up? On heel height? On jewellery? On hairstyles? On nail polish or gel nails? On religious symbols or designer logos? A scruffy workforce is not going to present well to the outside world. If it's a mental health care setting or small home for people with learning disabilities, jeans and loose hair may well be acceptable; dirty jeans and inappropriate slogans are never acceptable, regardless of the setting.

Hello, My Name is...

A campaign for more compassionate care

Kate Granger was a consultant geriatrician working at Pinderfields in Wakefield.

The original idea for her campaign for more compassionate care came out of a personal tragedy when she was being treated for cancer and realised how dehumanising and impersonal the whole process could feel for patients. It had been a porter called Brian that helped her have her 'lightbulb moment' – as he had arrived to take her somewhere in a wheelchair, he had simply said "Hello, my name is Brian". This gave Kate back a sense of being acknowledged as a person; many other healthcare staff hadn't felt it necessary to introduce themselves.

Kate and her husband, Chris Pointon, started the 'hello my name is' campaign in August 2013, asking frontline NHS staff to introduce themselves to their patients.

They used a blog and social media to share her experiences and gain support for #hellomynameis. Over 400,000 health workers from across the world now back this initiative for more personalised care. Chris continues the work.

https://www.hellomynameis.org.uk/

There are many ways on the website through which you can support the campaign, but I suspect the most important way is to embed the practice throughout your service.

If you go into hospitals in England now, chances are you will see staff with badges or lanyards that say #hellomyname.

I am saddened that the campaign ever became necessary and that staff needed reminding to introduce themselves. As a nurse and regulator, I am embarrassed that healthcare professionals should need reminding of basic courtesy. It is a fantastic but indicting campaign.

I don't think I should need to tell you why staff should almost always introduce themselves. I am certain the badges and lanyards raise awareness and make us stop and think, but they aren't enough. Each staff member needs to take responsibility for ensuring they are courteous towards patients, visitors and other staff. The setting is immaterial. You cannot possibly be aiming for an 'Outstanding' rating if people are treated with the disdain that a lack of an introduction demonstrates.

The values of the campaign are ones that nobody could argue with and which everyone aspiring to deliver a good service should adopt. These values create a positive first impression, but the impact goes well beyond this. Their website is comprehensive in setting out why it is so important and what staff can do to make care provision more person-centred:

- See me as a person first and foremost before a disease or bed number. Individuals are more than just an illness, they are a human being, they are a family member, they are a friend etc. and we should all remember to see more of an individual than just the reason they are using healthcare.

- "No decision about me without me." These words ring true in healthcare as the most important person is the patient and everything should be done with them in mind.

- Little things really do matter – they aren't little at all, they are indeed huge and of central importance in any practice of healthcare and in society. This could be someone sitting down next to you rather than looming over you or holding the door open for someone coming through.

- Communication is of paramount importance. Timely and effective communication which is bespoke to the patient makes a huge difference and starts with a simple introduction.

There will be the odd acceptable exception – a resuscitation team, perhaps, or a scrub nurse in an operating theatre. In a small care home for people with learning disabilities where the staff and service users know each other very well, you wouldn't do it every time you met, clearly. They should remain an exception rather than cited as an excuse for why it isn't a cultural norm.

There is no service this couldn't or shouldn't apply to. It doesn't have to be restricted to hospitals. Indeed, internationally it has been adopted by organisations as diverse as the Pharmaceutical Society of Australia, Tasmania, The Johns Hopkins Hospital, Baltimore, USA, NHS North Derbyshire Clinical Commissioning Group, School of Nursing, Midwifery & Social Work, University of Manchester, Public Health Wales and Healthcare Improvement Scotland.

It would transfer very well to GP services, care homes, sexual health clinics, prison healthcare services, dental practices, screening services and just in everyday life. It doesn't take long to say, "Hello, my name is". Knowing each other's name puts the relationship on a more equal footing.

I was in my own GP practice very recently – it's a fabulous practice with a skilled and dedicated team who often go 'above and beyond'. Perhaps I am more attuned, having written this: maybe the campaign to introduce the 'Hello My Name is' approach to the Commission by two of the talented inspectors, Catherine Dale and Matt Preston, has heightened my awareness. Anyway, the practice nurse who was assigned to take blood from me was pleasant and courteous enough. She came to the waiting room and called, "Mrs. Salt".

I followed her to the treatment room. She smiled and said, "Sit down and roll your sleeve up, please". No introduction, no handshake. Nothing. I thought of Kate Granger and said, "Hello, my name is Terri". She looked a bit bemused and said, "It says Teresa on the form, but never mind, roll your sleeve up, please". Clearly there is a bit more work to be done to spread the word and ensure all healthcare professionals have the courtesy to introduce themselves – even in some very good services.

How can you build on the good practice rather than castigating poor practice? All sorts of ways.

Maybe start with presentations about the campaign at a local level. If, for example, your accident and emergency reception staff understand the possible impact of this simple act, they might be more willing to take the time to say hello as frightened people approach them for help. They are often the first contact people have with a hospital and should be an exemplar to other teams.

The last trust I inspected that was given an inadequate rating had a problem with front of house staff not understanding the importance of the way they greeted people. I sat in their emergency department and watched staff not looking up from their computer screens as they checked people in. It was a monotonous litany of "Next", "Name? Address? Date of Birth?… Take a seat". No real communication at all. No reassuring smiles. No connection with their patients. They were busy and working under pressure, but saying hello and looking at the patients might have saved a few significant problems that emerged as I was in the department. It might have made them more approachable and the parents of an extremely sick new-born infant might have not sat for an hour waiting to be called. They might have realised how poorly the baby was and how worried the parents were and summoned help. That the parents were not confident English speakers made the need all the greater; they were made to feel like they had done something inconvenient by seeking help. They weren't going to make a fuss. Smiling and saying hello, seeing the people in front of them would undoubtedly have made their job more pleasant too. How much better to be able to go home and say you helped get rapid treatment for a very sick baby and could reassure the parents than to have to admit to yourself that failing to see the people in front of you resulted in a delayed response and worsening of a baby's condition?

Role modelling might also help embed practice. Do senior staff introduce themselves to new staff, to agency staff, to service users or relatives? Is it part of the induction programme for your Resident Medical Officer if you run a private hospital? Do you introduce yourself to everyone that visits a travel clinic?

Do you ever audit whether it happens in practice? A formal programme of audits would be evidence but even simple records of observations which are discussed at team meetings can be a useful tool for supporting practice improvements.

No time for audits or observations? Find volunteers, explain about the campaign, provide a checklist so they can simply record whether a staff member introduced themselves. In a GP service, members of the patient participation group might be keen to help, try Healthwatch, students on work experience or placements, a relative of a care home resident, someone from the local branch of a related charity (perhaps shop volunteers could extend their role with appropriate vetting and training).

Auditing and observation needn't be about castigating individual staff members, but are useful ways to highlight good practice of those who invariably introduce themselves and to raise awareness where there is scope to improve on introductions.

I also have a particular dislike of staff who say "Hello, my name is Mr Consultant" but then assume it is acceptable to alter the balance of power, in what should be a partnership, by using my first name – particularly if they use the name printed on the form and not the one I use.

A CEO's secret

I hope he doesn't mind me revealing his secret too much. A new CEO arrived to take over leadership of a trust when it was not in a good place, culturally. Inappropriate and boorish behaviours of a few senior staff went unchallenged and staff felt they couldn't raise concerns or that their concerns would not be acted upon.

I visited after he had been in post only a short while and went to speak, as I always do, to operational staff in various wards and departments. They were all effusive in praise for him and there had been a tangible shift in morale and self-belief among the staff groups. The story was the same wherever I chose to wander: the new CEO had visited their ward or department. The staff felt that he listened and understood. They were really, really impressed that he had not only taken the time to visit but that he had also bothered to learn every single person's name. He apparently knew all about them and what they did. They felt valued and respected. Indeed, they were. The CEO spoke proudly of the achievements of his staff and talked about 'Our trust' and 'Us' rather than 'The trust' or 'My trust'. He accepted no responsibility for the improvements but was careful to attribute all success to the frontline staff.

Still impressed by how he could possibly have learned so many staff names so quickly, I visited at a later date and toured the newly opened Surgical Assessment Unit with him. It was true. We walked onto the unit. He approached the ward housekeeper, shook her hand and said, "Hello, I am the CEO. You must be Sandra. I've heard so many good things about your work". She was absolutely delighted to have been acknowledged.

When we returned to his office, I asked him how he managed to learn so many names so quickly. He told me his secret was that he didn't learn all the staff names, just a few key people's before he visited a ward. Those key people tended to be the housekeepers, the ward clerk or the healthcare assistant he was likely to meet that day. He said that if you knew the names of a few junior members of staff, the senior staff would assume you knew theirs too. It worked brilliantly. It wasn't cheating; he was genuinely interested in all his staff but understood if his cultural changes were going to work, he had to ensure they were recognised and appreciated by staff working at all grades. He is a role model that sets a cultural norm of saying "Hello".

So, how can you try to improve here? Ask for feedback at local level, perhaps? When you do a local survey, you could ask people whether staff introduced themselves by name. You can benchmark this quite easily and share results with the teams, so they know how well they are doing. Encourage observations from an independent person, maybe? You could get a volunteer or staff member from another site or another service to just sit and listen. The observer fades rapidly into the background and they can simply log how many times staff members said, "Hello my name is... How can I help you?" against how many times they didn't: a straightforward 58% of times staff did versus 42% when they didn't. This would be very simple to do in a multitude of settings and the results could demonstrate service improvements and could also provide evidence for the caring domain.

It can be left as that, a straightforward reminder, but there is potential for that to be considered naming and shaming, a touch punitive, if it was just a monthly graph of consecutive results or numbers pinned to a noticeboard. Staff might resent it and then the best intentions will have created negativity towards something that should be entirely positive. How much better to share the results in a team meeting, group supervision or study day?

Now perhaps I'll tell you about someone who got it very, very wrong because they wanted to create the 'right impression'. It feels so far beyond the norm, even for the time it happened, that it is almost humorous.

The provider used to own three care homes in a seaside town. They weren't called care homes but rather 'Hotels with discreet care'. They had sweeping staircases, deep, good-quality carpets, stained glass panels in the front doors of large Edwardian seaside villas. They were beautiful buildings certainly, and had an air of slightly dated grandeur; they conjured up mental images of Miss Marple or Jeeves and Worcester on holiday.

What they didn't have was appropriate care for guests. They were definitely guests, not service users, patients or residents.

When we inspected, we found that they were sending people who were living with quite advanced dementia to wander the streets without any support. When we asked about the risk, we were told that it was fine, as they wanted to go out and had a card in their pocket with the person's name, the hotel name and the phone number on it. Apparently, the local police were always helpful in returning anyone that did get 'a little lost'. We also found they had replaced hospital issue walking sticks and walking frames with much more tasteful umbrellas to "save embarrassment" and not make it too obvious when someone had a bit of a mobility problem. They had decided against providing institutional handrails for the staircases. The building was three stories plus a basement. There was no lift. One of the reasons we were inspecting was because several people had sustained serious injuries following falls. The injuries included a person losing the sight in one eye when they had fallen, and a sharp object had pierced their eyeball. To further avoid the establishment feeling like a care home they had decided not to employ night staff. We were told nobody needed overnight assistance and they had someone sleeping in on call, in case of an emergency. The guests had no way of contacting the person who was sleeping in. One elderly man had been found in the morning with hypothermia and a fractured neck of femur.

We found one woman who was being cared for in a reclining chair, as she was too heavy for staff to lift into the hotel type divan bed provided in her room. There were no hoists and no height adjustable bed. There was no provision for pressure area care. The woman was very cheerful and brave saying it was her own fault that she was too big to move and that the staff were all kind. She'd been sitting in the same chair, in a basement without any view from the tiny window, for over two years.

We stopped all further admissions with immediate effect but were told that was impossible as the hotel already had guests booked to arrive on Christmas Eve, the following week. I remain incredibly proud of the team at the time who, to a person, offered to give up part of their own family Christmas to go and check on the elderly people at the home and to ensure there had not been any further admissions.

The homes were shut by the regulator at the time – but not without a battle. First impressions are important but not at the cost of high-quality care.

Equality as the root of excellence

"I will, from this day, strive to forge togetherness out of our differences. We need to reach that happy stage of our development when differences and diversity are not seen as sources of division and distrust, but of strength and inspiration."
Josefa Iloilo (president of Fiji, 2000-2009)

Your service can never be 'Outstanding' without a deep and embedded commitment to ensuring equality is threaded through all aspects of the service.

The Equality Act 2010 legally protects people from discrimination in the workplace and in wider society. The Act replaced preceding information and made the law easier to understand and strengthened protection in some situations.

Full details of the Act and associated guidance can be found on the Equality and Human Rights Commission website.

Equality in terms of the current legislative framework is defined as ensuring individuals or groups of individuals are not treated differently or less favourably, based on their specific protected characteristics, including their race, sex, disability, religion or belief, sexual orientation, pregnancy and maternity including breastfeeding and age.

I would suggest that for an 'Outstanding' service there should be recognition that equality for all is far more than is covered by the legislative requirements of the Act. Equality is about ensuring that every individual has an equal opportunity to make the most of their lives and talents. It is also the belief that no one should have poorer life chances because of the way they were born, where they come from, what they believe, or whether they have a disability. Unless everyone is equal, nobody is.

My own understanding of equality as a force for good was awakened during my late teens. As I mentioned before, I think it is essential to reflect on what has formed our views and really understand our own position, being honest with ourselves, if not more publicly. Education around equality and diversity is essential for all organisations but if it's tokenistic or insufficiently challenging, nobody is going to have their deeply ingrained opinions modified. We all have prejudices and we all stereotype people; what's important is to understand and modify our behaviours and strongly held views to adapt towards seeing the individuals beyond our bias.

Between leaving school and starting nurse training, I spent the summer volunteering at summer camps for disadvantaged children from the Greater London area with a children's charity that was originally set up as a 'fresh air mission' to improve the health of Victorian children living in slums. Little did I know then that I would meet my future husband, make lifelong friends and continue to volunteer with the charity for over 15 years. Among the other volunteer staff was a real champion of equality who ensured that what are now termed 'protected characteristics' were respected and catered for.

Edith

The Post Office in London used to raise funds for the charity and sponsored individual children's holidays, alongside allowing some staff two weeks' community service time to attend the camps. We were truly fortunate that Edith was allocated to our camp, forgave our youthful ignorance, and continued to join us for many memorable years. She herself had been a child on one of the charity's camps a long time before; her memories were mixed with a view that her horizons had been widened, she'd met people who encouraged her to do well but who had no understanding of what growing up as a black child in 1960s London meant. She wanted to give back and help other children to have a fantastic holiday in the country or at the seaside.

We all met at Paddington station. British Rail were very tolerant of 60 children and about a dozen young adults turning up to register and make introductions. We travelled by coaches that were permitted to pull right into the station. Chaos was an understatement with last minute lavatory trips, children disappearing to spend all their pocket money in the sweet shop before we'd even left, some weeping and frightened at leaving their mothers, and others climbing where they weren't meant to climb.

Edith arrived and looked less than pleased. She introduced herself to the group of adults who were being very tolerant of loud and excitable behaviours; we were all young and all very inexperienced (although we failed to recognise this at the time). Her first words to us all were, "Am I the only person like me going? Am I the only black adult?" She was indeed. The charity's recruitment at that time was a phone call to the main office and the camps' organiser deciding whether you sounded nice or not. It wasn't actively seeking out staff who were reflective of the group of children we were taking with us – it assumed gap year students who had been in the Red Cross, army cadets or scouting/guiding, were probably the best fit. I was recruited because I held a current lifesaving qualification, a first aid certificate and claimed to like children.

Fair play to Edith, she didn't simply walk away but climbed aboard to travel to Somerset with us. She sat by herself and watched carefully. On arrival we all went to the main hall to establish order and gain a semblance of control. The leader was giving out lists of the groups each supervisor would have under their care. He gave Edith her list of allocated little girls with a smile and a slightly patronising, "They shouldn't be too difficult". She looked at the list, looked at the leader and said, "No. That's the wrong list. I am having the older boys since none of you know how to get the respect from them. Look at them, you've let them be all over the place". She was quite scary in her conviction and the leader relented. Edith picked her own team that year and every subsequent year. She usually had a larger group than other supervisors as she said she needed enough to play football properly and they were older lads, predominantly black, who she ruled with unfailing kindness but steel-like firmness.

She set incredibly high expectations (or so we thought); she said it was normal expectations, just relaxed a little for the holiday. She taught us that black skin needed creaming with cocoa butter daily, that black children could sunburn and that it was not acceptable to 'suck your teeth' at an adult. She helped us understand that many of the children's mothers' expectations would be that their sons were neatly turned out, in clean clothes and well-groomed. She washed their t-shirts while they played football and was disapproving of particularly 'mucky activities'. We thought rolling in mud was fine and she taught us to consider that these families had scrimped and saved all year to ensure they didn't 'bring shame' by turning up with old or scruffy clothes. She questioned what gave us the right to be dismissive of that effort and hardship by letting the children destroy their clothes. Her boys set the tone for the camp and their trainers stayed white. Edith ensured they arrived at meals with clean hands, sat politely at the table and had a total ban on swearing. They adored her. They knew and understood her expectations; she would always ensure that they were well cared for and felt secure, in a way the rest of us didn't initially understand.

She also taught us how to manage girls' hair when extensions fell out or they'd undone cornrow plaits that a relative had put in for the holiday. She strongly discouraged the other supervisors from allowing cornrow to be undone, explaining how long it took (or cost) and why parents chose to send their daughter away with hair tightly plaited.

The other gift Edith brought was to teach us that we had a responsibility to provide a supportive challenge to outsiders. She taught us all not to accept the racism (often hidden as 'teasing') that we regularly came across when you had large groups of children from different backgrounds in rural middle England in the 80s. If a camp cook refused to offer vegetarian food for a child, Edith went into the kitchen to make something for the child herself instead of trying to take the ham off a pizza, as perhaps the rest of us would have done. If people made loud inappropriate comments to their friends at the park or on a beach, Edith approached them and asked what they meant? She didn't let go until she had an apology. If we had forgotten to react to something, she prompted us with, "Aren't you going to say something?" She was never rude in her challenge, never visibly angry, always courteous in the face of extreme provocation. She simply would not accept racist behaviour; this alone gained her enormous respect and credibility with both the children and other supervisors.

While we supported and respected her stance we weren't as aware; new supervisors were often heard to say that they treated everyone the same when they arrived, but Edith patiently educated and helped us all understand that treating people fairly and equally does not always mean treating people the same. When we introduced training and formal selection weekends a few years later, we offered a session on equality and Edith came along to co-facilitate the session. She always refused to lead and felt very strongly that racism would never be addressed until it stopped being a black person's problem.

Charles West School of Nursing and Professor Alan Glasper

At the time I trained, schools of nursing were attached to hospitals and not to universities. Great Ormond Street Hospital was affiliated to the University of London, but students were appointed to the school of nursing. I remember the Director of Nurse Education talking to a small group who had arrived for an interview telling us she was always reluctant to accept girls from South Wales as they invariably got homesick and left before completing training. We were surprised at such open prejudice, as we had a Welsh girl on our course. Unfortunately, the Welsh girl did leave after about ten months; sometimes people do fulfil stereotypes, but this doesn't mean that all girls who grow up in South Wales will never leave the valleys.

I also remember one of our tutors, Alan Glasper, who was then quite young and ambitious (but who has now recently retired from his post as the Foundation Professor of Nursing at The University of Southampton). He was talking to us about something and went off on a slight tangent and posed the question, "What are the main differences between the children in the private patient's unit and the children who are admitted to Queen Elizabeth's?"

Queen Elizabeth's was a sister hospital to Great Ormond Street. The Hospital served the East End and all nurses training at GOS were required to rotate and spend some time training there. It was an eye opener as the community served was a local community, rather than a global one, and usually quite poor. It was almost the opposite of Great Ormond Street: no grandeur, no rarefied atmosphere, just a large hospital serving the children who came through the doors. You could literally walk in the door and be seen in the Accident & Emergency Department. It was a genuinely open-door policy, whoever you were and wherever you came from – and people travelled quite a way to have their child be seen at the hospital.

The answers to Alan's question were shouted out, as answers to a game.

"They wear much nicer clothes."

"They might not speak English."

"They eat different food."

"They are foreign."

"They don't want the chaplain to visit."

"You have to chaperone the mother."

"Only the father can sign the consent form."

"Their parents will need an interpreter."

"The East End kids have snotty noses."

He must have had about 30 answers which were all accepted with a "Yes, they might"

Then he left a pause (he always liked a touch of drama in his lessons).

"You've all identified differences in how their parents choose to raise them, where they come from and how they live. You've made assumptions about their wishes. What you haven't done is look beyond the different clothing, the accent, the prayer mats or the family customs to see that every child is an individual.

Each of you wants to be a paediatric nurse. You chose GOS because you want to be the Crème de la Crème. To be a good sick children's nurse you must not only look but you must see the child and their family and understand what their needs are. Children, rich and poor alike, need the same basic things to thrive but also sometimes want or need different things. Each child is an individual who needs special consideration. As much as each child is different, so each child is the same; learn where the differences sit and respond to each child as an individual outside of your own misconceptions."

This might not be quoted word perfectly, but I have hung onto that message throughout my career and hopefully I continue to not only look but to see.

Stella and Michaela

A few years later I was employed as a part-time lecturer and tutor in Childhood Studies in an EU-funded project which aimed to enable women living in rural poverty to gain employment through childcare. The idea was that women could be supported to gain accredited qualifications and would then become more confident and more employable. It was a fantastic way to bring equality of opportunity to women living in rural poverty. It also supported other women through better childcare provision.

As I had my own young family, I didn't want to commit to too many hours and tended to opt to lead the shorter, more accessible courses. I agreed to tutor the Diploma in Childcare and Education which ran one day a week for an academic year. There were no entry requirements except a personal statement and a current role in an early years setting.

On my first day, I explained the course content, the assessment criteria and support offered. Most women were nervous, but introductions revealed a warm and enthusiastic group. This was a big deal to many of them; they wanted to learn but were not convinced of their ability to do so.

Two women stood out.

Stella was already a grandmother and close to retirement age. She had left school at 15 with no qualifications. She'd raised her family and now helped with her grandchildren and volunteered on the local play bus that toured rural villages and traveller sites. During the introductions she had shared that her family thought she was daft to even consider doing a course as she was too old; on that first day she hadn't told them that she was starting, as she was worried that they would put her off.

Michaela had a quite different story and told the assembled group of about 30 women that her boss had made her come along but that she was "too thick to pass", so it was a waste of everyone's time. Her boss has said she could continue to work at the nursery, which her little girl attended, but she needed to work towards qualifying and this course was a start. Michaela was shaking when she introduced herself. She said she was "rubbish at everything": she said she had missed lots of school because she wasn't clever enough for exams. She then showed us a photograph of her little girl, Emma, who was four and starting to prepare for big school. Michaela warmed up as she spoke about Emma's dancing, singing action songs together and helping her learn to put tights on. Michaela was only 19-years-old herself.

I shared a reading list and looks of horror crossed their faces. I talked about reading anything – literally any reading at all to get themselves into the habit. We talked about the importance of reading to children and the lovely books they could share with them. A few confessed to avoiding the reading corner, sadly. I suggested they stop panicking about the reading list and gather some magazines – either professional ones related to childcare or general ones that had articles about children in. We agreed that each person would read one article in the coming week and come back next week to share what they had felt or learned in small groups. Everyone left with my phone number and the phone number of the special school where we lived at that time, in case they needed to contact me. This was a time before we all had mobile phones.

The following week I discovered that, after the last week's study day, Stella had asked Michaela if they could meet for a coffee. They had discussed the course and formed an alliance that was committed to working together to try and pass; they both stood slightly apart from the rest of the group as one was significantly older than most, and one was significantly younger.

At the next session, I had prepared to discuss a few articles from childcare magazines and discuss something non-contentious. I went around the groups, and topics such as positive behaviour, weaning, reins and suchlike were being debated. It felt good, there was a real buzz in the room. Then we came back together and agreed it was good to share and hear other viewpoints.

Nothing unexpected then… until Stella put her hand up and said, "We didn't really discuss it much, but I read *Dibs in Search of Self* and there are some bits I'm not sure I understand properly". Now, *Dibs* was written in 1964 by a child psychologist, Virginia Axline. Dibs is a young boy who is silent and a mystery to his parents and teachers. He is a troubled child who hides under tables and lashes out at other children. Some think he's incapable of learning and interacting in a regular classroom. Some think he's emotionally disturbed. The book has its challenges and wouldn't necessarily be the first thing I would have suggested reading to someone who is out of the habit and lacking confidence.

My mind was somersaulting but I was about to answer when Michaela chipped in: "I tried to read it like Stella suggested but I haven't had time to finish it yet. We have a little boy like that at nursery; I just sort of sit alongside him and make sure he knows I am there. He doesn't often say much but sometimes he hands me things and then I'll dig a bit in the sandpit with him. He likes the sandpit but gets cross if others want to use it, so I brought in Emma's old baby bath and he has his own sandpit now."

The only thing I could suggest was that they come around to my house during the week and we discuss it in more detail then, as the rest of the class was beginning to disengage. They did turn up that week and every following week, having usually read yet another weighty tome. They wanted to debate and discuss everything. They loved learning and our Thursday afternoon session continued with Emma becoming a playmate to my children and Stella always bringing a new interesting activity for them all. They had an insatiable appetite for learning and while Stella initially had better literacy skills, Michaela had an innate understanding of child psychology. Neither woman was really the person they presented to the group on the first day.

I was so proud when the moderation process confirmed they had both gained distinctions. I was even more proud when they each told me they had been accepted onto a degree course, a few years later. Stella went on to complete a master's in childhood studies – just for fun and to prove she could. Michaela is now a lecturer in Midwifery. I learned so much from those two women and use professional reading and reflection in my work still.

So how does this link into lessons about equality? I think, partly, it is about understanding the difficulties some people face because of protected characteristics (although this was before the Equality Act 2010 was enacted). Stella's own family thought she was too old, that it was silly and a waste of time. Michaela felt isolated from her school friends who didn't have children; she couldn't go out clubbing but had no desire to do so; her pregnancy and need to care for a child limited her work and study options.

More importantly, perhaps, is the message around treating everyone fairly, according to their needs and preferences and that isn't necessarily treating everyone the same. These two women were enthused by learning and wanted to widen their knowledge; the core curriculum of the course wasn't enough for them. Did they get preferential treatment? I think the answer must be no. Others on the course wanted to work at the level that was set by the accrediting body. They weren't interested in the additional learning, for whatever reason. A real injustice would have been done if, because these two wanted to stretch themselves, everyone else was made to feel bad. It would not have been fair to have everyone sit through long discussions about the impact of antenatal trauma on attachment when they wanted and needed to focus on the play curriculum. Similarly, if anyone else wanted to join the group (as two others occasionally did) they would be very welcome.

The Equality Act 2010 requires employers to have systems in place to eliminate discrimination, harassment and victimisation, and promote equal opportunities. This means employers should consider those protected under the Act when designing and delivering statutory and mandatory training. The employer should consider what adjustments can be made for staff with a disability. This could be to ensure the times and locations and delivery of the training is suitable and accessible. The employer should remove any physical barriers, or provide extra equipment or aids where required.

The earlier idea of using a fresh eyes approach to your environment, your policies and your work norms can help identify and address areas where you or your service are acting outside of the legislation – and so prevent the costs, stress and disruption of tribunals.

Many larger organisations have networks such as Black Minority Ethnic (BME), Lesbian, Gay, Bisexual, Transgender+ (LGBT+) or Disability networks that can be a genuinely useful and wise critical friend, working with the executive team and providing advice from the perspective of those affected by the shortfalls. Most of these work well to support the service in improving their equality outcomes for both staff and people using the service. Where there is executive level collaboration with a well chaired and inclusive group, it can reap huge benefits in building a positive culture. It won't work so effectively if it's just about being able to tick the box that says you have a network group; it must be a true commitment. My only word of slight caution would be to ensure that your networks are representative and open to all. A small group who have the validation of being an officially recognised network but who are selective in who can be active within the group may do more harm than good. I've certainly known one formal network group had evolved to a point where meetings were held in a church and Christian prayers were said before the meeting started. Many people felt this group did not represent them and was exclusive to a small subgroup.

Smaller providers may feel they do not have enough staff to form an official group but can (and should) still consult with staff who work for them and talk about equality and diversity. They should still look at whether their staff are representative of the population they serve and whether their leadership team is representative of their staff group.

True consideration of equality and access to services sometimes reveals the reality that reasonable adaptations are anything but. Able-bodied staff making assumptions about people with limited mobility or who are reliant on a wheelchair may not identify the barriers. Involving people who are most affected is the best way to see if adaptations work in practice. There has recently been a programme of inspections of diagnostic services (stand-alone MRI scanning services, for example). The reports are presented at a quality assurance panel and often talk about a ramp or level access as evidence of adaptations for people who use wheelchairs. What the reports invariably fail to consider is what support or adaptation there is for a person to get from the wheelchair to the scanning couch.

Likewise, most reports mention a telephone translation service for people who use English as an additional language or who do not speak English. They generally don't mention what translation services are available to deaf people. The following excerpt from the Disability, Pregnancy & Parenthood website shows how pregnant deaf women are failed by our services.

"I waited in the Antenatal clinic. All the other pregnant women were reading their magazines. Me? I wanted to do the same, but I knew I couldn't. I had my eyes glued to every nurse walking in and out of the doctor's room. For two and a half hours I was like this until a nurse came to me for my name. She had called my name two hours earlier! I never heard her. At last it was my turn. I went in to see the doctor. I was really dismayed to see he had a huge beard. I couldn't see his lips – I couldn't understand him at all so all these questions I wanted to ask were wasted. I went home tense, tired and miserable – and still no wiser about what I wanted to know."

"I was giving birth – it was hard work, watching the midwife telling me what to do. She was good at her job, but I did not understand her very much. When the baby was finally born, I was elated, though absolutely shattered. The midwife was handing over to me my new-born baby and tried to say something to me. I was too doped and tried to lip-read. After a few minutes I realised what she was trying to tell me – I had a baby girl. All that communication hassle – why didn't she just show me her sex?"

Our approach to equality and human rights in regulation strengthens our focus on the equality and human rights of people using services – and also covers workforce equality in providers.

Why do we need to consider equality and human rights in regulatory work?

To fulfil our purpose, we want all people using services to receive safe, effective, high-quality care. There is also increasing evidence of the link between workforce equality and good quality care. This is why looking at equality for people who use services and for staff in our regulatory work is important. Equality for people using services is included in our regulations – and equality for people using services and for staff is covered in our assessment frameworks.

The human rights principles of fairness, respect, equality, dignity and autonomy are also fundamental to good care. Many of the most serious failings in care services have been human rights breaches. Human rights principles are built into our regulations and assessment frameworks. Having a shared understanding of what these principles mean in practice, building on human rights law, and then acting to protect and promote these rights is necessary for us as a regulator. This is why human rights are important.

(CQC February 2019)

Colin Powell once said, "Good leaders are almost always great simplifiers. Who can cut through argument, debate and doubt to offer a solution that everybody can understand?" Colin Powell was the first African American appointed as the US Secretary of State, and the first to serve on the Joint Chiefs of Staff. His understanding of the importance of simplicity of message and actions are both profound and obvious. It can be a very lengthy wait until a committee or action plan is created to start considering how to make a service equal for all. It can become very bureaucratic when large organisations start to talk about succession planning and aspirations, about skills gap analysis of the board members; to debate about how best to celebrate Eid and whether it was appropriate to do so in a Methodist care home.

Some people, some leaders, some staff, might feel that equality and diversity is something that isn't necessarily relevant to them because they serve people who are mainly from a similar background. The assumption being that if you don't have people who speak another language or have a different faith, then you don't need to consider them. You are unlikely to ever be 'Outstanding' when you have a staff group who think equality is not something they need to really consider. A great leader will role model a holistic and simple view of equality; that it is everyone's responsibility and that all people should be treated in a way that considers their individual needs and preferences.

All action toward greater fairness is positive, but there shouldn't be a perception that staff must wait until someone imposes an Equality Strategy. This is true partly because the strategy is never going to be embedded in practice if it is imposed without collaboration and consultation. In a truly outstanding service, everyone would have ownership of equality and everyone would understand that equality is the true basis of exceptional care based on individual needs and preferences. There is an awful lot of tokenism in demonstrating an awareness of diversity, but a sign saying Ramadan Kareem in the window is wasted if a GP practice doesn't support women who wish to see a female GP. Equality is not about signs in windows, it is not about banning all signs of difference, it is about recognising and accepting and being comfortable with difference. A strategy and policy bought on the internet is unlikely to make you 'Outstanding' and won't raise your Workplace Race Equality Standards survey results.

Equality and action taken to support fairness towards the workforce is likely to feature more prominently moving forwards.

From April 2015, the Workforce Race Equality Standard (WRES) became mandatory for all NHS trusts and for most independent healthcare providers. In the case of the independent healthcare providers, CQC currently looks at implementation of the WRES as part of the well-led lines of enquiry within the inspection framework at location of service level. →

Workforce race equality survey results are included in all assessments of how well-led these services are. Looking at race equality for staff in NHS is also one the CQCs equality objectives.

Northamptonshire Healthcare NHS Foundation Trust

Northamptonshire Healthcare NHS Foundation Trust (NHFT) started as a mental health trust before expanding to incorporate both physical and mental health community services. Their performance in the WRES had improved over a four-year period and was now showing results in the top few trusts nationally.

The data provided by the WRES showed a marked improvement with a staff engagement score, the 7th best score across the country. The number of staff recommending the trust as a place to work increased from 62% in 2015 to 76% in the most recent survey.

The numbers of BME staff believing the trust provided equal opportunities for career progression improved from 68% in 2015 to 80% in 2019. BME staff experiencing discrimination was an area which had significantly improved. In 2015, 25% of staff reported experiencing discrimination but by 2019 this had been reduced to 11%.

The Chief Executive had set up an equality steering group which was co-chaired by the BME network. This helped improve trust between senior leadership and staff and lead to co-production of action plans. The Board had regular papers related to equality to scrutinise and provide direction.

The WRES action plan was co-produced with BME staff and because of this plan, a reverse mentoring initiative and staff led focus groups were implemented. The executive all participated in a reverse mentoring programme. They spoke emotively and powerfully about this and it informed their planning and practice. The National Director for WRES had recently visited the trust and praised the culture and approach. The right culture provides the 'building blocks' to improve the whole workforce experience, which in-turn improves patient experience and outcomes.

West Midlands Ambulance Service

This is one of those examples where 'Outstanding' doesn't mean perfect. The West Midlands is culturally diverse – in some areas 15% of the local population are from BME backgrounds. The trust staff make-up did not reflect the cultural make-up of the population it serves. For example, as of March 2016, WMAS workforce included 5.12% Black, Asian and Minority Ethnic (BAME) employees, while 91.61% of staff described themselves as white and 3.26% of staff chose not to state their ethnic origin. 39.9% of the workforce was female compared to 60% male, and 5.19% of staff described themselves as disabled.

The trust had recently recognised this, and the executive team were able to describe some of the steps they had taken to address this. For example, the Equality Diversity and Inclusion (EDI) steering group undertook an analysis to identify barriers to women progressing beyond a band 6 (majority of women were in pay bands 3-6). Proactively encouraging people from BME backgrounds to apply for posts and offering additional support during the recruitment process and a mandatory training session put in place for all PTS control staff to cover the importance of diversity monitoring information.

The trust had engaged with local BME communities through a range of local initiatives such as visiting local Mosques and holding focus groups.

The trust also found innovative ways of engaging with the local population, for example the Youth Council and the Youth Cadet scheme, the aim of which was to encourage a commitment to young people who wish to have a career in the NHS including the West Midlands Ambulance Service.

Although these initiatives were in the early stages, they had already been shown to have had a positive impact.

How can services promote equality for all?

You can promote equality and diversity by:

Treating all staff and people using the service fairly: This is clearly not the same as treating them all the same. People are all different and understanding that care needs to address the individual needs by ensuring a fair service is key to providing not only equality but better care for all. Maybe use those fresh eyes again or a patient participation group to walk the journey of a patient or group of patients with needs. Look at your access for someone with reduced mobility – which might be about something more than a door that is wide enough for a wheelchair. If you run a GP service or an outpatient or an emergency department, look at the environment from the viewpoint of a parent with an autistic child who is stressed by sensory overload. Would it be better for all to find a quieter space where they can wait without the child going into a meltdown? Children in meltdowns are rarely easy to treat.

Creating an inclusive culture for all staff and people who use services: A positive culture is key to an organisation moving towards becoming 'Outstanding' – and I don't just mean in terms of ratings. There is a strong link with organisation improvement. In December 2018, Lucy Wilkinson, equality, diversity and human rights manager at the Commission, said in discussion with Joan Saddler, associate director at the NHS Confederation and co-chair of the NHS Equality and Diversity Council, "Firstly, there is a body of academic work now that shows that when staff are treated equally and feel valued and included, this is very positively correlated with care quality – and the converse is true. So, looking at workforce equality through a range of areas such as the WRES is a particularly good signifier for us as to the culture of a trust. Secondly, while staff on the frontline can do a lot to improve equality for patients, this also needs leadership attention to look at trust-wide issues and to ensure good engagement with a diverse range of people using services."

She went on to say, "Part of our purpose is to encourage services to improve. We were finding outstanding health and social care services – of all types – that were using equality and human rights-based work to improve care quality. Often these approaches are relatively low cost, for a big improvement, so this is an approach which can reap rewards even in times of financial constraint."

Talk to people: Engagement is shown to be particularly important: having significant associations with patient satisfaction, patient mortality and infection rates. The more engaged staff members are, the better the outcomes for patients and the organisation generally. The extent of positive feeling – exemplified by good communication, involvement of staff, and an emphasis on quality – is a predictor of both staff outcomes (absenteeism and turnover) and patient outcomes (satisfaction and mortality).

Where there is less discrimination, patients are more likely to say that, when they had important questions to ask a nurse, they got answers they could understand and that they had confidence and trust in the nurses.

Where staff surveys in NHS trusts showed that staff reported high levels of discrimination, patients felt that:

- doctors and nurses talked in front of them as if they weren't there
- they were not as involved as they wanted to be in decisions about their care and treatment
- they could not find someone on the hospital staff to talk to about their worries and fears
- they were not treated with respect and dignity while in hospital.

Analysis of many data sets relating to hospital trusts shows that not only does a positive and more equal culture improve patient outcomes, it is also cheaper and can improve organisational finances (West *et al*, 2012).

According to the 2009 Boorman Review of NHS Staff Health and Well-being, NHS staff are absent from work on average 10.7 days each year, losing the service a total of 10.3 million days annually and costing a staggering £1.75 billion. Total absenteeism equates to the loss of 45,000 whole time equivalent staff annually. High levels of staff engagement correlates with much lower absence rates than low or moderate levels of engagement. A positive culture undoubtedly saves money and is something providers cannot afford to dismiss.

Ensuring equal access to opportunities to enable all staff to fully participate in the learning process. Training and time for training should make your staff feel valued, confident and more able to do their work effectively. I tire of reports that show a 93% completion of mandatory training rates but with staff who cannot remember the content of the training or for whom it was just another chore completed in a coffee break. That is never going to be enough to enthuse and engage your staff. Learning should be so much more than staff skipping to the simple assessment page of an online course and ticking a few boxes to prove they have been trained.

Good training provides challenges and encourages staff to ask questions of themselves and their colleagues and leaders. It opens eyes and allows opportunities for individual and organisational development. Why would you exclude anyone from this? What impact would it have on the member of staff who was unable to get up the stairs in your GP practice to attend the lunchtime training session held in the conference room? How would the member of staff who is deaf feel if the training were a video without subtitles?

Training must fit in around the needs, dignity and well-being of those that rely on the staff team and must meet the expectations and aspirations of your staff. What is the effect of offering staff training every other Friday if you have four staff who work a nine-day fortnight? Far from improving those members of staff skills and commitment, you are likely to demotivate and discourage them because they either have to miss out on training or attend on their day off.

Do you consider the religious or cultural practices of your staff? If you offer training on a Friday and have Jewish staff, would you consider an earlier start and finishing in time to allow staff to get home in time for Shabbat? Could it be offered in two half sessions? Sunset in November in London is just after 4pm, so a 4:30pm finish time would make observance of an important religious practice difficult for observant Jews.

If the staff are given the correct tools and empowered to problem solve, there will be a rise in morale and motivation. Work ethic will improve and, as a result, so will the quality of care offered.

Look at your senior leadership team and board. Are they representative? If not, are there plans to make the board and leadership team more diverse?

Enabling all staff to their full potential

Having a diverse workforce means that organisations can tap into a wide range of ideas, skills, resources and energies, to give themselves a greater chance of success. There is a much wider pool of talent available to the organisations that embrace diversity. Diverse organisations also reap the benefits of a broader recruitment pool, improved productivity and a raised profile within the community.

The benefits of actively encouraging a diverse workforce include:

- Local people have local knowledge, and a diverse workforce that is more representative will enable better planning to meet the needs of the local community.

- Most people want to work for an employer with a good track record of equality and where people are supported and promoted on merit and potential not skin colour or gender, for example.

- Where people feel comfortable, they are likely to remain in employment. This means a wider recruitment pool and more opportunities for 'growing your own' senior staff.

- A representative staff group will be better able to provide for a diverse service user group; there will be a greater understanding of diversity and cultural needs within the staff group. Shared learning will spread that understanding.

- Staff may feel more able to challenge inequality and discrimination in their work environment, meaning you stay within the law and allow concerns to be raised.

Services that encourage diversity tend to be better employers. Better employment practice costs less and offers better service delivery.

- Staff become comfortable with difference.

- Different views are encouraged and respected. This improves team working and can improve productivity and outcomes for people using the service.

- Staff morale is improved, which raises motivation, which means better outcomes, which improves morale…

- Staff attrition rates are reduced. Good employers keep staff. Investment in staff training is worthwhile and there is a greater likelihood of recruiting good people to senior posts.

- The workplace becomes a joy to work in. Staff are happier and more tolerant.

The example below is an exemplar of good practice and support for a diverse workforce.

First Community Health and Care CIC

We saw an exceptionally strong commitment to equality and diversity across the organisation. The CEO worked part-time and there were effective arrangements to allow this to succeed. It provided a good model of the way the service considered and responded to the diverse needs of individuals.

Two administrative staff with learning disabilities who were employed on the same terms and conditions as other staff but given high levels of support to fulfil their roles, told us that the employment, "Had transformed their lives and was the best job ever".

One of the members of staff sat for over an hour waiting to speak to us (we didn't realise he was waiting for us). After the interview, we went to speak with the executive directors to find the staff member was engaged excitedly in conversation with the CEO and chief nurse about what they had told us; they were hugging the CEO and she was reassuring the staff member that they had done very well with the inspectors and should feel very proud. The staff member was employed for one session a week to assist with laminating, photocopying non-confidential information and stapling papers together. They had been working at First Community since it was set up and were a well-known and much valued member of staff employed on the same terms and conditions as other staff.

A member of staff who had worked in palliative care felt unable to return to this role after her husband died. The organisation had sponsored and supported her to retrain as a clinical nurse specialist in another role and to transfer to another job that was not focused on end of life care.

We met with BME staff but were told that each of them felt they were simply members of staff doing their jobs in a supportive organisation. The organisation had considered the Workforce Racial Equality Standards (WRES), was monitoring and considering how best to meet the needs of BME staff, but also felt it was more about meeting each member of staff's individual needs.

There was role modelling with a BME Deputy Chief Nurse who had been supported to join a BME Aspiring Director of Nursing Network to enhance their development opportunities. A WRES audit had been carried out and there was an action place to address areas where improvements could be made.

Ensuring policies, procedures and processes don't discriminate

Employers can make 'reasonable' dress code demands. They must give their employees time to meet those demands but can dismiss members of staff that don't follow workplace dress codes. Different work environments require different ways of dressing; sometimes it is about health and safety requirements (hi-vis jackets or hard hats), sometimes it is about infection prevention and control or patient safety (static risk where oxygen is used, for example) and sometimes it is about corporate image. They are all perfectly legitimate reasons for dress and uniform requirements. What isn't acceptable is saying that female nurses must wear dresses or that administrative and reception staff must wear corporate uniform shoes with a 2" heel.

You can insist that no religious symbols are worn at work but that might be much more complicated than it seems, and you should seek proper advice about the wording of your policy if you don't wish to find yourself in a tribunal.

Victoria Atkins, Parliamentary Under Secretary of State for Crime, Safeguarding and Vulnerability, is quoted as saying, "Discrimination in the workplace is not only completely unacceptable but also against the law. We will not stand for it. We live in an integrated and cohesive society with a proud tradition of religious tolerance and I want to see that reflected in workplaces across the country. As long as it doesn't interfere with someone's work, they should just be allowed to get on with the job."

The Government website, GOV.UK, shows that under the Conservative and Liberal Democrat coalition government (2010–2015) Eric Pickles, the then Secretary of State for Communities and Local Government, responded to misleading media reports that the Government favoured banning the wearing of Christian symbols in workplaces. He said, "We should be concerned about any move to strip individuals of their right to celebrate who they are. For some Christians, wearing a crucifix or cross or carrying a rosary is very much part of their faith, although it is a personal choice and not a formal requirement of their religion. The issue is not whether faith perspectives and religious voices should be included and tolerated in the public sphere, for that right is incontestable, but the way such a right is exercised and any restrictions that may be necessary to impose on that right. It is reasonable, and lawful, for Christians to wear a discreet symbol of their faith if this does not get in the way of their work. Indeed, given the massive contribution of Christians to our country over centuries, it is to be welcomed. Where religious symbols do not physically interfere with a person's work, but employers have instituted dress codes prohibiting them, employees have good grounds to ask for the code to be reconsidered. We urge employers to be flexible." This guidance stands.

What you absolutely cannot do is allow someone to wear a small crucifix on a chain but make someone else take off their tiny Palestinian Sunbird necklace or their Star of David earrings. Your dress code would have to ban all necklaces.

The report below doesn't formally refer to what many people perceive as equality and diversity but does show how the care provided is personalised in accordance with individual preferences and needs. That shows a real commitment to equality and valuing of individuality. How much nicer for staff to be able to offer something that the person really wants and will (hopefully) enjoy.

Arcot House Residential Home

"Staff were very responsive to people's individual needs. A person who liked to lie in was having a late breakfast in the dining room and had two separate mugs of tea in front of them and toast with an extra thick layer of butter."

Other services have considered how they meet the needs of the individuals – both staff and people who use services.

The Sussex Beacon

"The particular needs and preferences of all patients were identified and respected. Patients were seen very much as individuals. This meant that whilst the needs of LGBT and BME patients were recognised and addressed there was little in the way of planning to meet the needs of these patients as groups. The culture was to promote personalised care not cohort care."

"The unit admitted and cared for pregnant women, when necessary; they offered HIV related support and not pregnancy support. All pregnant women were under the care of the specialist HIV consultants and midwives at the local hospital. If there were any concerns during the admission, the patient would be medically reviewed and transferred to the maternity unit."

Concord Medical Centre, Bristol

"The practice was sensitive to people with poor mental health. They offered them greater flexibility regarding access to and duration of appointments, including offering them appointments at the end of morning surgery or during quieter times. The practice felt this was well received by patients, providing individualised care in a quiet and supportive environment. This was intended to reduce potential stress for the patient and reassure them they would be treated without fear or prejudice."

The practice had also recruited a mental health nurse consultant following a review of their patient needs.

Benenden Hospital

"Staff gave us examples of action they had taken to meet individual patients' complex needs, such as learning disability and dementia. On Bensan Ward, staff gave any patients with dementia a room adjacent to the nurses' station. The ward allowed family members of patients living with dementia or learning disabilities to stay overnight in an adjacent room. In theatres, staff gave us an example of a patient with learning disabilities whose parents came into the anaesthetic room with them before surgery. The parents also waited in recovery to greet the patient when they woke up from general anaesthetic."

Royal Berkshire NHS Foundation Trust

"The Polish community is the largest Eastern European community living in Reading. Polish translation services are the most frequently requested language translation service in Reading. Instead of relying on translators, the maternity service at the Royal Berkshire Hospital offered Polish speaking clinics."

Some providers have also responded to support the public anger and protests following the killing of George Floyd by a US Police Officer in Minneapolis. Undoubtedly, there is much work still to be done to ensure equality of opportunity and equality of outcomes for non-white people across the globe.

The Coronavirus statistics provide evidence of significant differences in the mortality rates for black and white people. The Institute for Fiscal Studies has said a higher proportion of people from ethnic minority backgrounds live in areas hit harder by Covid-19 but, as they are usually younger on average, they should be less vulnerable. Unfortunately, the report found that despite being younger, people from black, Asian and minority ethnic groups were experiencing much worse outcomes. After accounting for differences in age, sex and geography, the study estimated that the death rate for people of black African heritage was 3.5 times higher than for white Britons. We don't yet understand fully why this is, but it is unlikely to be genetics alone; socioeconomic factors and social inequalities almost certainly influence the figures. It's hardly surprising that communities are so very angry about the police officers' action in the US and the public celebration of people linked to the oppression and killing of people from non-white communities throughout modern history.

Guy's and St Thomas' NHS Foundation Trust

The trust has removed statues depicting Robert Clayton and Thomas Guy from public view. Both were actively engaged in the slave trade. Clayton was a former Lord Mayor of London with links to the Royal African Company, which transported slaves to the Americas. The Royal African Company had a monopoly on the transportation of slaves to the Caribbean because of the Navigation Act (1660) which only allowed English-owned ships to enter colonial ports. Between the 1670s and 1680s, the Company captured and transported an estimated 90,000 to 100,000 slaves to British-held colonies.

Thomas Guy invested in the South Sea Company, which was also involved in the slave trade. The company was a private/public company set up to address the national debt. In order to generate income, the company was granted a monopoly to supply African slaves to the islands in the 'South Seas' and South America. The slaves were often supplied by the Royal Africa Company and the company transported more than 34,000 slaves.

In Britain, many investors were ruined by the share-price collapse but that is probably little consolation to those left questioning why such people would be feted. A statement from the trust said, "Like many organisations in Britain, we know that we have a duty to address the legacy of colonialism, racism and slavery in our work. We absolutely recognise the public hurt and anger that is generated by the symbolism of public statues of historical figures associated with the slave trade in some way. We have therefore decided to remove statues of Robert Clayton and Thomas Guy from public view, and we look forward to engaging with and receiving guidance from the Mayor of London's Commission on each."

Equality is everyone's business. Equality for staff is more likely to mean fair treatment for people using services. Sadly, there is still a long way to go, with the NHS Confederation reporting in 2019 that the proportion of board chairs and non-executive directors from a non-white background recruited or re-appointed during 2017 was 8% of a total of 1,603 appointments. That is down from 12% in 2009.

Evidence or opinion

"Facts are stubborn things; and whatever may be our wishes, our inclinations, or the dictates of our passions, they cannot alter the state of facts and evidence." John Adams (Second president of the USA, 1797- 1801).

Often when staff are being interviewed, we ask what they feel is a real strength of their service or part of a service; what they are proud of as managers and leaders or what is it that makes their service special. Almost without exception we are told either "Fantastic teamwork" or "The staff always go the extra mile". More rarely it is simply "The culture". Even quite senior leaders can be very vague.

Inspection teams want services to show us their good side. We want them to do well. We enjoy hearing about exceptionally good care. Sometimes getting that as evidence we can use is like pulling teeth from a tiger. Invariably we ask for more specific details or examples of what that means in practice. The conversation usually goes something like this:

"Gosh, we've been talking for 50 minutes already, so we'll have to wind up our discussion. Last question, can you talk to me about what makes you smile when you think about your work, what are you most proud of, what do you do very well?"

"Oh, um, let me think; teamwork, definitely the teamwork."

"Excellent, what particularly about the team working? Any really good practices, any good examples?"

"Oh, um, just it's a really good team. They all work well together."

"In what way?"

"Just that they are all really committed to working as a team."

"Excellent, can you think of an example when they've been really supportive of each other?"

"Um, oh, nothing specific really but just really good teamwork."

It's good to hear that the team works well; I usually believe the person telling me, but it's not something I can write in a report; it's not evidence. It's simply the person saying what they think; it's an unsubstantiated opinion.

Now, think about how the conversation could have gone.

"Gosh, we've been talking for 50 minutes already, so we'll have to wind up our discussion. Last question, can you talk to me about what makes you smile when you think about your work, what are you most proud of, what do you do very well?"

"I'd say teamwork was a real strength."

"In what way? Do you have examples?"

"Yes. In our recent internal staff survey, which included all of the staff in the practice staff and partners, 96% of staff reported that there was a strong culture of team working."

"Excellent, anything else?"

"Well, recently when it snowed, we had problems with people getting into work as many staff live in villages on the moors. One of the receptionists, who lives close by, offered to come in on her non-working day to provide cover. One of the HCA's husbands is a farmer and she persuaded him to pick up two of the GPs in a specially adapted four-wheel drive vehicle which he has for seeing the livestock out on the hills and he took them home at the end of the day. The practice nurses all live in town, but they helped see patients from the other practice in town, where the nurse lives more remotely. One of the nurses brought a huge pan of warm vegetable soup and home-made bread, for all the staff to have for lunch. The GP registrar turned up wrapped up for the Arctic and offered to walk to all essential home visits."

I'm sure that you can see the second example gives more depth and readability to the idea that it is a good team. We could check out the amount of snow and where the doctors lived but we didn't need to – it contained enough detail that we knew it was true. Just by telling us a story, we had evidence that this team really did work well together.

Ratings judgements cannot be based on vague opinions. We can't necessarily see all the good work that is going on in a service. This is particularly true in areas such as leadership, culture and caring that are somewhat harder to capture using data alone.

Stories are important to creating an understanding of the experience of staff and people using services. They humanise and create a sense of what the service is genuinely like in a way that data alone can never quite replicate. They are also an important way of sharing and building a positive culture. The inspection team often won't collect some of the powerful narrative evidence unless someone tells us about it. That isn't cheating; it's helping your staff reflect and celebrate what they do particularly well and when they have truly gone above and beyond a 'Good' level of care. In particularly good services, it can be a learning tool, a means of disseminating good practice. How difficult is it to share a positive (and specific) story about the good work of your team at each team meeting or with the board? Use concrete examples rather than platitudes. Then when the inspection team turn up and ask for examples, your staff will be able to retell the story.

Caring is a particularly hard domain to evidence as 'Outstanding'. If you are in the NHS, then there is the Friends and Family Test scores, you may have local survey results, but nothing beats a good story.

Sussex Community NHS Foundation Trust

Sussex Community Trust has a 'Book of Good' held on each ward at their community hospitals. Nothing fancy, just a small notebook. It was because of these notebooks that we saw the exceptional level of caring and personalised service that was offered to patients on their inpatient wards. It was such a simple idea. Staff wrote a note when they had seen another member of staff going above and beyond expectations. There were lots of entries that were nice statements about someone being kind – much too general to use. However, among those were some truly lovely to read examples of staff 'going the extra mile' and working beyond their job descriptions. We could talk to staff about these and when they were asked, they all validated the entries and remembered the example and sometimes a few more – because they understood what we were looking for.

Staff throughout community inpatient services had an overwhelming pride in the service and level of care they delivered. Staff across all locations demonstrated providing care in excess of what would be expected to their patients. We were given examples of staff accompanying patients to outpatient appointments when family members were unable to attend. Staff ensured a patient's pets could visit them at the end of their life. Staff arranged new furniture to enable a patient to return home. It was not uncommon for staff to take patient's washing home, if they had no one to do this for them. Staff had organised a wedding blessing for a patient unable to leave the ward.

At one location the staff had set up a trolley with donated toiletries so that patients who were admitted without anything could be provided with what they needed for their stay. Staff in a community hospital regularly 'popped across' to a local shop, in their own time, to purchase newspapers, sweets or snacks or toiletries for patients.

Western Sussex Hospitals NHS Foundation trust

The provider has a lot of trust Ambassadors, from all groups of staff and at all grades, from porters to radiographers, from receptionists to consultants. Their primary role is to spread positivity and they do, when asked (or at any other convenient time), open their mouths to speak and suddenly it's like Mount Etna erupting with loveliness. They approach inspection team members (but not only inspection team members) and offer help, volunteer to show you the way, and then talk to you of good works and tell nice stories as they escort you. It's clever, very clever. These are people with a huge sense of pride in their trust, who are supported and given a platform to talk to people and create a joyful culture. It was in part due to these Ambassadors that the trust received its 'Outstanding' rating for caring. If the Ambassadors had not been so open and had not been so knowledgeable about the good work being done we would not have been pointed in the right direction to see what some of the staff were doing, in a quiet unassuming sort of way, as part of their everyday practice. A couple of examples given to us by the trust Ambassadors follow.

"We saw many examples of compassionate end of life care. Several members of staff talked to us about the chaplaincy services and told us how they had helped reunite an elderly, terminally ill patient with their baby that had died many years previously. The patient had asked the Patient Liaison service to find out where their baby that had died during childbirth at the hospital many years previously was buried. Records were searched but no clue found so PALS talked to the chaplain about it. The chaplain made contact and started searching in their own time, visiting local authority records departments, the registry office, local funeral directors and eventually located where the baby was buried in an unmarked grave. The chaplain escorted the patient to the grave and then provided ongoing support as they finally came to terms with losing their baby. The story spread, and the chaplains have helped several other families who have 'lost' babies to be reunited."

We would never have known about this had the Ambassadors not told us about this story; the chaplain was far too modest to have told us themselves.

"The trust carried out 'Sit and See Observations' to observe the care and compassion of staff towards patients. The principles of the tool were to safeguard people through recognising that the absence of compassion was one of the first indicators of a failing environment. The scheme also celebrated and spread good practice that was observed and enabled staff to see care through the eyes of a patient. This was a simple but highly effective way of involving non-clinical staff by allowing them to see the impact of their work and share ownership of patient care".

Western Sussex had provided two types of evidence that we could use in the report: the ambassador scheme itself showed an organisational culture that had 'buy in' from staff at all levels and we could follow up the stories that the Ambassadors mentioned. Win, win. The Sit and See wasn't expensive to run but allowed those 'fresh eyes' that staff working on a ward or in a hectic department are so often too busy to stop and see. This would be so easy to do in most settings where regulated activities were provided. It might be difficult in a mobile MRI scanner, but it would certainly be possible in a GP practice, independent hospital or termination of pregnancy clinic, to get a fairly objective person to sit and observe in waiting areas to see what the people using service saw. A regular 'Sit and See' session by different staff with a record of those observations would form quite powerful evidence about understanding the patient perspective.

Find ways to show exactly what having staff who go the extra mile really means.

At the opposite end of the spectrum, I recently instigated enforcement action against a provider who could easily have avoided such a negative report and a warning notice had they considered the patient's perspective. That was around the physical journey for children on a surgical pathway where nobody had stopped and considered what it must feel like for a frightened five-year-old to walk, in a hospital gown, down long corridors with lots of scary equipment, strange smells, loud beeping noises everywhere and adults in scrubs rushing around. The better providers would have walked the journey with the child's eyes. The ideal would be to get a child who was not facing surgery to walk it with their parents and tell you what they saw and how it made them feel. Western Sussex has a toy-sized electric Rolls Royce for the children to drive to theatre; it just needs staff to be open to seeing and understanding the patients' perspective.

> "Evidence is anything that you see, experience, read, or are told that causes you to believe that something is true or has really happened.
>
> Evidence is the information which is used in a court of law to try to prove something. Evidence is obtained from documents, objects or witnesses."
>
> Collins English Dictionary

The other key thing about evidence is that it should be current when published and that is something providers can use to their advantage. The Commission sometimes don't have the most up to date information about the service and won't necessarily have anything to update nationally recorded information unless the provider gives it to the inspection team. Some providers are better at maintaining up to date information about their service than others. That is true of all sorts of services. It is not necessarily the case that large NHS trusts are all very data competent while a small home for people with learning disabilities doesn't really use data.

There are several points during the inspection process where you can ensure that the report that is published and the information provided is most reflective of your service. The first is when submitting PIR (Provider Information request) responses.

From the CQC website:

"The PIR is an important element of our new inspection process. We are asking for this information under Regulation 10(3) of the Health and Social Care Act 2008 (Regulated Activities) Regulations 2010.

Please provide the information we require using this form. It will help us plan our inspections by asking you to provide us with data, and some written information under the questions:

■ Is the service safe?

■ Is it effective?

■ Is it caring?

■ Is it responsive?

■ Is it well-led?

The information you include in your return will help inspectors decide on the areas they need to look at during their visit. Some of the content may also be used to inform national reporting. When we use information in this way, it won't be attributed to any provider. You might find it helpful to use the return as part of your quality assurance process and as a way of understanding and reviewing how well you are meeting the five 'key questions'."

The PIR return is factual but is also an opportunity to sell yourself and show the good work that you or your staff are doing. It asks seemingly quite simple questions. If you respond in a minimal way, the inspection team will form a view and may think (not unreasonably) that this response is indicative of the care that you are providing. It seems so obvious, but so often PIR returns are rushed, inaccurate and give the shortest possible response with barely any evidence to support assertions.

Under the 'Safe domain' you might be asked, "Do you currently administer controlled drugs at the location?" The easiest response from a provider of adult social care or a private ambulance service might simply be, "Yes". That is not wrong, but it tells the inspection team very little, except that they need to look at how controlled drugs are managed. What about:

"Yes, we maintain supplies of morphine sulphate, midazolam and diazepam which are prescribed as anticipatory medicines for all patients identified as approaching the end of their life. We developed our anticipatory medicines policy in consultation with the local specialist palliative care team and the GP who service the home. Our registered nurses are all trained by the local hospice in recognising and managing end of life symptoms. Audits of end of life care for all patients who died within a six-month period showed that 94% of patients had effective pain management (according to their individual records and feedback from relatives). Our monthly controlled drug reconciliation and audits completed by a third-party pharmacist showed that we managed our controlled drugs very well but that we needed to replenish stock in good time to avoid the potential risk of shortages over bank holiday weekends. We have now addressed this by having a fortnightly review and order, if necessary, rather than waiting for a low stock level to be identified."

How much more evidence of 'Good' (or even 'Outstanding') practice does that submission give compared to a simple 'Yes'. Even better if you send the documents to support what you write, as evidence of what you've done.

Analytics

The Commission is constantly improving the use of service analytics to inform and monitor risk. Insight dashboards are now available to staff to help determine risk levels and, consequently, inspection frequency and timings. For some services (such as the NHS) there is far more data available from national and local sources. Independent healthcare hospitals data is becoming more visible, as they increase the amount of NHS contracted work they provide. Adult social care risk profiles are now available to Commission staff and providers.

You can't change some of the data, but you can certainly ensure that the risk profile is accurate and that the level of risk showing is a true reflection of your service by taking a few simple steps to reduce the number of 'red flags'.

It makes sense to ensure you have appointed a registered manager, if that is a condition of your registration. Failure to do so is an offence and you might find yourself with a fixed penalty notice unless your service is dormant or there is an application being processed. Long delays in appointing a new registered manager after someone has left will increase your risk score. There is good evidence that services without a registered manager perform less well.

Regulation 5 of the Care Quality Commission (Registration) Regulations 2009 requires the Commission to impose a registered manager condition on the registration of most providers. The exceptions are NHS providers, and individual providers who have been assessed as fit to carry on the regulated activity, and who intend to be in full time charge of the running of the service.

It's wise to send in your statutory notifications in a timely way. The chances are the Commission will find out. If it is a death notification, they may find out via the coroner, for example. If they haven't been notified it will increase your risk score and there is a possibility of enforcement action. If the Commission inspects and discovers unreported occurrences, then that breach of regulation is likely to limit your rating to 'Requires Improvement' in at least one domain.

Registered providers must notify the Commission about certain changes, events and incidents that affect their service or the people who use it. It is an offence not to notify CQC when a relevant incident, event or change has occurred.

NHS bodies (only) can submit some notifications through the NHS Commissioning Body's National Reporting and Learning System (NRLS – the system run previously by the National Patient Safety Agency); this does not apply to providers of adult social care, independent healthcare, primary dental care and private ambulance services.

Under- and over-reporting via the Statutory Notification process can impact on your risk score. A comparison with similar services over the preceding four months and 12 months is made to benchmark accurately. It pays to educate yourself and your staff about the requirements and sort of things that should be reported (it's not every incident or near miss, as a commercial incident reporting system would be).

Under-reporting is suggestive that a provider or manager isn't aware of the requirements, or worse, is hiding something. Deaths are required to be reported, for example. Deaths, however sad, aren't necessarily an indicator of poor care and may not be unexpected. What would interest the Commission staff might be a spiked increase in deaths related to falls in a community hospital, for example.

Over-reporting also suggests that the provider or manager aren't confident with the regulatory requirements and could increase the risk score if it persisted.

Honesty and integrity

"Atticus, you must be wrong."

"How's that?"

"Well, most folks seem to think they're right and you're wrong…"

"They're certainly entitled to think that, and they're entitled to full respect for their opinions," said Atticus, "but before I can live with other folks I've got to live with myself. The one thing that doesn't abide by majority rule is a person's conscience."

Harper Lee, To Kill a Mockingbird

The dictionary suggests that 'honesty' is being truthful or able to be trusted; not likely to steal, cheat, or lie, or (of actions, speech, or appearance) showing these qualities. 'Integrity' can be defined as the quality of being honest and having strong moral principles that you refuse to change. It can also mean wholeness and unity – something essential to successful teams.

Organisations that aspire to an 'Outstanding' rating need to develop an open, trusting and honest staff body that acts with integrity. It is a regulatory requirement when things go wrong, but it goes beyond that and should be embedded in all aspects of individual and organisational behaviour.

The duty of candour came into effect for all non-NHS bodies registered with CQC (including all General Practices) from 1 April 2015. This is Regulation 20 of the Health and Social Care Act 2008 (Regulated Activities) Regulations 2014, which sets out Fundamental Standards. It aims to ensure that providers are open and transparent with people who use services and other 'relevant persons' (people acting lawfully on their behalf) in general in relation to care and treatment.

It also sets out some specific requirements that providers must follow when things go wrong with care and treatment, including informing people about the incident, providing reasonable support, providing truthful information and an apology when things go wrong.

Introducing Regulation 20 was a direct response to the Francis Inquiry report into Mid Staffordshire NHS Foundation Trust, which recommended that a statutory duty of candour be imposed on healthcare providers. It applies to organisations rather than individual clinicians. In interpreting the regulation on the duty of candour, CQC uses the definitions of openness, transparency and candour used by Sir Robert Francis in his report:

- Openness – enabling concerns and complaints to be raised freely without fear and questions asked to be answered.

- Transparency – allowing truthful information about performance and outcomes to be shared with staff, patients, the public and regulators.

- Candour – any patient harmed by the provision of a healthcare service is informed of the fact and an appropriate remedy offered, regardless of whether a complaint has been made or a question asked about it.

There may be significant consequences for providers who fail to uphold the Duty of Candour. The Care Quality Commission fined Bradford Teaching Hospitals NHS Foundation Trust £1,250 for failing to apologise to a family in a reasonable period. The Commission issued a fixed penalty notice to the trust because it had failed to comply with the Duty of Candour. In this case, a baby had been admitted to Bradford Royal Infirmary in July 2016 but there were delays in diagnosing his condition and missed opportunities to admit him to hospital. Although the trust recorded it as a notifiable safety incident, the family were not informed and did not receive an apology until October. The action taken by the Commission against Bradford Teaching Hospitals did not relate to the care provided to this baby, but to the fact that the trust was slow to inform the family that there had been delays and missed opportunities in the treatment of their child.

Integrity is one of the core values of the Care Quality Commission. All staff are expected to 'live the values' and ensure that everything they do is underpinned with integrity. Most do a pretty good job at this and where there are serious concerns about integrity then staff may find themselves being asked whether regulation is the right place for them. It would be unthinkable to have a regulator that providers thought was corrupt, who believed their success was dependent on currying favour, or worse.

As staff are generally honest and demonstrate integrity, relationships within the organisation are, overall, good. For most staff, it's a nice place to work. The most recent full staff survey showed that 91% of staff felt that the CQC values were relevant to their work. If only the operational, directorate staff are considered, then the level who felt the values were relevant rose higher. A similar 91% of staff felt that the work that CQC does with providers improves the quality of care and encourages improvements. That can only be true if the relationships between the regulatory staff and providers is based on honesty and the impartiality of the inspection teams. As an aside, the lowest scoring question was around rewards for CQC staff being comparable to similar roles in other organisations; that scored a lowly 38%, which suggests the main driver for most staff within the Commission is not money.

I suspect most people working in health and social care feel they are honest, too. Interestingly, a study at the University of Massachusetts (Feldman, 2002) found around two thirds of people lie at least once during a ten-minute conversation, with many of them telling two or three lies in that time period. Most people would recognise that they do tell lies for a variety of reasons and often justify it by saying they were trying to be kind or didn't want to stand out from the crowd; they succumb to peer pressure and may agree to something they didn't really want to. The study also found that the type of lies told by men and women varied, although the frequency did not. Women were more likely to lie to make the person they were talking to feel good, to tell them they liked their new haircut or that they looked young for their age. Men were more likely to lie to make themselves look more impressive, to falsely claim responsibility for achievements or ideas.

So, does it matter in health and social care settings? A few white lies? Isn't it better to agree and not rock the boat? I would assert that even the small lies we see as benign can hurt us or others. My husband tells me my greatest virtue and biggest challenge is my tendency to honesty, at all times. I find it difficult to let injustice or falsehood lie quietly. In the workplace, lies tend to come around and create problems further along for the person who lied and those who were lied to.

I can think of a few examples where people have said daft things as part of an inspection (myself included) and have seen the impact and angst these seemingly innocuous untruths can cause. Quite recently I had to respond to the fallout where a very experienced member of staff had told a provider, during feedback at the end of a three-day inspection that, "If they were taking their driving test, they would have passed".

This was not true as:

- The Commission doesn't pass or fail providers – it gives ratings.
- The Commission doesn't agree ratings at the end of a site visit; inspection teams need to consider all the evidence and take the suggested ratings through a quality assurance process.
- There were potential breaches identified that were not fed back to the provider at the end of the site visit.

It left the provider and staff feeling that they were on track to receive, at worst, a 'Good' rating. Unfortunately, their draft report landed on their desks for factual accuracy checking with an indicative rating of 'Requires Improvement' and several requirement notices to address the breaches of regulations.

The leaders of the service were, unsurprisingly, unhappy about this and challenged it vociferously. We had to do what was right and fair, rather than simply hold fast to our report. This meant meetings, independent review of the report and the factual accuracy responses, submitting the report to a further quality assurance panel and time spent trying to rebuild the damage to the relationship with the provider. There were no winners because of a silly momentary lack of integrity when giving a difficult message. I suspect that, had we been more circumspect in our feedback, we would not have had the same degree of challenge.

Another example occurred a good few years ago in a nursing home. We had been contacted by the daughter of an elderly resident who had been badly scalded by excessively hot soup that they had accidentally tipped into his lap. The daughter had visited three days later and was concerned that he had not been seen by a GP or specialist nurse but had just had some antiseptic cream put on the large, angry blisters. The daughter was clear that the resident needed a lidded beaker to be able to manage soup for themselves and that this was a recorded part of their care plan. The Head of Care at the home had told the daughter she wasn't on duty and had only just found out about the scalds but hadn't had a chance to look yet. The daughter contacted the regulator at the time, and I spoke with her.

As the daughter was so distressed and getting nowhere with the home, and because I didn't like to think of anyone being left with untreated serious burns, I phoned the home and spoke with the registered manager who was very evasive. I was told it was the resident's fault as they pulled the soup over themselves. They denied any care plan that suggested a lidded beaker was needed. They also said the GP had refused to visit but had suggested antiseptic cream. They also told me that as a nursing home they were not entitled to advice from a tissue viability nurse. I telephoned the daughter to discuss this and she remained clear that the beaker was essential, and this was recorded.

Obviously, the priority must be the welfare of the patient. Despite being somewhat outside our remit, I couldn't leave an elderly person in pain and with untreated scalds across their thighs and pelvic region. I spoke to the local GP practice and asked for a GP to visit – they had not refused; they had never been contacted. The local (now 'Outstanding' rated) NHS acute trust immediately agreed to their tissue viability nurse visiting with the GP to provide expert assessment and ongoing advice in the management of the wounds.

We carried out an unannounced inspection a few days later, on a Saturday morning at about 11am, just before lunch was served. What we found rather compounded the lack of honesty and refusal to accept any responsibility. Despite a person being seriously injured, the manager and organisation refused to take any responsibility or learning from the situation. We found:

■ Soup was still being served at 92 degrees centigrade in open bowls to frail, elderly people. It takes just one second for liquids at over 68 degrees centigrade to cause a significant burn to a healthy adult. The catering staff recorded the temperatures for assurance around food hygiene regulatory compliance, but nobody had used this information to consider the safety of residents.

■ Open bowls were used because there was only one agency member of staff for over 30 residents in the dining room. They simply didn't have time to look at the individual records and just gave everyone the same soup in an open bowl.

■ The scalded resident's personal care records showed that nobody had checked his wounds for two days. He had large, open blisters with dressings caked in antiseptic cream stuck to them. No pain killers had been given.

■ The head of care and manager who both denied knowing about the scald had both been on duty in the home at the time. The head of care had left her shift to go and check on her dogs, leaving a single, agency member of staff in the dining room. The manager had, ironically, been hidden away in the office updating policies, in case of a CQC visit.

■ No attempt had been made to assess the wounds or to seek expert advice.

■ The elusive personal care plan had managed to find its way into the back of the home's staff diary, which was kept in a desk drawer, rather than in the person's individual record. It specifically mentioned that the person needed a lidded beaker for all fluids.

■ The relatives had been lied to.

There was more – lots more – around staffing, training, governance and all the basics that should be in place. The manager kept telling us she had only been in post eight months and couldn't do everything. As well as taking enforcement action against the provider, I referred her to the Nursing and Midwifery Council, as I believed she was in breach of her professional code of conduct. The head of care also faced an NMC disciplinary hearing. Had the truth been told, had they acted with integrity, the poor man would have been treated much sooner and his daughter would have been upset about her parent's injuries but nowhere near as angry as she was. Had the manager been honest on the phone, we might not have inspected; I was seeking assurance that appropriate care was being given and that the risk of recurrence was minimised. I heard defensiveness, a refusal to accept responsibility and a total lack of integrity. The manager and head of care both lost their careers because they put self-preservation above the needs of the resident and the truth.

I could write at length about the problems caused by a lack of integrity, but I suspect that if readers stop and reflect, most will be able to think of their own examples in which not doing the right thing, not telling the truth, being defensive or minimising situations has created more problems than it has solved.

Now I want to focus on the good and outstanding practice, the benefits of creating a culture where staff feel strongly that honesty really is the best policy, where individuals and organisations learn from mistakes and how they do this.

Carmen

Having mentioned reflecting on our own experiences, I stopped to consider where my firm belief in integrity and honesty originated from. It's certainly deep-rooted and probably begun at some point in my childhood. The one moment where I think I began to understand that integrity was more than telling the truth – it was standing up for what is right – was from those summer camps when I, along with lots of other volunteers, took large groups of children from the greater London area on holiday to the countryside for two weeks.

I was the deputy leader to my, now, husband at a field study centre in the Somerset hills. We had 45 children that we'd met for the first time at Paddington station, along with ten adults. It was a beautiful centre with a swimming pool, large sports hall and fields and a wonderful dining room on stilts, looking over the valley. It was idyllic and we had the late Arabella Churchill, granddaughter of Sir Winston and a founder of both the Glastonbury Festival and a children's charity called Children's World, bring her play bus, her huge inflatables and access to Longleat. We had tea with Lord Bath, which was fun with 20 children. They loved his interesting murals! Apologies, my reflection has become reminiscence...

We had a girl called Carmen on camp; a lively, energetic, bright, witty and generally charming 12-year-old who had an edge to her tongue, if crossed. We also had local volunteer cooks who were, generally, late middle-aged, middle-class women who did wholesome food using homemade and homegrown supplies whenever possible. Sadly, many of the children had limited experience of locally sourced, organic produce and preferred pizza to cassoulet.

Carmen was one of those who preferred almost everything to what was on offer. She was not used to food that was representative of rural Middle England. She liked pizza, goat curry or rice and peas. When she returned a fish pie that had only been moved around the plate, the lead volunteer, called Bunny, enquired, with a voice that shot out pure sulphuric acid, whether there was anything wrong with the food. Carmen said she didn't like it and was asked why. She said, "It's nasty". Not the best response, perhaps. It resulted in Bunny telling her to sit down, as she couldn't have any pudding because, "Undoubtedly, that will be nasty too". She then made an overtly racist comment about girls 'like her' being ungrateful and 'not eating normal food'. Carmen flashed, called her a very unfortunate name and stormed out. Bunny was upset and could not see that she could, as the adult, have avoided this. She demanded an apology before the next meal, or nobody would be served any food. I rather suspect she meant it; she was a bit scary.

We found Carmen and calmed her down, she was tearful and slightly contrite about the swearing. She wasn't in the least contrite about exploding at Bunny. She had a point. She had been picked on unfairly and the reaction from the volunteer to her not eating fish pie had been harsh. The comment about 'girls like you' was entirely unacceptable. Somehow we had to ensure that 50 people were fed and that required a degree of diplomacy – but we also wanted to do the right thing. In the end, Carmen agreed to apologise for using a swear word and for upsetting Bunny; she was definitely the bigger person. Her words were, "I am sorry that you felt I was wrong when I called you a ****. I was terribly upset at the way you spoke to me, it felt like it was because I was not white".

Bunny looked quizzical and toddled off, coming back later to speak to me and ask whether that was really an apology, as it felt like she was being cast as the one in the wrong. She wondered whether Carmen had deliberately avoided giving a full apology and should be made to do so. We could only suggest a forced or insincere apology was not really an apology and that perhaps we had all learned a little in the process. Carmen demonstrated absolute integrity and stood her ground about something she knew was right. She didn't waver under pressure from the other children or some staff. She knew that while swearing wasn't right, it was the lesser wrong.

So, what exactly are the benefits of developing a culture of honesty and integrity? Is it not better to avoid airing our dirty laundry in public? Should we minimise mistakes to avoid censure? Will the Commission look at meeting minutes or incident reports and think that, because the staff report concerns, you are a bad provider? Absolutely not. High reporting or no or low harm incidents is a positive sign. It suggests a culture that wants to get things right. High reporting of moderate and serious harm incidents is a different matter altogether but looking at near misses or trends of low harm incidents might just prevent something more serious occurring.

To act with integrity is to ensure that every decision made is based on ethical and moral principles. Organisations that are clear that they have an expectation that staff will always act with integrity, in the best interests of patients and carers, also tend to be the organisations that treat their staff with respect and where leaders are honest and open. Trust, respect, honour and honesty are key elements to the concept of integrity. In the workplace, employees that act with integrity will always tell the truth, are accountable and reliable, and treat co-workers, stakeholders and customers with respect. They will do the right thing, even when no one is watching.

Despite being an absolutely essential element of good organisations, integrity is difficult to foster. There are several main hurdles to integrity. First is the innate human ability to rationalise behaviour. Despite our knowledge that we should always do the 'right thing', humans have an inbuilt ability to justify their behaviour when they do the 'wrong thing'.

Think back to the Massachusetts study, women tell lies 'to be kind'. A woman might make a comment that a dress looks lovely, to provide reassurance, but the truth is that it is a colour that makes their friend look jaundiced and the shape is very unforgiving of middle-aged curves, with clingy material that outlines underwear and rides up to expose cellulite and thread veins. Is it kind to allow that friend to collect an award on stage with the audience smirking at their outfit or to allow them to attend an interview in something that is so unsuitable? We all justify such lies as kindness, but it's not really kind, is it? While small white lies and untruths persist, then the relationship lacks honesty and will undermine trust. If the inappropriately dressed woman hears two people talking about their dress in the lavatory, how will they feel about the advice you gave them that it was 'lovely'?

If this is then translated into health and social care settings, we can see that the 'small lies' really are the sand on which a poor culture is built. If staff justify acceptance of poor care, then there will be no improvement. I have seen fabulous, high-quality care delivered in run down or cramped environments without complaint and I have also seen other staff blame the environment for poor care.

The second roadblock to integrity is the unclear definition of what it means. Not everyone envisions integrity in the same way. In care of the elderly, for example, some people see 'doing the right thing' as protecting the patient or resident from all risk, making sensible decisions rather than decisions the person necessarily wants made for them. Do domiciliary care workers support a frail elderly person to smoke in their own home, if the person has capacity to make the decision but is physically unable to purchase their own cigarettes? Does the perceived fire risk outweigh the person's right to live their life as they want to?

Another roadblock is the perception of blame and feeling that mistakes will be penalised; staff not trusting others in their organisations to focus on improvement and see shortcomings as learning opportunities. If you know you'll be summoned to your managers office to be given a firm dressing down because you gave the wrong patient an antibiotic tablet, you might not feel inclined to own up to the mistake. If, however, you know that your manager will show you how to respond to ensure both patients' safety and will then come with you to speak to the patients concerned before discussing how it happened, you are much more likely to tell them, aren't you?

Dorothy House

Dorothy House is a hospice located just outside of Bath. It is registered for ten beds and provides specialist palliative and end of life care for adults with life limiting illness or complex symptom management needs.

The CQC report published following an inspection in September 2016 said, "Staff were open and honest with people when things went wrong and were committed to learning from people's experiences. The provider information showed two complaints had been received in the past year. Full explanations were given about the investigation, its findings and any actions being taken to address concerns. Responses offered unreserved apologies where any aspect of care fell below the standard expected. For example, in the information submitted by the provider prior to inspection, the service had highlighted how the service had reviewed the way food was provided for visitors following a concern raised by a relative."

Clarity and shared understanding

"If you can't explain it to a six-year-old, you don't understand it yourself."
Albert Einstein

"There is no greatness where there is not simplicity, goodness, and truth."
Leo Tolstoy

I write this as the book nears completion; I've come back to it while writing about 'well-led'. I was going to talk a little about it under 'Vision and Values', but thought a bit more and realised it is one of the key considerations in any relationship, any organisation and all communications.

The word 'simple' pops up quite a few times throughout this book, because simple things are generally easier to understand. The very best do not need complicated explanations. Those who understand most on a subject can allow others to share their understanding through a clarity and simplicity of language. Jargon and complexity lead to misunderstandings and creates conflicts that could easily be avoided. Long words and incomprehensible jargon might impress a few people but is more likely to lead to errors and arguments.

I remember sitting through the first hour of an interview where the person I was speaking with just talked about their initiatives and methodology. They were hugely enthusiastic and just spouted a stream of incomprehensibility, wrapped up as technical excellence. I could have been impressed if they had been able to tell me the impact or explain it in basic language. As it was, I didn't understand a word of what they were saying, it could have been spoken in Arabic or Greek for all the information that I gained from the discussion. I had to stop them and ask them to speak more simply, so I understood what they were telling me. They clearly thought I was a jobbernowl (lovely word) and incapable of assimilating the information they wished to impart.

I rather think that problem may have been their lack of true understanding, they were simply parroting the protologism from some course they had been on; they were invented words created to sell something without any great substance. When I asked for tangible examples of where it might have made a difference to my hypothetical

Great Aunt Maud, they weren't able to say. When I asked about any data to show that it had brought about improvements, they weren't able to say. It might have been fantastic work they were doing but I couldn't fathom out what they were trying to tell me. I've always enjoyed the story of the Emperor's new clothes, and some of the technical jargon used when people want to impress is just that.

I was reading an article on quality improvement that suggested it was a good thing to "Facilitate Adoption Through Participatory Intervention Projects". Just nonsense, isn't it? Much better to say, "Staff are more likely to agree to ideas that improve quality if they are involved in real projects".

When we lack clarity and are insufficiently explicit, we create a void that can be filled with mistakes.

- There is scope for errors, such as vague instructions about which implant might be preferred by an individual surgeon that could lead to a Never Event.
- Lack of clarity can create conflict if, for example, everyone thought a general request for weekend cover had been responded to by someone else.
- Lack of clarity can cause confusion about responsibilities. Imagine if nobody was sure who was in charge when the fire alarms went off unexpectedly.
- Lack of clarity can lead to behaviours we might consider inappropriate or not in line with the organisation's values.

If we set a rather vague objective such as, 'Be a sustainable organisation' and don't clarify what we mean, what sustainable looks like, how can we expect staff to join us on the path to being sustainable?

If we ask a new member of staff to, "Help sort out Mr. Bloggs", how can we complain when we see Mr. Bloggs has a fresh glass of water but his hearing aids are still on the table?

If we ask a team member to organise a social event without setting any boundaries, how can we be dismayed when a member of staff complains that they feel excluded because the planned event is a bar crawl during Ramadan?

I know full well that some of the people I have worked with on inspections think my very explicit expectations, that I make clear at the outset, is a bit of 'teaching granny to suck eggs'. When I talk about the consumption of alcohol and explain how I will react if someone overindulges in the hotel bar, or when I talk about being respectful to the providers' staff at all times, or that we hold discussions not interrogations, I suspect some of the team think it's a bit basic and that people should know this anyway. I am sure most do know and have similar expectations themselves. It is not for them; it's for the odd person who forgets to behave professionally, who takes a step outside of acceptable behaviour. I can hardly step in and ask someone to leave a hotel bar for being rowdy, if I have not set limits, if I have not said that a glass of wine with supper is acceptable but when the amount consumed disturbs others, it is too much.

I think the risk of someone being momentarily affronted that I am telling them not to smoke within sight of a service we are inspecting is better than finding a member of the team puffing away outside the emergency department, in front of a No Smoking sign.

"We're a bit short this weekend and could do with someone extra on the early shift," is far too woolly to guarantee cover. It's more likely to lead to a short staffed shift, with staff cross that they have had to work much harder and stay late to finish, a cross manager who felt unsupported by the staff, and ill feeling among other staff who feel a sense of blame. Far, far better to approach someone and say, "Carol, I know this is short notice, but Jack is going to be off for a fortnight and I need someone to change their rota to cover the early shift on Saturday. Are you able to do that?"

Kindness and woolliness are not the same thing at all. Ambiguity is unkind and leaves people not knowing what is wanted; it makes it much harder to deliver and succeed.

Clarity is not the same as micromanaging and being overly directive. Perhaps the most important time to be very clear about what is required is when delegating something. Clarity allows people to succeed rather than setting them up to fail.

First Community Health and Care, Surrey

First Community Health and Care is an employee-owned social enterprise, providing community healthcare services to people living in east Surrey and parts of West Sussex.

They have a very kind culture with one of their values being:

"First-rate people

We are caring, conscientious, compassionate and approachable people, supported to develop our potential. We are respectful and listen, to understand what is important to others. We are effective at communicating with confidence and authenticity. We are flexible and adaptable to our community and its requirements of health care services."

That's quite explicit. Its stronger than 'First-rate people' alone. The provider had taken it a step further and produced a set of core behaviours that were the basis for all staff and patient communications, including during supervision and appraisal. The framework set out very explicitly and in detail the expected behaviours of the staff and maintained a patient focus at its core.

Their behaviour framework was effective because it was both simple and balanced; it gave clear direction about positive behaviours (such as making eye contact when speaking and contributing ideas at staff meetings) balanced against indicators of less positive behaviours. It set the tone for how staff were expected to behave and this meant that those in more junior positions could, if needed, challenge more senior staff who were felt to be behaving inappropriately. It wasn't left to individuals' interpretation of what appropriate behaviour looked like.

Part 3: Ratings and the five key questions

Ratings

Social media is full of providers and services displaying their green 'Good' ratings with, perhaps, excessive pride. I understand that staff should feel proud that they are continuing to deliver good care routinely, in difficult times – particularly if they have moved on from a lower rating. However, there is a significant part of me that says 'Good' is the minimum acceptable level of care and treatment and not something to shout from the rooftops.

It's also important to remember that the CQC rating is not the sole indicator or protector of quality. As the King's Fund has said, regulators cannot alone ensure quality and can only ever be the third line of defence against poor care – the first line of defence being frontline staff, and the second being the leaders and boards of organisations.

That word 'regulator' is critical. The Commission's primary purpose is not to provide a good marketing tool for health and social care services – that's a by-product. The statutory purpose is to make sure health and social care services provide people with safe, effective, compassionate, high-quality care and we encourage care services to improve. Realistically, that means finding and addressing poor practice as the primary function. Identifying and sharing good practice, uncontroversially, takes second place to this.

Ratings are an indicator not an absolute. A 'Requires Improvement' rating does not mean that you don't provide good care or treatment to most people most of the time. An 'Outstanding' rating does not mean everyone gets a perfect experience, all of the time. Mistakes still happen in the best of services – it's how services react and learn from those mistakes that distinguishes them.

One hospital trust rated 'Inadequate' in 2018, still had people posting on the NHS choices website very positively about their care at the time. Just as CQC found serious concerns (and they were serious) some patients were saying:

■ "Yesterday I had an operation. I was taken through the Surgical Day Assessment Unit where all the nurses and doctors were fantastic. I was then taken down to theatre and other than a short wait in recovery due to a lack of beds on the ward, everything went really smoothly. Once on the ward the nursing staff were amazing and really caring. Absolutely fantastic service. I am very pleased!"

■ "From the reception team through to the medical staff including doctors, nurses etc. I found all the staff very friendly, caring whilst very professional.

I would like to thank them all for making my visit as pleasant as they could under the circumstances."

That doesn't mean CQC got it wrong, or that the report was inaccurate, but rather it demonstrates that ratings are not the entire picture and not what the driving force should ever be. High ratings are a bonus, the ambition must be high-quality care and treatment. The ratings are useful for all sorts of reasons, but they are only part of the picture.

There are rules for aggregating ratings. There is an option to vary but that is quite a rare thing. It is always a very carefully debated and considered decision and must be underpinned by good reasoning. I've only seen it happen a couple of times. Once was due to a breach of regulation about statutory notifications that was an oversight by a previous registered manager in an otherwise exemplary service – the breach was still recorded as such, but the decision was that they would be rated at 'Good' despite this, as it was a different management team and there had been system improvements to prevent a recurrence. Without the breach they might have been rated 'Outstanding', but we'll never know as the discussion was whether to step outside the rules about the limiting effect of a breach.

Far better not to rely on a possible variation to the aggregation rules and get the basics sorted, to ensure a 'Good' rating.

Ratings rules

These vary slightly dependent on sector, but the principles apply to all.

For each of the key questions (domains) of safe, caring, effective, responsive and well-led, the aggregated rating (for the provider or location) should consist of:

- **An aggregation of the underlying service ratings.** Where more than one core service is inspected, the ratings from the different core services will be aggregated together to give the overall rating for the key question. In non-CQC speak, this means if, as part of the inspection, patient transport and urgent and emergency care were both inspected separately with one rated as 'Requires Improvement' for safety and the other as 'Good', then the overall rating for the provider for safety would be 'Requires Improvement'. Even if four core services were inspected with three rated as 'Outstanding' for safety but one was 'Requires Improvement', then overall the rating would be 'Good'.

- **An assessment of any relevant evidence.** The quality assurance processes are quite stringent. The Commission doesn't always get it right (more about that later) but generally speaking there is much improved consistency in awarding ratings and fairer representation of the services inspected. The regulator is maturing and evolving; →

part of that is moving away from the, very burdensome, comprehensive inspections that were necessary to set a benchmark and to assess the quality of care being provided nationally by various sectors. An approach to regulation based on risk is developing and improving as data becomes more readily available and technology allows for easier sharing of the information. That means a far greater emphasis on accuracy or evidence and proper consideration about whether the evidence is sufficient to allow a fair assessment of the service in order to provide a rating.

Evidence is critical if services want to challenge or secure a positive rating at any point in the process. That means evidence supplied by the provider where the Commission has not been sighted on it (despite it being available). It means evidence that has been collated over a period of time being shared with the inspection team. It means national data sets. It means balancing observations with documentary evidence. It means considering the validity of evidence supplied and what that says about the service.

The five key questions are all equally important and should be weighted equally when aggregating:

- Is it safe?
- Is it effective?
- Is it caring?
- Is it responsive?
- Is it well-led?

There are clear guidelines where the total number of ratings given is balanced with the number of each level of rating to come to an overall rating for each core service, for each domain, and at location or provider level.

This means that, where there are between 1 and 3 ratings given (or carried forward from previous inspections), then there must be at least one 'Outstanding' rating for the overall rating to be 'Outstanding', assuming the other two ratings are 'Good'. If there are between 4 and 8 ratings given (or carried forward) then two 'Outstanding' ratings are needed to tip the overall rating into 'Outstanding'.

Breaches

Where a breach of a regulation has been identified and we issue a requirement notice, the rating linked to the area of the breach will be limited to 'Requires Improvement' at best.

Where a breach of a regulation has been identified and we take action under our enforcement powers, such as issuing a Warning Notice or imposing a condition of registration, the rating linked to the area of the breach will be 'Inadequate'. →

Well-led (Adult social care only)

For the question is it well-led?, there are principles taken into account when judgements are made about the rating.

The four principles below show events and circumstances that mean that the well-led key question can never be rated better than 'Requires Improvement'.

■ The location has a condition of registration that it must have a registered manager, but it does not have one, and satisfactory steps have not been taken to recruit one within a reasonable timescale.

■ The location has any other condition of registration that is not being met, without good reason.

■ Statutory notifications were not submitted in relation to relevant events at a location, without good reason.

■ When the Provider Information Request has not been filled in and submitted within the agreed deadline, or has not been updated in the last 12 months within the Provider Information Collection or any other information has not been completed when requested by the Commission or supplied in another format, indicating that the service is unable to demonstrate an understanding of the importance of keeping and using management information to deliver a good quality service.

An example of aggregation might be where a new private hospital provides two core services – surgery and outpatients. Surgery is rated 'Outstanding' for caring and outpatients is rated 'Good'. Overall, the rating for 'caring' for the hospital would be 'Outstanding'. This rating carries forward into the overall rating for the hospital; there are five domains (safe, effective, caring, responsive, well-led) and if only 'caring' was rated 'Outstanding' then the overall rating would be 'Good'. If, however, they'd been rated as 'Outstanding' for responsiveness in outpatients because of the fantastic work they were doing for patients living with dementia and people with sensory impairments, then the rating for responsiveness overall would be 'Outstanding' (as one out of a possible two). This would carry up into the overall hospital rating and the two 'Outstanding' ratings for caring and responsiveness would give them an overall 'Outstanding' rating.

Ratings for primary medical services such as GP practices are done slightly differently. In all inspections of GP practices, the Commission rates the population groups for 'effective' and 'responsive' only, aggregating these to an overall population group rating. They no longer award ratings for safe, caring and well-led for the population groups. This means that following a next phase inspection, all previous ratings for population groups for safe, caring and well-led will be removed from the new ratings grid for that practice.

Moving forward, as inspections are increasingly risk based and focusing more on the highest identified risk levels, it may be harder still to move from a 'Good' to 'Outstanding' rating. Inspections will be streamlined, and fewer core services will be inspected at any one time for the better services. Historic ratings will be aggregated into the overall rating for providers or locations.

This means, for example, that if you are an NHS community trust that has been rated as 'Good' overall, based on ratings of 'Good' for adult inpatient, community children and young people and community adults, and sexual health services, but with a 'Requires Improvement' for end of life care; you may find that the next scheduled inspection is only looking at the leadership (all inspections in NHS consider leadership) and end of life care as the service where the rating indicates a heightened risk (from the previous inspection). Even if end of life care has improved significantly and achieves an 'Outstanding' rating, based on 'Outstanding' ratings for caring and effectiveness, the overall rating for the trust will remain the same. There are five underpinning ratings for the five core services and only one is now rated as 'Outstanding', which means the overall trust rating stays as 'Good'. It could feel like an awfully long journey towards 'Outstanding'.

My view is that providers should believe that the Commission is wanting to encourage and support the dissemination of good practice. There is now a much greater emphasis on engagement with providers and a commitment to building positive relationships. Recognising and rewarding good practice is the best way to spread the message; to show that there is a shared understanding of 'what good looks like' and a commitment to see the very best practice spread to improve care and treatment for everyone. Certainly, in regulatory planning meetings and more informal discussions, the subject of ensuring that we continue to be a conduit for supporting excellence is often raised. As engagement practice moves forward and monitoring systems for soft and hard intelligence evolve, it will become clear where there have been improvements in services, such that they deserve an opportunity to be re-rated. That will then become a trigger to include that service in the next inspection.

Full details of the ratings rules and characteristics are on the Commission website. https://www.cqc.org.uk/guidance-providers

What are the characteristics of an 'Outstanding' rating

There are slight differences between the sectors, but in general the Commission is looking for the same things regardless of sector. The way they assess the rating may differ, there may be consideration of different evidence, but the characteristics are remarkably similar. I have used the hospice characteristics because this is statistically the highest performing group of providers and probably where everyone should be aiming. A provider does not have to meet every element of the rating characteristic to gain that rating, and clearly some criteria are less applicable to some provider types. Obviously, a dentist doesn't need to provide a varied and nutritious choice of meals.

Safe

The hospice rating characteristic for 'Outstanding' in safe reads:

"There is a high level of understanding of the need to make sure people are safe.

People who use the service and staff tell us they are actively encouraged to raise their concerns and to challenge when they feel people's safety is at risk. They tell us there are no recriminations for doing this and it is seen as part of day-to-day practice.

Staff have exceptional skills and the ability to recognise when people feel unsafe. Staff and their mix of skills are used innovatively to give them the time to develop positive and meaningful relationships with people to keep them safe and meet their needs.

The service is creative in the way it involves and works with people, respects their diverse needs, and challenges discrimination. It seeks ways to continually improve and puts changes into practice and sustains them.

Staff show empathy and have an enabling attitude that encourages people to challenge themselves, while recognising and respecting people's lifestyle choices.

There is a transparent and open culture that encourages creative thinking in relation to people's safety. The service seeks out research, including that around the use and management of medicines and current best practice and uses this to drive improvement.

The service uses imaginative and innovative ways to manage risk and keep people safe, while making sure that they have a full and meaningful life. The service actively seeks out new technology and solutions to make sure that people have as few restrictions as possible.

The service sustains outstanding practice and improvements over time."

Effective

The hospice rating characteristic for 'Outstanding' in effective reads:

"For a good service to be rated 'Outstanding' there are additional key characteristics that make the service exceptional and distinctive. People's feedback about the effectiveness of the service describes it in these terms. →

The service has innovative and creative ways of training and developing their staff that makes sure they put their learning into practice to deliver outstanding care that meets people's individual needs. The service works in partnership with other organisations to make sure they are training staff to follow best practice and where possible, contribute to the development of best practice.

The service sustains outstanding practice and improvements over time and works towards, and achieves, recognised accreditation schemes. There is a proactive support system in place for staff that develops their knowledge and skills and motivates them to provide a quality service.

Staff confidently make use of the Mental Capacity Act 2005 and use innovative ways to make sure that people are involved in decisions about their care so that their human and legal rights are sustained.

There are champions within the service who actively support staff to make sure people experience good healthcare outcomes leading to an outstanding quality of life. People experience a level of care and support that promotes their well-being and means they have a meaningful life.

When people have complex/continued health needs, staff always seek to improve their care, treatment and support by identifying and implementing best practice.

There is a strong emphasis on the importance of eating and drinking well. Where the service is responsible, innovative methods and positive staff relationships are used to encourage those who are reluctant, or have difficulty, to eat and drink and this significantly improves their well-being.

There are excellent links with dietetic professionals and staff are aware of people's individual preferences and patterns of eating and drinking. These preferences are sustained over time, as their health allows.

People say that the mealtimes and the quality of food and choice are exceptional, their individual needs are met and staff go out of their way to meet their preferences."

Caring
The hospice rating characteristic for 'Outstanding' in caring reads:

"For a good service to be rated 'Outstanding' there are additional key characteristics that make the service exceptional and distinctive. People's feedback about the caring approach of the service describes it in these terms.

The service has a strong, visible person-centred culture and is exceptional at helping people to express their views so they understand things from their points of view. Staff and management are fully committed to this approach and find innovative ways to make it a reality for each person using the service. They use creative ways to make sure that people have accessible, tailored and inclusive methods of communication.

People value their relationships with the staff team and feel that they often go 'the extra mile' for them, when providing care and support. As a result, they feel really cared for and that they matter. →

Staff are exceptional in enabling people to remain independent and have an in-depth appreciation of people's individual needs around privacy and dignity.

The service also focuses on people's well-being and develops innovative ways to support and help them, both psychologically and practically. Family support is also seen as key to people's well-being and the needs of people's families are also supported.

Staff will be highly motivated and inspired to offer care that is kind and compassionate and will be determined and creative in overcoming any obstacles to achieving this.

Bereavement services are tailored to individual needs and may be provided over a significant period of time after death. The service continually strives to develop the approach of their staff team so this is sustained.

People receive outstanding care from exceptional staff who are compassionate, understanding, enabling and who have distinctive skills in this aspect of care. Staff also care for and support the people that matter to the person who is dying with empathy and understanding."

Responsive

The hospice rating characteristic for 'Outstanding' in caring reads:

"People tell us staff have outstanding skills and have an excellent understanding of their social and cultural diversity, values and beliefs that may influence their decisions on how they want to receive care, treatment and support. Staff know how to meet these preferences and are innovative in suggesting additional ideas that they themselves might not have considered. This means that people have an enhanced sense of well-being.

People's care and support is planned proactively in partnership with them. Staff use innovative and individual ways of involving people so that they feel consulted, empowered, listened to and valued. For people in transition, specific support groups are available and in children's hospices, links are made to antenatal services to support families where unborn babies have life-limiting conditions.

Professionals visiting the service say it is focused on providing person-centred care and it achieves exceptional results. Ongoing improvement is seen as essential. The service strives to be known as outstanding and innovative in providing person-centred care based on best practice.

The service is flexible and responsive to people's individual needs and preferences, finding creative ways to enable people to live as full a life as possible. The service uses innovative ways to support people in the community when they are not with them. Where required, there is a rapid response to people's changing care needs and advice on care and support is available round the clock.

Where the service has a responsibility, the arrangements for social activities and, where appropriate, education and work, are innovative and meet people's individual needs. →

There are specific staff with the skills to understand and meet the needs of people and their families in relation to their emotional support and the practical assistance they need with day-to-day life.

The service takes a key role in the local community and is actively involved in building further links. People who use the service are encouraged and supported to engage with services and events that have a positive impact on their quality of life. Input from other services and support networks are encouraged and sustained.

People are actively encouraged to give their views and raise concerns or complaints. The services sees concerns and complaints as part of driving improvement. People's feedback is valued, and people feel that the responses to the matters they raise are dealt with in an open, transparent and honest way. Investigations are comprehensive, and the service uses innovative ways of looking into concerns raised. This includes using people and professionals who are external to the service to ensure an independent and objective approach.

There are specific staff with the skills to understand and meet the needs of people and their families in relation to their emotional support and the practical assistance they need with day-to-day life.

The service takes a key role in the local community and is actively involved in building further links. People who use the service are encouraged and supported to engage with services and events that have a positive impact on their quality of life. Input from other services and support networks are encouraged and sustained.

People are actively encouraged to give their views and raise concerns or complaints. The services see concerns and complaints as part of driving improvement. People's feedback is valued, and people feel that the responses to the matters they raise are dealt with in an open, transparent and honest way. Investigations are comprehensive, and the service uses innovative ways of looking into concerns raised. This includes using people and professionals who are external to the service to ensure an independent and objective approach."

Well-led

The hospice rating characteristic for 'Outstanding' in well-led reads:

"For a 'Good' service to be rated 'Outstanding' there are additional key characteristics that make the service exceptional and distinctive. People's feedback about the way the service is led describes it in these terms.

The service has a track record of being an excellent role model, actively seeking and acting on the views of others through creative and innovative methods. They have developed and sustained a positive culture in the service encouraging staff and people to raise issues of concern with them, which they always act upon.

There is a strong emphasis on continually striving to improve. Managers recognise, promote and regularly implement innovative systems in order to provide a →

high-quality service. The service sustains outstanding practice and improvements over time and works towards, and achieves, recognised quality accreditation schemes.

The service finds innovative and creative ways to enable people to be empowered and voice their opinions.

The vision and values are imaginative and person-centred and make sure that people are at the heart of the service. They are developed and reviewed with people and staff and are owned by all and underpin practice. The service recognises the ongoing importance of ensuring these are understood, implemented and communicated to people in meaningful and creative ways.

The service has innovative ways of communicating with staff who work in the community to make sure they are informed of changes and can share views and information.

The service works in partnership with other organisations to make sure they are following current practice and providing a high-quality service. They strive for excellence through consultation, research and reflective practice. They can also show how they sustain their outstanding practice and improvements over time."

Are they safe?

Key messages

- All the incredible research and highly specialist treatments in the world cannot offset a culture of poor safety and inattention to basic care needs.

- An organisation that doesn't want to learn, that is complacent or accepts 'good enough', is never going to reach or stay atop the pinnacle of excellence.

- Safety is everyone's business.

- Safe practice saves money and saves pain.

- Safe practice is nicer for staff to deliver.

- Efficiency and asset stripping are not synonymous.

> By 'safe', we mean people are protected from abuse and avoidable harm.
>
> Abuse can be physical, sexual, mental or psychological, financial, neglect, institutional or discriminatory abuse.

Fundamentals First

"In the field of human relations nothing is so important as safety, for safety applies with equal force to the individual, to the family, to the employer, to the country. Safety in its widest sense, concerns the happiness, contentment and freedom of everyone. There is no mystery in safety. The important thing is to think a situation through and then apply common sense."

(Bill Jeffers, 1945)

The 'Safe' domain is the aspect of a service that is least likely to be rated 'Outstanding' and yet it should be the most straightforward to get right. Safety continues to be the biggest concern across all the services that are inspected. The Commission rated over one in 10 hospitals (13%) and a similar proportion of adult social care providers (10%) as 'Inadequate' for safety.

I have led inspections of large teaching trusts (with attached medical schools); they should be the flagship hospitals of our country, offering highly specialised services and research programmes alongside more commonplace treatments. Some have been disappointed not to be given the top rating and appealed based on the incredible work they are doing for people with rare disorders – and there is no doubt that if you have a rare condition then some of these are the hospitals where you would want to be treated. They retain and deserve their world-class status. What it sometimes takes a while to understand, however, is that we are a regulator and our assessments are trust wide and focus on quite mundane, but important, things. One CEO understood and put it very eloquently as being necessary to 'make sure the floors were swept before swinging from the chandeliers'. In other words, to join the elite group of providers with an 'Outstanding' rating for the safe domain, it is necessary to ensure that the basics of patient safety are in place before adding on the exceptional.

I talk in the caring section (see p177) about that being the most important domain to focus on as a stepping stone to excellence. This doesn't change that view. Caring staff will ensure that they wash their hands and don't increase the risk of their patients developing a post-operative infection. Compassionate staff will understand that not reacting appropriately to a patient showing the early signs of sepsis is beyond unkind and places them at significant risk of serious harm or even death. You cannot be kind and yet choose to deliver poor, unsafe care.

It is possible to have very structured and carefully monitored safety systems that deliver consistent care to all patients with the same condition, but they won't work very well without a compassionate culture where staff understand why they are important. Staff who understand why something needs doing and can see what their role or actions do to improve patient outcomes are more likely to adhere to the correct processes. Staff who receive praise for completing things properly are more likely to sustain the quality of care. Consistency of process and equipment is important to maintaining safety and preventing harm; valuing and educating staff is how you get them to want to do things properly.

It's quite hard to find services rated as 'Outstanding' for safe. I suspect the reasons are multifactorial, but it's perhaps related to showing that what you are doing is truly exceptional – maybe a care home collating evidence to show a reduction in falls or maybe a reduction on medicines errors through a programme of staff education and improved systems. It could be a psychiatric service demonstrating a reduction in the number of deaths from suicide from an early intervention model they created, or perhaps the use of a psychiatric early warning scoring system they have developed. It might be an ambulance provider who is monitoring outcomes for patients who aren't transferred to hospital and using the information to improve patient safety through focused staff training. There is no single answer to what a service with an 'Outstanding' safety rating does; it is unique to that service.

There is also untested potential that this is the area of the inspection the team focus on most. In many services it is the easiest aspect to inspect while on site; the easiest to observe. I can see whether care home residents have appropriate footwear and their glasses have been cleaned. The pharmacist can scrutinise medicines charts to check for correct completion. A theatre specialist can observe whether the World Health Organisation's guidelines for safer surgery are being implemented. In a GP service it is quite simple to see whether the practice has trained staff to recognise and react to signs of abuse. The trouble with these things being easy to evidence is that it is also extremely easy to see where there are shortcomings.

I'm not entirely convinced that reporting is always entirely proportionate (but that is very much my opinion); I dislike seeing a commentary about seeing two individual patient records missing one minor detail. I think this undermines the usefulness of regulation in driving improvements and would far rather that inspections focus on the impact on patients rather than very minor errors. The Commission has definitely improved in this area, with more stringent quality assurance processes and better benchmarking. The default position is that a service is good, but it is easy for an inspection team to find shortcomings in the processes designed to help staff deliver safe care.

My suspicion is that sometimes inspection teams are so focused on collecting evidence to write their reports that they fail to collect the evidence that really matters. I reiterate, this is just my opinion and many within the Commission would have a different perspective. Overall, they collect and record evidence very well but sometimes that is to the detriment of actually looking and observing the quality of care. It is much easier for a person who is new to regulation to collect the results of the audits against the National Specification for Cleanliness in the NHS than to say how they know patients in a ward are comfortable and free from pain. It is much easier to look through personal care plans in a home for people with learning disabilities than to spend time talking about and observing whether those care plans are being implemented fully. It's much simpler to write about the documents than describe the care provided, which can be subject to greater challenge than an entirely factual and data-based comment in a report. Inspection should always be about the care and treatment people receive and how the regulator and providers can work in partnership to improve this. Don't get me wrong, the records and the documents are important, but they can never be as important as the care that people actually receive. The wise provider will supplement documentary evidence with evidence of the quality of care people receive. Think carefully about how you can demonstrate you are offering safe care which meets the fundamental standards, and that you can present evidence of this.

It is sad if a service is held at 'Requires Improvement' because the leaders cannot evidence that everyone has completed the appropriate level of safeguarding training. The guidance is out there and available free on the intranet. It is explicit about what level of training various staff in different types of services need to complete. The idea that staff must complete the appropriate level of safeguarding training and have refresher training, that policies must be up to date and reflect latest national guidance and that (most importantly) they understand how to recognise and act when they identify potential abuse isn't a secret.

If it is so difficult to get an 'Outstanding' rating for safety, what can you do? Is it ever attainable? It is possible but it's not easy. Proving you do more than deliver safe care is a tough ask. Is no attributable grade three pressure damage indicative of 'Outstanding' care or something that should be expected?

As a first step, the absolute basics need to be right. Nobody is going to get an 'Outstanding' rating because of reduced mortality figures if their lavatories are filthy and commodes are soiled.

I might suggest that, as part of the overall journey towards an 'Outstanding' rating, providers ensure that the safe domain was at least a solid 'Good'. A *good* 'Good'. An understanding of the ratings aggregation used by the Commission is key to knowing that you need a 'Good' rating in safety for an overall 'Outstanding'. Any breach of regulation identified at inspection limits you to a 'Requires Improvement' rating. Any 'Requires Improvement' rating on the ratings grid limits the overall rating to a maximum of 'Good'. That's quite a key message to think about.

Allowing staff to deliver or accept shoddy practice and shortcuts – or doing so yourself – poses risks to people using services and, consequently, risks your overall rating. It is definitely worth understanding the ratings aggregation rules and perhaps focusing on the areas that will make the most difference. Consider working towards eliminating all the yellow 'Requires Improvements' from the grid – this has numerous benefits. There is a regulatory requirement for the ratings to be displayed and it has to be better to be displaying a grid that tells the world how good you are.

It should mean the care and treatment people experience has improved. That's the main reason it should be happening.:

■ A green and blue grid (or just a green grid if it has been amber and red previously), is a real morale boost for staff. It validates and reinforces the work they have been doing to bring about improvements.

■ It provides reassurance and encourages people to look differently at your service. It's an incredibly good marketing and recruitment tool.

Of course, one should aim for an 'Outstanding' across the board but there are only two NHS trusts in the country that have achieved this – one a specialist trust and one a trust providing district general hospital services. Coincidentally, they achieved the rating within a week of each other. Both providers did exceptional work but also got the basics right.

Royal Papworth Hospital NHS Foundation Trust

"There was the use of ultraviolet decontamination in the respiratory/ cystic fibrosis unit to ensure the environment was as safe as possible for vulnerable patients. In the outpatient department the systems and processes to minimise the spread of infection were outstanding. The air filtering and ultraviolet cleaning systems were innovative, and precautions to protect patients particularly prone to infection were well thought out and fully embedded."

All very well, but most providers don't offer such specialist services, so is it a fair comparison? Other areas of the report demonstrate the point that the basics have to be right before the 'swinging from the chandeliers' provision is considered. The following are reasonable expectations of a good service, surely?

- "Staff kept detailed records of patients' care and treatment. Records were clear, up to date, stored securely and easily available to all staff providing care."

- "Staff completed and updated risk assessments for each patient and removed or minimised risks. Staff identified and quickly acted upon patients at risk of deterioration. The service used systems and processes to safely prescribe, administer, record and store medicines."

Western Sussex Hospitals NHS Foundation Trust

The executive team at Western Sussex were clear about their vision. They were clear about what services they offered. They had no aspiration to provide heart lung transplants or neurosurgery. They wanted to be the best district general hospital in the country. They knew that getting the basics absolutely right, with the patients as the focus of everyone's work, was the only way to achieve this.

- "The trust had sustained an improvement in the level of deaths related to septicaemia, more than halving the observed rate since April 2017, providing evidence of effective staff support and training."

- "The provider has a sustained track record of safety supported by accurate performance information. There was ongoing, consistent progress towards safety goals reflected in a zero-harm culture. The service used safety monitoring results well. Staff collected safety information, and shared it with staff, patients and visitors. Data was used to drive improvements both locally on wards and across the trust. Performance was closely monitored, and action taken if themes or variance from the target trajectory were identified. All safety data was considered inside the Patient First framework and there was a commitment to holding steady to the key improvement objectives whilst maintaining sufficient flexibility to adapt to changing priorities."

- "Safety thermometer information and ward dashboards were used to drive local improvements. The number of patients who suffered no new harm during their inpatient stay at the trust was 98.7%, as reported to the board in July 2019." (The national average in November 2019 was 94.1%)

The example below is one where I am sure many providers will think 'well, we do all that'. I would ask you to reflect and think whether you really do… Having the personalised risk assessments is one thing; implementing them consistently is quite another. An additional step would be measuring the effectiveness of the fall's prevention work. Falls cost a huge amount in personal misery, pain, loss of mobility, loss of independence and increased mortality. Falls are the most common cause of death from injury in the over 65 age group and cost the NHS over £2bn a year and over 4 million hospital bed days. One in three people with a hip fracture dies within a year (although not necessarily as a direct consequence of the fall). It is much, much more caring and much cheaper to implement effective falls prevention work. Cleaning glasses and checking hearing aids really is cost effective. Multidisciplinary reviews of elderly people's medicines might also reduce falls. Can you evidence these for people using your service?

Falls reduction

In 2016, the American Hospital Association's Health Research & Educational Trust published a report, *Preventing Patient Falls: A Systematic Approach from the Joint Commission Centre for Transforming Healthcare Project*, which showed that hospitals that had the most success with reducing patient falls share two common traits:

- They measure and analyse specific contributing factors that led to falls.
- They have a culture that supports 'zero falls'.

Five hospitals participated in the study and between them they reduced patient falls with injury by 62% and patient fall rates by 35%. Based on those results, a 200-bed hospital that followed the same approach could expect 72 fewer injuries and reduce costs by over a million dollars.

Bassett Medical Centre, New York

This 180-bed, acute care inpatient teaching hospital achieved a 435% reduction of fall through their 'Call, Don't Fall' campaign. The campaign focused on human factors such as patients who were reluctant to ask for help with toileting and staff who wanted to protect the patient's right to privacy so didn't proactively assist with toileting. The hospital put up signs in patient rooms, reminding patients to call for help before getting out of bed or up from their chair. Their falls prevention team held two daily huddles to identify patients at high-risk of falls and then made sure staff helped these patients to use the lavatory every two hours. The result was a significant reduction in falls, especially during the night.

University Hospital Southampton NHS Foundation Trust

This was among the first trusts to implement a now more widespread Bay watch scheme in their hospitals. In 2016, the trust piloted the initiative on two medical wards in an attempt to reduce the number of falls. The practice, or modified versions of it, is now used in many hospitals and has significantly reduced falls. It would not be difficult to introduce it into other settings such as care home sitting rooms or conservatories, elderly care wards in psychiatric hospitals, independent hospital outpatient department waiting areas or supported living communal lounges. GP surgery waiting areas even.

Bay watch falls prevention model:

- The nurse in charge can designate any bay on the ward a 'bay watch bay' and must review at least daily which patients would benefit from this care.

- A bay watch bay must always have a 'bay watcher' who provides observation within the bay to prevent falls both during the day and night. The bay watcher must be a member of UHS staff as often as possible. The bay watcher must not be a staff member doing a drugs round.

- The bay watcher must position themselves in the bay to ensure maximum observation of all patients (e.g. moving to ensure they do not have their back to patients).

- The bay watcher must risk assess if it is safe for them to provide care behind curtains and either minimise the amount of time they spend behind curtains or request other staff members to support them to ensure that observation within the bay is not reduced.

- The bay watcher must be identifiable at all times by wearing the bay watch lanyard. The member of staff holding the lanyard is responsible for falls observation within the bay at all times until the lanyard is handed over to a colleague

- Where appropriate, the bay watcher should rotate every hour according to the rota unless clinical exceptions arise. The bay watch rota should be drawn up at the beginning of the shift.

Another trust that has introduced the scheme reported excellent results with 82 fewer incidents over a 12-week period compared to the same period the previous year.

Arcot House Residential Home, Sidmouth

Arcot House is a residential home for older people who are physically frail and require help with personal care, it does not provide nursing care. The home is a grade two listed Georgian manor house set in lovely gardens.

Their report says:

"Risks for people were anticipated, identified and proactively managed to maximise people's continued independence. For example, when a person experienced difficulty getting up from their chair, a staff member spent time reminding the person of the techniques the physiotherapist had taught them for getting in and out of their chair safely. They patiently prompted the person through the steps they needed to take, in accordance with the person's mobility care plan, which enabled the person to get up independently.

Where a person was unsafe to manoeuvre a regular wheelchair, staff referred them to an occupational therapist who arranged for them to have a tailor-made wheelchair. This meant the person was able to move safely around the home and enjoy time socialising in communal areas.

A member of staff, referred to as a 'Falls ambassador' had a lead role and worked with the local falls team to implement best practice and minimise people's risk of falling at the home. They shared practical advice and literature on how best to support people to age well and maintain their independence. They ensured staff followed The National Institute for Health and Care Excellence (NICE) guidelines on 'Falls in older people: assessing risk and prevention of falling.' Staff implemented good practice tips about the environment, such as how chairs and beds should be positioned in people's rooms in ways which minimised people's risk of falling.

Personalised risk assessments identified ways in which staff could promote people's safety. For example, by ensuring people had good fitting footwear and were familiar with their surroundings. Staff made sure the person had everything they needed to hand, such as their drink, glasses and TV remote control. Where people were particularly at risk because of their frailty, staff did regular 'comfort rounds' to anticipate their needs. For example, checking if they wanted a drink, or needed anything and by offering the person help to use the toilet. Environmental risk assessments showed measures were taken to minimise risks. For example, making sure areas were well-lit, avoiding trailing leads and keeping corridors clutter free to prevent trip hazards."

Mandatory training

All too often I have completed or seen examples of online mandatory training that simply tick a box and offer assurance that providers won't be sanctioned. I have even known staff admit that they don't do the training but simply go to the end and do the assessment that consists of a few questions that gives them a pass and marks them as having completed the training.

I understand why this might be. In the hospital reports there is a specific section on mandatory training where the level of compliance is recorded as a table using information supplied by the trust to the analysts. It is separated into nursing staff and medical staff and lists the subjects offered by the trust, as part of their mandatory training requirements, and the target achievement level set by the trust themselves. The level of compliance for each area and each professional group is given as a percentage and then a column shows whether the target is met or not in green or red. It is, at best, arbitrary: if you want to appear to be better at educating your staff you simply lower your target from 95% to 90% and, 'hey presto!', you have improved. It is a measure that is a quick win for providers but it is not really a true indication of whether the staff have gained any significant improvement in their understanding of infection prevention and control or conflict resolution. It is also quite easy to spot and any regulator worth their salt will look at a green grid of completed mandatory training and ask, "Why is the target set so low when they are telling us they are committed to excellence?"

Perhaps if you want to be a provider of excellence, a service that wants to be among the very best, rather than setting a lower target for completion, you might be better providing mandatory training that is interesting, that engages staff and actually helps them do their jobs more effectively.

Going off at a tangent, and perhaps because of my name, the expression 'worth their salt' originated because salt, as a preserving agent, has always been a valuable commodity. The word salary comes from the Latin salarium which was an employees' salt allowance. I digress.

I probably shouldn't say this, but sometimes the data is a little wayward too (always check on factual accuracy that the right numbers are showing as either the provider or the Commission can and do make mistakes). I've just looked at an evidence appendix and smiled to see a very neat table showing details of the numbers of eligible staff and the number of staff completing mandatory fire safety training. Eight staff had completed the training out of an eligible nine, which, given as a percentage in the table, was 88.9%... What it is also important to note is that one member of staff was the reason for a big red-filled square on the table.

What a huge pity that this opportunity for improvement is not fully used in a more effective way to drive improvement in practice. The Care Quality Commission guidance is quite vague. There is no requirement in legislation that says how training must be delivered and what must be covered.

Health and Social Care Act 2008 (Regulated Activities) Regulations 2014: Regulation 12

Regulation 12 states, in part:

1. Care and treatment must be provided in a safe way for service users.

2. Without limiting paragraph (1), the things which a registered person must do to comply with that paragraph include:

   ▪ (c) ensuring that persons providing care or treatment to service users have the qualifications, competence, skills and experience to do so safely.

The guidance for provider about the regulation says:

Staff must only work within the scope of their qualifications, competence, skills and experience and should be encouraged to seek help when they feel they are being asked to do something that they are not prepared or trained for.

Staff should be appropriately supervised when they are learning new skills but are not yet competent.

Only relevant regulated professionals with the appropriate qualifications must plan and prescribe care and treatment, including medicines. Only relevant regulated professionals or suitably skilled and competent staff must deliver care and treatment.

Most providers do offer Mandatory training and most staff complete it. Some have improved the way they deliver training and offer face-to-face sessions or have broadened the subjects that they include. How much better to go beyond and deliver mandatory training that improved outcomes, that engaged staff, and which could reduce errors or complaints and therefore costs?

Children's Camps Charity

I mentioned previously that I met my husband while we were both doing voluntary work with children living in poverty in inner city areas. When we started, the recruitment process consisted of a phone call or visit to a tiny office in London. There was no training at all. If you had a RLSS Bronze medallion, you went to somewhere with a pool or a beach. If you could drive, you were handed the keys to an ancient transit minibus with bench seats. Everything else was down to luck and we saw some pretty poor childcare practice over the first couple of years. There were several camps where the behaviour management was erratic with arbitrary, and sometimes inappropriate sanctions and rewards were used. The physical care wasn't always good. Given that the majority of staff were students or other young adults, with limited experience, it was hardly surprising.

As a student teacher and a paediatric nurse in training, we wanted to share our very extensive knowledge and improve the way things were done. We had been training in our respective professions for about two years, so felt pretty expert, when we set up tighter recruitment processes and introduced a training programme for all potential group leaders and other camp staff. Even at such an early stage in our careers we could see there was room for significant improvement and that some shared learning opportunities might improve the experience for children and other adults.

We introduced a series of residential training and selection weekends that all prospective staff were required to attend. It wasn't universally popular with other people who ran camps, there was talk of 'over-professionalising' the holidays and taking away the fun. I'm not sure we ever understood the concept of 'over-professionalising' and we certainly didn't want to reduce fun, but we did want the holidays to be safer, to offer a positive experience and to ensure staff could recognise the limits of their expertise. The training weekends started up, improved and expanded. They continued for about 15 years, altogether.

Our own children still look back fondly to weekends in London, playing in the Bishop's Palace Gardens, a lovely park just beside the residential centre we used. They were terribly spoilt by a lot of child-friendly adults who let them eat ice cream and chocolate cake all weekend, despite our protestations that they were not allowed them.

We offered mandatory training that was fun, interactive and an opportunity for people to say, 'on reflection this isn't for me'. We weeded out a few unsuitable applicants. It meant the group leaders turned up better prepared, knowing what to expect and understanding the benefits of positive behaviour management. They gained some understanding about how to recognise an unwell child and how to treat headlice. They knew what behaviours were and were not acceptable from adults working with children.

One of the most important aspects of the training was learning a little about child protection and what needed to be escalated. We were surprised there had been so much resistance from a couple of 'the old guard' about this and although we understood that they didn't want us to frighten people away, we felt it was important that any potential abuse should be recognised and reported. Just how important and effective the session was only became apparent a couple of years later when two of the 'old guard' were arrested and charged with historic criminal offences. Had we not made it the right thing to do to report any concerns and given staff ways of speaking about issues to someone other than the leaders, then other children might not have been protected.

Safeguarding training has statutory requirements around the level of training that is required. There are national guidance documents that are explicit about the level and content of safeguarding adults and safeguarding children training. Some providers offer a higher level than the statutory minimum.

Mortality

The most important issue for people using services is around their mortality. There is little point offering six flavours of ice cream or a decent Sancerre with supper if people are suffering from avoidable harm and even dying. Mortality is everyone's business. Every member of staff, every service, should be playing their part in reducing avoidable mortality.

In 2017, there were more than 140,000 (almost one in four) deaths that could be averted or delayed through timely, effective health care and which were therefore considered avoidable. Cancers were the leading cause, followed by cardiovascular diseases, injuries, respiratory diseases and drug misuse.

This statistic is relevant to all health and social care practitioners, all practitioners in physical or mental health services, all grades of staff.

In 2018, there were 6,507 suicides registered in the UK.

In 2018, of all deaths among children and young people aged 0 to 19 years in the UK, 1,720 deaths out of 4,883 were considered avoidable.

In 2010 there were 2,843 deaths from falls (excluding falls on building sites, ladders or off cliffs).

2013 data shows 11,458 avoidable deaths related to infections, 40,805 related to cancers, and 11,745 related to respiratory disease.

There were 18,765 avoidable deaths related to injuries in 2013.

It's not difficult to think of examples where people have died unnecessarily and quite easy to see how, while the provider remains accountable for safe practice, individuals can do their part to reduce the risk of people dying unnecessarily.

An elderly patient died after drinking cleaning fluid because it was in a water jug on the ward. It is easy to think it couldn't happen to us, but I've been around several hospitals subsequently and seen the same cleaning fluid out on cleaning trolleys on elderly care and children's wards. It was an acute hospital trust; it could just as easily have been a care home or psychiatric unit.

Reducing mortality is everyone's business. It could come under outcomes in effective, but I put it under safety because all services can improve how they attend to basic safety measures and as a consequence reduce avoidable mortality. Reducing mortality is not just something for those working in elderly care.

Saving Babies Lives Care Bundle

The Morecambe Bay Investigation report was published in 2015 following a scandal at Furness General Hospital involving the deaths of several mothers and new-born babies during the 2000s at Furness General Hospital in Cumbria. Concerns dated back to 2004, with a number of major incidents occurring in 2008. The tragic death of Joshua Titcombe and a suppressed report by the Morecambe Bay NHS Trust brought Furness General Hospital to the attention of the nation.

The government report provided details of five serious incidents during 2008: a baby damaged by the effects of shortage of oxygen in labour; a mother who died following untreated high blood pressure; a mother and baby who died from an amniotic fluid embolism; a baby who died in labour due to shortage of oxygen; and a baby who died from unrecognised infection.

All five incidents showed evidence of similar problems of poor clinical competence, insufficient recognition of risk, inappropriate pursuit of normal childbirth and failures of teamworking.

In March 2016, NHS England published an initiative called, Saving Babies' Lives, a care bundle designed to reduce stillbirths. The guidance was supporting the delivery of safer maternity care, as described by the National Maternity Review in Better Birth.

Saving Babies' Lives is designed to tackle stillbirth and early neonatal death. It brings together four elements of care that are recognised as best practice:

■ Reducing smoking in pregnancy.

■ Risk assessment and surveillance for foetal growth restriction.

■ Raising awareness of reduced foetal movement.

■ Effective foetal monitoring during labour.

Has it made a difference? Professor Alex Heazell, Clinical Director of the Tommy's Stillbirth Research Centre, led an evaluation of the impact. He said, "This large scale evaluation of the NHS England Saving Babies' Lives Care Bundle shows that the interventions to reduce cigarette smoking, detect small for gestational age babies, inform women about reduced foetal movements and improve monitoring of babies during labour, have been increasingly implemented in the early adopter maternity units. Over the same time period stillbirths have fallen by 20%, meaning 161 fewer stillbirths in the participating units."

Royal Surrey County Hospital

Royal Surrey County Hospital was the winner of the 2017 HSJ Patient Safety Award and also picked up the Quality Lead of the Year for the same initiative.

A consultant identified that the mortality rate for emergency surgery was far too high. After some research, he determined that in some hospitals the mortality rate was as high as 30%. Using best practice that had been published by various bodies such as The National Confidential Enquiry into Patient Outcome and Death (NCEPOD), the Royal College of Surgeons and the Royal College of Anaesthetists, the 5-point evidence-based care bundle was formed:

■ Early recognition of sepsis and antibiotics within an hour.

■ If appropriate, early surgery within 6 hours (including next slot CT scan using 'Code Laparotomy').

■ A consultant anaesthetist and consultant surgeon.

■ Directed fluid therapy during the operation and for 6 hours post-op.

■ Intensive care for all patients post-operatively.

Using this evidence-based care bundle, the initial four hospital projects dropped crude mortality by 25% and risk-adjusted mortality by 42%. Patients were dying less.

As a result of the initial project, The Health Foundation awarded a Scaling Up award to increase the scope of the work from four hospitals to 30 across the South of England. The project lead was tireless in his determination and ensured that consultant surgeons and anaesthetists would attend any emergency laparotomy operation at any time of day or night.

The four original hospitals maintained low mortality rates.

It was subsequently shown that the evidence-based care bundle was more cost effective than 'normal care.' The Scaling Up Project took this one step further and reduced the length of stay by 1.5 days. This resulted in over £1 million pounds in savings. As ever, improved care brings financial rewards.

Harm Free Care

"The very first requirement in a hospital is that it should do the sick no harm. The symptoms or the sufferings generally considered to be inevitable and incident to the

disease are very often not symptoms of the disease at all, but of something quite different - of the want of fresh air, or of light, or of warmth, or of quiet, or of cleanliness, or of punctuality and care in the administration of diet, of each or of all of these."
(Florence Nightingale)

In *What is preventable harm in healthcare?*, Nabhan *et al*'s systematic review of definitions suggest that, "Patient harm is PREVENTABLE if it occurs as a result of an identifiable modifiable cause and its future recurrence can be AVOIDED by reasonable adaptation to a process or adherence to guidelines".

It seems very obvious to me that providers of health and social care services should do no harm to the people they serve, and yet around one in 20 patients are affected by avoidable harm, according to a UK study that estimates the cost to hospitals in England each year would pay for more than 3,500 nurses. The research, published in the *British Medical Journal* in 2019 found that 6% of patients had been affected by preventable harm, causing permanent disability or death in 12% of cases.

My intention is not to describe in detail best practice in respect of specific care and treatment. There is enough already published and far greater expertise than mine readily available in trusts, clinical commissioning groups, professional organisations and suchlike, that offer detailed guidance on areas such as tissue viability, falls prevention, surgical safety and infection prevention and control. My intent is to persuade you that harm-free care is both possible and a marker of good care. It should be the norm and the expectation.

Most incidents of preventable harm in hospitals relate to drugs, therapeutic management of patients and invasive medical or surgical procedures, and were more common in surgical and intensive care units, the study found.

More than 40% of emergency admissions from care homes could be avoided. Hospitals are often not the best place for most frail elderly people. Nurses in the community, working in care homes and GPs are probably the solution.

Researchers from the Improvement Analytics Unit – a joint initiative between NHS England and the Health Foundation who studied NHS data found that 41% of admissions were potentially avoidable because they were for conditions that could have been prevented or treated in the community or were the result of poor care or neglect.

They were surprised to find emergency admissions were particularly high in residential care homes compared with nursing homes where residents are generally more seriously ill and require care from registered nurses. There were 0.77 emergency admissions per resident per year from residential homes compared with 0.63 admissions from nursing homes.

The impact of providing enhanced support for care home residents in Rushcliffe

A briefing written by Therese Lloyd, Arne Wolters and Adam Steventon reported on the impact of a package of enhanced support for older people living in care homes. The enhanced support was introduced in April 2014 and was developed by a local partnership of general practitioners, patients and community services.

The authors point out that in order to be effective, improvement efforts require access to robust and timely information on the differences that changes are making to the quality of the care provided to people using services.

An enhanced support package for care home residents was offered to 24 care homes caring specifically for frail older residents. The strategies they put in place included:

■ Alignment between general practices and care homes.

■ Advocacy and independent support.

■ Enhanced specification of general practice care for frail older people living in care homes.

■ Improved support from community nurses for nurses employed within care homes.

■ A programme of work to engage and support care home managers.

The overall aim was to improve the residents' care, including more involvement in decisions about their care, and their quality of life. There were specific aims to reduce secondary care utilisation, including the numbers of accident and emergency attendances and emergency hospital admissions.

The Impact analytics unit collected and analysed data from the project r group and from a comparator group. There were seven measures including:

■ Attendances at A&E departments (which might not result in a hospital admission).

■ Emergency admissions (occurring through A&E departments, or via direct and urgent referrals from GPs and other healthcare professionals).

■ The subset of 'potentially avoidable' emergency admissions, based on a list of conditions considered to be manageable in community settings or preventable through good quality care.

■ Outpatient attendances.

■ The number of nights spent as a hospital inpatient following either an emergency or elective admission.

■ The percentage of deaths that occurred outside of a hospital.

The results from data analysis showed that older people living in care homes that participated in the enhanced support programme attended A&E departments 29% less often than a matched comparison group, and were admitted to hospital as an emergency 23% less frequently.

The key message is that new ways of working can impact on safety and that multidisciplinary approaches can transform care and the experience of people using services. Setting up new ways of working is a positive step but doesn't, in itself, demonstrate excellence. Providers need to collect data to evidence that any changes they introduce lead to safer care.

Acute hospitals are generally well set up to collect and consider data around patient safety. Other services may want to consider how they can use data to provide evidence that safety initiatives result in more harm-free care.

Sunrise Senior Living's Care Homes

Sunrise has 25 care homes in England and Wales and more in other countries. One of Sunrise's general managers states that their homes have a clear falls reduction strategy:

"At Sunrise, we have a 'whole team' approach to checking the surrounding environment on a daily basis, ensuring that there are no trip hazards in any of the residents' rooms, such as rugs and clutter which could risk an incident. The general manager of the community also checks the overall building during their daily walks around the community to catch up with residents and staff members.

"Ensuring that appropriate footwear is worn at all times by all residents is also essential in preventing falls and keeping safe, and every resident has a regular review with their GP to reduce and monitor any medications that may contribute to falls, as well as indicating when and where residents may need additional support or assistance."

The Alzheimer's Society offers other falls reduction actions which include:

■ Adapt the physical environment to include handrails, sensory lighting and bold colours.

■ Use slip resistance flooring and provide suitable footwear.

■ Check the positioning of furniture.

- Avoid trip hazards.
- Keep objects within easy reach.
- Label the environment.
- Provide multiple and accessible seating areas both inside and out.
- Offer daily exercises and physical activities.
- Arrange regular visits from opticians, GPs and chiropodists.
- Train staff to manage and reduce the risk of falls.

Dementia increases the risk of falls and trips; services caring for people living with dementia should therefore be experts in falls reduction if they are providing good care to their residents. That care starts with the environment and means that staff should ensure uncluttered premises, handrails, plain coloured flooring that is non-slip and good lighting. Beautiful table lamps, mahogany coffee tables and patterned rugs might look nice, but they are likely to increase the number of falls people sustain.

How do you know if you are reducing the number of falls? How do you review incidents and near misses relating to falls so that future falls risks can be reduced? What evidence can you provide that you are committed to providing safe care, if you accept falls as 'something that happens' when people age?

Can you show that people have had a medication review to ensure that they are not at increased risk of falls from sedating medication or drugs that reduce their blood pressure too far?

Can you show people have their eyesight tested?

Do you ensure people are supported to maintain mobility?

For providers who are neither acute hospitals nor care homes for the elderly, how do you contribute to falls reduction? As a GP service do you have a falls lead? Do you check your own premises? Do you work with care homes to reduce falls through medication reviews and general health assessments?

Where does podiatry fit into the picture? Healthy feet make mobility easier and more comfortable. Do only people in care homes who pay privately get foot care?

What about in mental health services? Do you focus on care of the mental health needs at the cost of the physical health needs? Are patient safety initiatives focused on mental health or do you include falls prevention and skin integrity?

Tissue Viability Team at Bassetlaw Clinical Commissioning Group

NHS England reports on a Tissue Viability Team at Bassetlaw Clinical Commissioning Group which led the development of the 'React to Red' resource to support the prevention of pressure ulcers in care homes and the community. This resource and programme of work significantly improved outcomes and the experience of people using services.

Pressure ulcers cause significant pain and distress. They result in unnecessary hospital admissions and contribute to longer stays. This in turn leads to an increased risk of complications, including infection. Pressure damage costs the NHS more than £1.4 million every day and yet many pressure ulcers are avoidable if simple knowledge is provided and preventative best practice is followed.

NHS Bassetlaw CCG is a member organisation consisting of 12 GP practices across the area. The group is committed to working with its partners and patients and the public to improve the commissioning of services.

The CCG's Chief Nurse met with families and residents affected by pressure ulcers, as well as care home staff, to identify the root causes of the ulcers as well as identify any lessons that might support improvements. The findings suggested that, unlike acute service staff, care home staff were not being supported or equipped appropriately with the knowledge and skills to take steps to prevent pressure ulcers from developing or support residents to minimise their risk of developing sores.

Care home staff reported having minimal access to pressure ulcer prevention education and training. Service pressures frequently meant they could not be released to access training and this was compounded by a lack of local training for them to access.

To gain a deeper understanding, tissue viability nurses undertook a scoping exercise with 28 care homes within Bassetlaw CCG and found that 47% of staff reported that had not had any pressure ulcer prevention training. Of those who had, many said it had been many years before, some had been shown by another carer and some said they had looked at resources online.

While initially concentrating on pressure ulcers, it was also apparent that staff were not recognising early skin damage and therefore early intervention and prevention was not occurring effectively. This led the team to consider the need to provide education and support more widely rather than just focusing on how to manage pressure ulcer care, but instead providing a more holistic, proactive and preventative approach to skin care.

The tissue viability nurses developed a 'Link Champion' network across all 28 care homes where staff were identified from each home who attended regular network meetings to increase their knowledge, gained updates, received support and channelled this information and best practice back to their respective homes.

An education and training programme were developed and rolled out across the prioritised care homes by the nursing leads. Although the training was welcomed following the initial training, it became apparent that due to high demand, the level of training the tissue viability team were delivering could not be sustained, and they looked to develop a bespoke care home training resource package to support this more widely.

This resource was called 'React to Red' and link champions could use this to cascade the learning across their care homes and support them to develop at their own pace, taking ownership and leading improvements within their homes with the support of the evidence base.

The team were able to evidence that the programme resulted in better outcomes. In the first 18 months there was an 87% reduction in avoidable pressure ulcers in the targeted care homes. There was also an 85% reduction in pressure ulcers deemed avoidable in community services and anecdotally pressure ulcers are much smaller in size and severity.

When the initiative first started there were nine care homes that had 0% care-home-acquired pressure ulcers in a year, and within two years this rose to 22 homes. A change in practice has been seen by all clinicians as the approach that pressure ulcer prevention is everyone's business has been taken.

As well as reducing distress for residents, the avoidance of pressure ulcers also reduced use and cost of dressings, with associated saved nursing time that would have previously been spent treating these.

Staff morale improved following the training and they report feeling confident to support residents to improve their skin health and prevent pressure ulcers occurring. How much nicer must it feel to be part of a project that improves people's lives – which, after all, is why most people go into health and social care work.

Safety thermometer

The Safety Thermometer was developed by the NHS as a point of care tool to provide a 'temperature check' on patient harms. It is often used in conjunction with other metrics to show performance and progression. Originally launched in

2010, the Safety Thermometer remains one of the largest and longest-lasting data collection exercises in NHS history.

It was game changing when introduced but more recent studies and feedback have shown that the data was often incomplete and did not represent an accurate picture of harm-free care. With inaccuracies in the data collection, it was unable to be used as intended, to show improvements over time and to allow benchmarking.

The response to a consultation supported ending the national collection of Safety Thermometer data from April 2020 and using alternative data sources to continue improving pressure ulcer prevention, falls prevention, venous thromboembolism (VTE) prevention and prevention of healthcare-associated infection.

While no longer used for the NHS (where there are alternatives put in place to collate date nationally), the idea still offers some practical use as an improvement tool in residential settings. The types of data collected were those where avoidable harm occurred; there were different types of safety thermometer for different types of NHS services (Maternity, Mental Health, Children and Young People, Medicine and Classic).

Could this form the basis of a dashboard that was reported monthly for each setting? Could it be used to show that either the service was performing well, or the service had used the information to identify a worsening of pressure damage in the setting and addressed it?

Larger providers could easily use a similar data set to identify whether the care in any of their services were offering care which resulted in higher levels of harm.

I think if I was running a residential service for older people I might include the frequency and level of pressure damage, the number of falls and the degree of harm, the number of urinary tract infections, the results of a hand hygiene and records audit, the number of people who have had a medicines review and the number who have been seen by their GP, plus the numbers of people subject to any deprivation of their liberty. I would want the number of verbal and written complaints recorded. If I wanted to stretch the team, I might think about recording the number of activities that offered opportunity for movement and the number of participants.

I think if I was running a residential service for people with mental health problems, I might want to record different performance indicators. Some would remain the same, particularly in mental health services for older people. I would think consideration should be given to pressure damage, falls, continence and infection control but also to opportunities for exercise and the frequency people were supported to be outside. Medication reviews and complaints would remain valid measurements but there might need to be a different focus in risk assessment to prevent self-harm or the use of restraint.

The key message is that by collecting safety performance data, you can demonstrate that you are providing safe care and that the service is improving. It may feel onerous and staff may feel they don't have time but it is much less time consuming than managing the harm caused by lapses in care.

The other key message is about honesty and being open. Using an in-house dashboard or safety thermometer only works to improve care if it is a true reflection of the care actually being provided. If staff feel that it is better not to mention that a pressure wound has worsened since admission from a hospital because it is 'not their fault, the person came with it', then they cannot realistically share the pleasure of seeing the wound heal and feel pride in their tissue viability work.

Kennedy ulcers

Acceptance of the term Kennedy ulcers has no place in high-quality care provision.

In the article 'The Death of the Kennedy Terminal Ulcer', Michael Miller says: "The concept of the Kennedy Terminal Ulcer has been ubiquitous in attempting to explain the development of pressure-based tissue injuries in patients with actual or presumed terminal conditions. The concept is problematic in that it uses factors other than pressure to explain the development and progression of pressure-based tissue injuries, specifically the presence of a terminal condition. Based on the most current understanding of how pressure-based tissue injuries develop and progress, the concept of the Kennedy Terminal Ulcer appears to be without physiologic basis and based solely on observation."

He goes on to say that, "The concept of Kennedy Terminal Ulcer relates only to presumed terminal status as the cause of the development of a pressure-based tissue injury without respect to pressure. The presumption that a terminal condition alone will result in a pressure-based tissue injury despite appropriate care (including turning, appropriate support surfaces, management of incontinence, etc.) is simply not a viable consideration based on the current understanding of the pathophysiology of how pressure-based tissue injuries develop."

I have been in an acute hospital where there was a growing incidence and under-reporting of pressure damage as the Chief Nurse described many grade three and four wounds as 'Kennedy Ulcers', and dismissed them as unavoidable. I suspect she was not alone in holding onto an outmoded term. This meant there was inaccurate SI reporting, no root cause analysis, an inaccurate consideration of the factors leading to the increase in tissue damage and reduced opportunity to improve pressure damage prevention care.

The Tissue Viability Society says that both avoidable and unavoidable pressure ulcers should be reported. For national reporting purposes, the Department of Health definitions for avoidable/unavoidable pressure ulcers should be used.

The key message is not to dismiss any pressure damage as 'unavoidable' and to consider, with honesty and transparency, all incidence of pressure damage to allow proper consideration of how well your service is performing. Teams caring for frail and vulnerable people that can post '100 pressure damage free days' on their website or noticeboard should feel proud. Hopefully, the recognition and knowledge they are doing well will encourage them to increase the 100 to 200. If they can get to 'One Year without pressure damage' someone needs to send each team member a personal thank you card and perhaps a tin of biscuits, or offer an afternoon off, as a reward and further incentive.

Infection Prevention and Control

"And whomsoever he toucheth that hath the issue, and hath not rinsed his hands in water, he shall wash his clothes, and bathe himself in water, and be unclean until the evening."
(Leviticus 15:11)

"Cleanliness and order are not matters of instinct; they are matters of education, and like most great things, you must cultivate a taste for them."
(Benjamin Disraeli)

Infection prevention and control is not a new idea; we should have got it well in hand by now, but preventable infections continue to cause pain and death. The financial costs are huge. This covers so many areas and impacts all services, which makes it almost too complicated to even begin to consider in a book such at this. Infection prevention and control has never had such a high profile as it does with the Coronavirus pandemic wreaking tragedy and mayhem across the globe.

As early as 500BC, hospitals recognised and used the benefits of fresh air, placing emphasis on space and using prevailing winds. I grew up near a hospital called The Royal Sea Bathing Hospital which still had walls that could be pulled back to allow patients to be 'out outside'.

There were notable early successes in the 18th and 19th Centuries in the challenge to reduce the harm from infection. Archibald Menzies, a Scottish Royal Naval surgeon introduced a programme of fumigating ships to reduce ship fever (endemic and epidemic typhus transmitted via body lice). Another Scottish naval surgeon, James Lind, not only cured scurvy using lemons but also joined the battle against typhus. He saw that, where patients were bathed and given clean clothes and bedding, they were typhus free. The incidence was extremely high on the lower decks where such hygiene measures were not in place. Lind recommended that sailors be stripped, shaved, scrubbed and issued clean clothes and bedding regularly. As a result, British seamen did not suffer from typhus, which meant the Royal Navy had a bit of an advantage over their French enemies.

Continuous improvements in public health and infection prevention and control continued and grew from the 1800s onwards with the work not only of Florence Nightingale and Mary Seacole, but also the discoveries of Lister, Pasteur, Ollivier and Simpson.

Vienna General Hospital in Austria

I find the history of hand hygiene fascinating; sad, but true. How can something first identified as key to reducing infection as a cause of avoidable death about 180 years ago still be something we need to work on continually nowadays? How can any healthcare or social care professional, knowing that hand hygiene is the most important measure in reducing the transmission of infections, not adhere to policy? How can anyone eat peanuts or pretzels in a bar?

The movement that encouraged women to give birth in hospital saw a significant increase in maternal deaths. Far from doctors decreasing the risks, they increased them; it was safer for a woman in labour to be attended by local, untrained midwives. Until the late 1800s surgeons did not scrub prior to surgery. They didn't wash their hands between patients. Doctors and medical students moved from dissecting corpses to examining new mothers without first washing their hands, causing death from puerperal fever. As dissection became more important to medical practice in the 1800s, the number of women dying increased. There were no antibiotics; Alexander Fleming only discovered Penicillin in 1928.

Ignaz Semmelweis was a Hungarian physician whose work demonstrated that handwashing could drastically reduce the number of women dying after childbirth. Using data collection and statistical analysis, Semmelweis determined where the problem lay and introduced rigorous handwashing rules in the maternity ward in Vienna. As a direct consequence, deaths were drastically reduced.

Today we know his work holds true, but we don't always follow his advice.

Florence Nightingale

It would be difficult to write of basic care and infection prevention and control without giving credit to Florence Nightingale, not only for her work at Scutari but also for her greater work in driving improvements in public health.

In her book *Notes on Nursing*, Nightingale says, "In these days of investigation and statistics, where results are described with microscopic exactness and tabulated with mathematical accuracy, we seem to think figures will do instead of facts, and calculation instead of action".

Many disagreed with her, she was, after all, a woman and a nurse and not a learned man, but had it not been for her contacts and the journalists on the battlefield, her strategies to reduce mortality might have been ignored.

In 1860, Nightingale wrote *Notes on Nursing, What It Is and Is Not* in response to the high infant-mortality rate in England, describing a strong link between hand hygiene and lower patient mortality. She wrote: "In almost all diseases, the function of the skin is, more or less, disordered; and in many most important diseases nature relieves herself almost entirely by the skin. Poisoning by the skin is no less certain than poisoning by the mouth – only it is slower in its operation. Every nurse ought to be careful to wash her hands very frequently during the day."

Despite global improvements in healthcare, key aspects of good care first identified by Florence Nightingale remain problematic. Florence identified that good hygiene was the single most important element in preventing disease and deaths. She suggested that there were five essential aspects of care that enhanced recovery: clean air, clean water, efficient drainage, environmental cleanliness and light. They all feel relevant today.

Poor air quality causes respiratory diseases, which remainsa major killer and are the leading cause of deaths worldwide. In one month in 1951 the London smog caused around 4,000 deaths and led to legislation on smoke pollution. It is notable that the incidence of acute exacerbation of asthma in major European cities has fallen as Coronavirus lockdown measures have resulted in fewer cars on the roads.

Dirty water spreads diseases such as cholera and typhoid. This was recognised by Florence Nightingale but sadly they continue to be the cause of many deaths still.

One of the Millennium Development Goals is access to safe drinking water, but in 2010 an estimated 780 million (11% of the world's population) still lacked safe drinking water. More people in the world have mobile phones than access to toilets; another sad but true fact.

A lack of hygiene, especially hand hygiene, is the leading cause of hospital acquired infections. Nightingale insisted that nurses scrub the ward clean. In the 1940s, nurses at the Royal Liverpool infirmary (and most other hospitals) were required to clean the wards still. Each week they had a deep clean: moving the beds and lockers into the middle of the ward, emptying every locker, cleaning inside, then putting it all back. In 2016, Nottingham University Hospitals NHS Trust reported that their nurses were having to clean their wards due to inadequate standards provided by a third-party contractor.

Maybe we should all take a leaf out of *Notes on Nursing* and ensure that the people we care for are offered the right to live and be treated by staff who have good hygiene standards and who support the people they are caring for or treating to maintain good hygiene too. At your next mealtime, just take a step back and ask yourself whether there has been opportunity and encouragement for people to wash their hands before eating? If you do have this as a policy, how do you know it is followed? Do you audit? Do you observe? Do you ask people?

Do all staff take responsibility for the cleanliness of the environment they work in? Do you think it matters less for someone with a learning disability or someone living with dementia?

Greater Manchester Mental Health NHS Foundation Trust

This mental health trust, currently rated 'Good' by the Commission, has run campaigns to encourage everyone to stop and clean their hands. Their campaign encourages staff, visitors and patients to practice quick and easy hand hygiene to reduce healthcare associated infections and help save lives.

Their website says, "If we all work together, we can make a difference. About a third of healthcare associated infections are preventable and the most effective way to do this is practicing good hand hygiene".

The campaign focused on making everyone aware of the hand hygiene stations across the hospital entrances and community centres, with eye catching posters featuring staff from across the Trust urging people to join the hand hygiene campaign. There were alcohol gel dispensers and posters showing the seven steps of effective handwashing technique at 'stations' across the hospital.

It maybe doesn't seem a big deal for acute hospitals but it's good to see mental health services also considering the benefits of good infection prevention and control, starting with the basics.

Providence Health & Services Alaska

Providence Health & Services in Alaska is a not-for-profit network of hospitals, care centres, doctors, clinics, homecare and affiliated services run by a religious order.

The group took top prize at an educational and humorous hand hygiene film festival. The competition, run by the Association for Professionals in Infection Control and Epidemiology, is in its seventh year and draws entrants from across the USA.

Providence Health & Services Alaska took top prize with a hip-hop production called "Look at Me (Hand Hygiene)". Complete with a helicopter shot showing off the hospital's helipad and a group of medical professionals backing up its lead rapper, the music video urged listeners to W.L.S.R.D (wet, lather, scrub, rinse, dry). Midway through the video, children from the paediatrics' department arrive on set to steal the show.

The conference chair said, "Utilising a music-video to provide an overview of hand hygiene best practices is a great way to disseminate our most important infection prevention intervention."

You can find the video on YouTube by searching 'Look at Me' (Hand Hygiene)'. Sometimes a bit of fun gets the message across…

The key message about infection prevention and control is that it really is important to get the basics right. Good hand hygiene, clean premises and equipment, good waste management and food hygiene underpin reduced costs associated with infections. Staff education and understanding about the impact of poor hand hygiene is imperative. Reflection is a good way to achieve this; nobody would clear up vomit and eat their own lunch without thorough handwashing, so how can it be acceptable to serve someone else lunch without handwashing?

Avoiding unnecessary admissions and reducing the length of hospital stays builds on the basics and is the responsibility of all providers and commissioners.

Good cross system working leads to better outcomes.

Learning from mistakes and near misses

Learning from mistakes is a basic way to prevent repetition and reduce the risk of harm to other people. A culture that avoids blame and works with staff to look at ways of improving how services are delivered is likely to have a better track record on safety. Where incidents are dismissed as one-off events, or where there is no consideration of trends, there is likely to be a greater risk of continuing harm.

Not reporting incidents and near misses makes it harder to identify risks and put measures in place to prevent it happening again. Hiding poor performance by not identifying and acting upon incidents is likely to result in even worse outcomes. Reporting incidents shows a staff team who want to improve the service they deliver.

It will come as no surprise, I imagine, that sometimes the Commission doesn't get it right. Providers are expected to identify mistakes, investigate, to apologise and try to make amends. In order to maintain any semblance of credibility, I believe it is also important that the regulator acts in a similarly honourable manner. The Commission values include Excellence and offers one of the defining statements as, "We are open to constructive challenge to enable us to learn from our mistakes and we agree stretching goals in our shared drive to be a high performing organisation."

I think few would argue that was right and proper. No organisation always gets it right. We should all be courageous enough to put our hands up and say sorry. That's not always easy or comfortable but it generally creates less of a fall out than trying to gloss over the chipped paintwork.

A while ago I took a call from a senior leader in a relatively large organisation. They were very cross on behalf of their staff and barely drew breath in their defence of the team. I didn't know the situation but listened and said I would look into the matters they were unhappy about. They calmed down and we managed to have a very reasonable discussion. They had received a very delayed report that they didn't feel was recognisable as their service. There were significant inaccuracies about the service they offered that raised concerns that someone had got in a muddle. They had a warning notice served for a seemingly insignificant issue that had not been raised at the time of the inspection. An uncomfortable challenge, certainly. I could do no more than promise to investigate and come back to them within a certain timescale.

As agreed, I did some digging and realised the report was indeed very late and was not well written. There were several reasons (not excuses) that became apparent, including staff leaving the organisation and a change of managers. It had basically slipped through a gap.

I said I would look at the factual accuracy response personally and would go through all the evidence that had been provided on the day and as part of the factual accuracy challenge. I did. They had a point and the report was changed significantly. The report was taken back to the national quality assurance panel to recalibrate the ratings. Instead of being an entirely paper-based exercise, we discussed the factual accuracies and shared the re-written draft report to ensure it was representative of the organisation. I agreed to visit the service and meet with leaders and staff to apologise personally. It was so sad that our mistakes and gaps in oversight had resulted in such distress to the staff; one cried when I spoke with her because she was so pleased someone had bothered to seek her out and say sorry. It shouldn't have been necessary but since it happened, we had an obligation to put it right.

Out of that shortfall came some real positives for our team. The managers tell staff until they are blue in the face that 'Getting it Right First Time', writing well and checking reports are in good order and delivered to time reduces stress and workload. It is cheaper, it improves provider/regulator relationships, and it builds trust. Generally, people listen briefly then start looking at their phones or talking about workloads. The provider very kindly agreed to bring a team, including the registered manager, to speak to the team about how it felt to receive a report they didn't recognise as their service and to have an unexpected warning notice drop into their inbox. It was powerful and personal. Far more powerful than any manager talking about KPIs. Our team could feel and hear how much distress the situation had caused. Nobody wants to upset people and listening to the speakers helped us understand the impact our actions sometimes have. I am certain that the provider's willingness to engage constructively has improved the way we work.

Imagine that a visiting healthcare professional trips over an electricity extension cable and falls but is uninjured. They pick up their belongings, look a bit embarrassed and say they don't want a fuss. Nobody reports it as an incident as it was so minor. Two weeks later, one of the staff trips over the same lead, when bringing around a tray of hot drinks. They aren't hurt just a bit cross they have to mop the floor and that two mugs have broken. They moan at the person who is using the extension to set up a fan in the reception area. The person apologises and they both agree no harm done. It is still very warm a week later when an elderly person comes to reception to book in. The fan is still whirring around cooling the reception staff. The elderly person turns and trips over the same extension lead. Unfortunately, they have osteoporosis and have sustained a fractured neck of femur. With a little thought, with the recognition that two incidents had happened because of the lead, the person might well not have fallen and needed surgery.

Are they effective?

Key messages

- Outcomes are important, improving outcomes even more so.

- Data should be collected for a purpose; unused data is of no value and is simply numbers or words.

- If you don't know how your service is performing when compared to similar services, or over time, you cannot know if it is providing good care or treatment.

- Some fundamentals of good care sit within the effective domain in the English inspection framework.

- Some of the major national enquiries into systemic poor care were as a result of failings that now sit under the effective domain.

- Good multi-disciplinary team working by competent staff improves outcomes and patient experiences.

By effective, we mean that people's care, treatment and support achieves good outcomes, promotes a good quality of life and is based on the best available evidence.

Are people's needs and choices assessed and care, treatment and support delivered in line with current legislation, standards and evidence-based guidance to achieve effective outcome? How does the service make sure that staff have the skills, knowledge and experience to deliver effective care and support? How well do staff, teams and services within and across organisations work together to deliver effective care, support and treatment? Is consent to care and treatment always sought in line with legislation and guidance?

Pain management

"The greatest evil is physical pain."

(St Augustine of Hippo)

"The art of medicine consists of amusing the patient while nature cures the disease."

(Voltaire)

"I think what worries me the most about pain is how it takes over and becomes the centre of your life. It shouldn't really be like that."

(Janet Allcock)

Nobody should be left with untreated pain – while some people will inevitably experience pain, it must never be ignored.

The National Pain Audit was commissioned in England and Wales between 2009-2013 and showed significant variability in access to specialist chronic pain management services. A joint working party report published in 1990 by the Royal College of Surgeons and the Royal College of Anaesthetists on pain after surgery recommended that every hospital should have an acute pain service to improve post-operative pain relief.

An audit of the way the report recommendations were carried out and published in the *Nursing Times* (2003) by Tarnia Taverner, a clinical nurse specialist – she found that patients had their pain managed well in the recovery room. At 24-hours post-operatively, patients rated pain management as less effective. At seven days post-surgery, 39% of patients had a pain score on movement of 5-7, while 8% experienced pain scored at 8-10. The scoring system used was a verbal self-report tool where patients reported the level of pain they were experiencing using a numeric rating scale where 0 is no pain and 10 is the worst pain imaginable. The audit found that the site with the best outcomes had a pain management team and unique to their clinical practice was the use of a prescription chart for all post-operative patients with analgesics and anti-emetics printed on to it, therefore ensuring that adequate drugs were prescribed.

The results also showed that pain management for post-operative patients was inadequate, especially for patients having Patient Controlled Analgesia (PCA). The author concluded that PCA is not effective for post-operative analgesia, although it fared better where patients received adequate education and staff received appropriate training.

We haven't really got pain management right for all yet despite it being shown that good pain management improves outcomes for patients and providers. Pain impacts on employment, activities, behaviours, relationships, mood, sleep and even coronary health.

Good pain management improves people's perception of the provider, is cheaper and improves patient flow. Pain delays discharges. Staff are less likely to experience verbal or physical aggression where pain is managed. There are straightforward cost savings and benefits to services managing people's pain well (over and above the humane and ethical position that people should not be left with treatable pain).

The effects of pain can easily be considered in terms of how pain management improves the efficiency of care and treatment. It is and should always be about the person receiving care, but with a recognition that better care offers significant benefits to staff and services.

- Pain causes poor wound healing, weakness and muscle breakdown versus managing pain well, which means less money spent on managing wounds, and a lowered risk of persistent and recurrent pressure damage.
- Pain causes reduced movement of the affected body parts resulting in an increased risk of thromboembolism and pulmonary embolism versus managing pain well, which means lower mortality risk and lower treatment costs.
- Pain causes shallow breathing and cough suppression, which can increase the risk of pneumonia versus managing pain well, which means fewer cases of chest infections or pneumonia and a lowered mortality risk.
- Pain causes increased sodium and water retention leading to swollen limbs and an increased risk of skin fragility. Professor Peter Vowden, from the University of Bradford, suggests that treating an average venous leg ulcer effectively within a year costs around £800. If the ulcer fails to heal within that time, costs can escalate up to £4,400 a year.
- Pain causes decreased gastrointestinal motility. How much staff time and money are taken up managing constipation?

We need to think particularly about pain management for specific groups. Older people are more likely to experience pain but less likely to complain about it and less likely to take their pain medication. Pain is under diagnosed and under treated in people with learning disabilities and dementia.

It is particularly important that staff working in social care settings understand that pain experienced by people with dementia is often poorly managed. Unmanaged pain can lead to further cognitive impairment, accidents and behavioural problems. The impact can be reduced if the pain is accurately assessed and managed.

Colm Cunningham's article, 'Managing pain in patients with dementia in hospital' published in the *Nursing Standard* in 2006 showed that people living with dementia receive fewer analgesics than any other patient group, but the likelihood of pain in this group is as high as in other older people.

My intention is not to tell people what prescribing algorithms should be in place and which drug protocol is most effective. That is beyond the purpose of this book. Suffice to say that all providers should have a pain or symptom management policy, that staff should understand it and that compliance against the policy should be monitored. Any such policy should be written with expert input and reviewed regularly. If you are a residential service, whether for elderly people or people with learning disabilities or autism, consider asking for help from your local hospice, your local GP services or the pain team at the local acute trust. I would hope psychiatric hospital services were already consulting with a pain specialist and ensuring mental ill health was not being exacerbated by unremitted pain.

Many factors unconsciously alter the degree to which pain is felt and reported, even though people all have the same anatomical structures to pass pain messages to the brain. Pain cannot be measured, only observed by one's behaviour to pain. As those who attempt to treat these patients, we need to recognise these factors and how they can influence our treatment and a patient's recovery.

There are also significant barriers to effective pain management including people 'not liking taking tablets', fear of addiction, fear of side-effects and patients worrying that it will be seen as a sign of weakness. Some healthcare staff still have concerns about the potential for addiction but there is better awareness of the need for effective pain control as part of the recovery process.

Recognising pain

Many hospitals I have been in and every report that I have ever read mentions the use of pain tools. That's a good thing, as it means people are at least aware that pain can be assessed using methods other than a direct question. Tools, however, are only tools. If they are not used properly, they are likely to be of little value. Ticking a box with a smiley face doesn't manage the pain. Pain assessment and management is a much wider process than writing a number 3 on a chart or asking if someone wants paracetamol.

Pain assessment for people who cannot effectively communicate the level of pain they are feeling (and also, perhaps those that can but who might want to be stoic) need to consider how pain can be seen in ways other than a verbal response to a simple question.

I think there is a ladder of pain assessment that should include:

- Verbal self-reporting. This would include a numerical pain measurement or a simple series of questions about the current level of pain.
- Non-verbal self-reporting. People who cannot talk can still offer some insight into their pain levels. That might be pointing to a picture, blinking a set number of times or squeezing a hand.

- A visual check on potential causes of pain as an integral part of the pain assessment. Have they got a foot in an awkward position? Has the sun moved and is now burning the back of their neck? Are they lying on a monitor wire?

- Consideration of behavioural changes such as insomnia, aggression, increased distress. It's no surprise that there is a negative correlation between pain recognition and the increased use of bank and agency staff who do not know the individuals well.

- Reporting by friends or family. Those who know someone best are more likely to identify changes that may be indicative of unmanaged pain. Staff should be listening to relatives.

- Direct observation of physical signs such as posture, facial expression, level of engagement.

- Physiological signs such as in increased pulse rate, increased respiratory rate, vomiting and increased blood pressure.

There are readily available tools to use but all health and social care practitioners should have training in recognising and managing pain, it's not complex if a process of reflecting on their own experiences of pain and how it impacted on them is used as a starting point.

If staff understand the physical and psychological impact of their own pain, the wanting to curl up in a ball, the grumpiness, the difficulty sleeping and the not wanting to do much, they might have greater empathy. If they consider how a hot water bottle or warm bath helped ease aching muscles or recall that getting up and moving helped their bad back, they might remember that there are strategies to employ as an adjunct to prescribed drugs.

Midwives are often experts in alternative pain management strategies and encourage the use of warm water, transcutaneous electrical nerve stimulation, relaxation, music, movement, hypnobirthing as well as the more traditional 'gas and air', opioids and epidural drugs. Maybe other directorates within hospitals and other services could think about what good maternity services offer and their approach to pain relief and use some of the ideas for other people?

I am not suggesting alternative ways are better than drugs to manage pain; I am suggesting there are highly effective strategies that can be used in addition to medication.

How do you know how well your service is managing people's pain? How does this work for people unable to tell you how well their pain is managed? Do you carry out 'non-verbal' pain assessment audits?

How often are you dismissing pain symptoms as challenging behaviour, anxiety, or normal for a particular individual?

Yannis

Yannis was an 11-year-old boy who joined us at a children's camp in Somerset back in the 1980s. It was a beautiful setting for the camp, a study centre in the Mendip Hills with several dormitories split into various levels and with half walls to offer children a degree of privacy, while allowing supervision. We exhausted the children with long days swimming and playing parachute games in the August sunshine. I've lost count of the number of daisy chain headbands I have made over time.

One evening Yannis, who was always lively and liked being the group clown, started screaming and jumping on his bed as the group leader was trying to settle the dormitory with a long and rather boring story. "I've got a wasp in my ear; I've got a wasp in my ear!" He wasn't particularly distressed, and it was assumed he was mucking around. The other boys were starting to mimic him, and everyone was laughing. It was only when the group leader 'got serious' and threatened to remove the first swim of the day that they all settled down… all except Yannis, that is. He was brought to me as the only person with healthcare credentials; I was a student nurse, after all.

When I asked why he thought he had something in his ear, he told me it was still buzzing. He denied any discomfort, just the noise. I did a perfunctory examination and couldn't see anything, but he was insistent and becoming upset that the wasp might eat his brain. I couldn't justify leaving a child with a wasp in their ear, however seemingly unlikely. He was repeatedly hitting his ear by this time, 'to stop the buzzing'. I found a driver and we set off to the nearest hospital at about 10:30pm. It was busy when we arrived, with people in various states of intoxication, and not an ideal environment for a child. We waited and Yannis became more tired and started getting upset. He was frightened, tired and beginning to become fractious.

After I did my best battle-axe to get him seen in a timelier manner, he was called in by a junior doctor and nurse. Nobody introduced themselves or explained anything. The nurse passed the doctor an auriscope and the doctor said, "Lets sort that ear of yours out then" as he grabbed Yannis's ear and the nurse grabbed his arms before I could say anything. Yannis freaked. Loudly and very physically. He started screaming and lashing out as he believed they were about to operate on him. Suddenly it hurt, and, if the noise was anything to go by, it hurt a lot. Pain is not a purely physical thing.

I asked them to wait and let me calm poor Yannis who by this time was sobbing. The doctor was already talking about an anaesthetic to have a proper look and an overnight stay. When you are working with a group of 40 children you don't know very well, you need to have various useful things up your sleeve (not literally) and my rucksack contained a variety of items to amuse bored children at short notice. Never have I been more grateful of Porky the naughty piglet and Chippy the Chicken – two puppets that lived among the packet of sandy marshmallows and rainbow-coloured tangle of embroidery thread.

Porky and Chippy came out and explained everything to Yannis, they talked about all sorts of nonsense and Indiana Jones; they told the most awful jokes ever. They calmed and engaged Yannis, so that he was willing to let someone look inside his ear. The pain dissipated. The jokes and custard pie style comedy really were that awful but were an effective distraction and distraction is a powerful tool when managing pain.

In the end we had to return three times, as there was disagreement among the emergency department staff about whether there was a wasp in his ear. Eventually an ENT consultant removed it while Yannis lay very still, listening to a story read by Porky in a suitably porcine voice. Yannis went back to camp proudly holding a dismembered wasp (named Weston) in a urine specimen bottle. As he had not needed an anaesthetic, his mother was happy for him to stay with us and he continued his holiday as a bit of celebrity.

Symptom control is not just about giving analgesic drugs. How often do you use strategies to ease pain and discomfort that do not just involve giving paracetamol? Drugs have their place but are not the only way to reduce pain.

"Even the smallest shift in perspective can bring about the greatest healing."
(Joshua Kai)

Beth Thorp: Living with, and managing, chronic pain – a patient's story

This patient story was published in the online magazine *Practical Pain Management*, aimed at pain clinicians in the US. I have not given the whole story here but two points about how Beth manages pain are useful in showing that listening to patients and using non-pharmaceutical methods of pain relief are important in managing pain. I think we often overlook the simplest cures and could reduce the need for drugs if we considered pain management more widely.

Movement and exercise

"This is probably my most important coping tool for a variety of reasons. Exercise helps in several ways, both physically and mentally. In my early adult years, I was very active, participating in ice dancing, skiing, and roller blading. Because of the pain, my exercise now involves mostly just walking and low-impact aerobics.

Even if I'm in pain, movement can help me to feel better. Physically, it loosens my joints, keeps me limber, and helps me to stay in shape. Mentally, it takes my mind off the pain, and it provides me with social interaction if I exercise with friends or in a class. If I'm in too much pain to really exercise, just changing positions – from sitting to standing, or standing to lying down – can help reduce my pain."

How often are people left sitting for long periods of time, and movement reduced because of fear of falling, staff being busy doing other things, or simply because of custom and practice? Are there ways you could increase the amount of exercise people get in your setting? I suspect a gym in a GP surgery is a step too far, but could you not run back injury exercise classes in a local village hall? It might just be cheaper and more effective than working up the prescribing ladder of ever stronger analgesics. Do people in your home sit in the communal area or their rooms with very infrequent movement from their seats? How uncomfortable must that be?

Change of scenery

"Even if I'm not really feeling up to it, getting out of the house, getting fresh air, walking around the block, doing an errand—anything that takes me into a different environment can help reduce my pain."

The enforced lockdown from Coronavirus will have had an impact on the number of people reporting increased pain, I am sure. I am truly fortunate to live in a rural village in a national park. We have been able to continue to get out and about, walking the dog along different routes, seeing first spring and now summer flowers emerging, fresh and bright. The lambs are growing rapidly, the wild garlic is in flower, the calves are sweet. The bluebells in the woods were stunning this year. In the evening we can sit and watch the bats swooping in an out of the adjacent 11th century church.

It's actually rather nice for us, but others, living alone in inner city flats, must be staring at the four walls with little to think about but their discomfort.

Could people using your service be helped to get a change of scene to help them focus outside of their discomfort? If they are a long-stay patient in a community hospital or even an acute hospital, could a relative be persuaded to push them into the grounds or to the hospital café or shop? Even with staff shortages it could be possible. What about using a volunteer scheme with trained volunteers using a wheelchair to take people for a wander to see what they can see? Your patients who are living with dementia might well be much calmer if they feel the sun on their face or the wind in their hair. In care homes, it should be the norm for people to be offered a change of scene – even if it is the garden rather than their room.

It has long been recognised how important play is for children and the adult health and social care world could perhaps learn much from good paediatrics – one is never too old to play. Maybe it's time for a campaign to encourage a change of scene and being out of doors, to supplement the PJ Paralysis campaign? I don't know, maybe, 'Outdoors for Better Outcomes'.

Play

Coram's Fields

Coram's Fields is a lovely oasis in the middle of London. I have very fond memories of taking children to play there when I was training and working at Great Ormond Street, which is just around the corner. Thomas Coram was a philanthropist who created the London Foundling Hospital to look after unwanted children in Lamb's Conduit Fields, Bloomsbury. The park now has accessible play equipment for all ages from toddlers to older children as well as two wide lawns for children to play.

They also have a sensory and music area, opened in association with Great Ormond Street Hospital, and a wheelchair-friendly play area. In addition, there are two large sandpits that are open all year round and a paddling pool that opens during the spring and summer months. As well as happy memories I also remember the sheer terror I experienced when a young patient with a tracheostomy ran off and into the sandpit.

Children loved the park; they were taken by staff and their families. It was space and time away from the stresses and discomfort of hospital treatments. It offered more than the familiarity of a few swings; it offered distraction, exercise, normality, the freedom to be children and to have fun. It wasn't unusual to see nurses taking their thick black tights off and holding their skirts up to enable children to paddle safely. As no adults were admitted without children, it was a very safe environment and there were always other doctors or senior nurses around to help, if necessary.

It was fantastic for pain management and symptom control without the patients realising it.

Thinking about it made me wonder which other hospitals have access to parks or playgrounds. I found some examples from across the world – clearly some providers understand the importance of play.

The Queen Elizabeth Hospital and Royal Hospital for Children, Glasgow

The two hospitals have access to a lovely play park that offers opportunities for imaginative Play with a shipwreck boat and familiar park equipment like 'springies'. There is equipment for teenagers too, including a trim trail to allow them to exercise despite being in hospital.

Leicester Royal Infirmary

The hospital opened a rooftop play area in 2008 which was bright, colourful and could be used year-round, because there was a heated conservatory. It shows that not having extensive green fields around a hospital is not a limitation on offering opportunities for a change of scene and play.

Harley Street Clinic, London

Another example of using the space you have to create an opportunity to get away from a clinical environment. They have a Flights of Fantasy rooftop play area for young patients.

Norfolk and Norwich NHS Foundation Trust.

The Jenny Lind Children's Hospital has a play area that provides exciting 'escape from reality' opportunities for their sick children. The facilities include playhouses, spinners, slides and integral play panels on the climbing equipment.

Every children's hospice that I have ever been to

I have yet to visit a children's hospice that does not have exceptional outdoor play spaces and 'escape from reality' opportunities. Just walking into the gardens of most makes you want to jump on a swing. They are all accessible for children with physical limitations but also sufficiently exciting to captivate healthy siblings and allow relaxed time for the whole family.

I would expect services providing care and treatment to children to have good play facilities, as it is such an integral part of paediatric care. Outdoor space is in some ways a bonus but services are unlikely to be judged poorly because their play spaces are indoors; how much better to offer something more?

Thinking about adults who are hospitalised for a long time or who live in a care home, I wonder how much less pain they might report and how much better their lives might feel if they had the same opportunities for a change of scene and fun that children often have?

I am not imagining octogenarians on zip wires (unless they particularly wanted to) but I do recall a Worthing care home (but sadly can't remember the name) where they had put a see-through panel in the perimeter fence, so that the residents could watch the children playing in the primary school next door. Some had 'made friends' with a couple of children, who regularly popped over to show off their merit badges and new shoes. This was long before the trend of children visiting care homes became a thing.

Would older folk in hospital not like a pleasant outdoor area to sit and chat with family? A few hospitals have somewhere for patients identified as being at the end of their life but I rather suspect that someone in hospital for a while, but who was not dying, might also appreciate a change of scene and opportunity to be outside in an area they could sit and watch the world go by. Care home residents might like somewhere they could easily access without support or supervision.

Then I thought about psychiatric provision. It's not my area of expertise but looking back to my training, we spent three months on placement in a large London psychiatric hospital with acres and acres of parkland surrounding the many institutional ward blocks. I don't ever remember anyone being encouraged to use those grounds. It made me look at the website for mental health services in the counties around where I live. The websites for many of the locations didn't mention a garden or easy access to outside space at all. I find that quite surprising. I think if I were in a hospital for a long time, I would feel much more responsive and engaged if I could relax in the fresh air and perhaps even take part in outdoor activities like yoga, tai chi or, dare I say it, swimming.

Frimley Park Hospital

The Time Garden at Frimley Park Hospital was funded through the Department of Health and the King's Fund grant as part of their Enhancing the Healing Environment programme, after the idea came from a patient.

It was a courtyard garden which was designed to enable easy movement of bed-bound patients and provide as much privacy for them as possible. There was a glass-fronted summer house that afforded shelter and which had tea and coffee-making facilities and a music system. It also has a separate small private garden area of its own providing even greater seclusion and privacy while still offering a view of the rest of the garden.

The staff across the hospital used it well and made every effort to ensure patients and families that wanted to use it were able to do so. It was about bringing families and friends together as they faced approaching death but is also a useful space to take people away from their pain, albeit briefly.

Sometimes we manage pain using non-pharmacological methods, without even realising we are doing it. How many of us have put frozen peas onto burnt fingers?

Visitors to care homes, Coronavirus and the legislative framework

The distant approach of Coronavirus towards the UK threw up some interesting situations with some care home providers. Well before any suggestion from central government or the professional bodies, some care homes were banning visitors to their homes. Sadly, sometimes social media showed a few providers and managers making unilateral decisions to 'close the home' from as far back as early February 2020 when the formal restrictions didn't come into place until late March 2020. While undoubtedly this was done with what was perceived as the best of intent (and possibly foresight), it was also done without due consideration of the wider needs of individuals and the legislative framework that applied at the time.

Care homes do have responsibilities to protect all of their residents, both those being visited and their fellow residents. If it is believed that a visitor may pose a risk to residents, they need to consider how to mitigate or reduce that risk. There cannot be an absolute 'no visitors' policy when most visitors were posing no greater risk than their own staff, delivery drivers or visiting professionals. Any condition applied should be proportionate.

A blanket approach was outside the principles of the Mental Capacity Act 2005, which includes:

- The third principle, which states that a person is not to be treated as unable to decide merely because they make an unwise decision. If a resident has capacity and chooses to accept the risk that a relative may be infected, they had a right to accept that risk, regardless of what home staff felt. Obviously, there should have been discussion and support to reduce the risk of transmission but stopping them meeting because staff felt it was unwise isn't in accordance with principle three.

- The fourth principle, which states that if a decision is made on behalf of a person who does not have mental capacity, then it must be made in their best interest. It may be the care home staff thought that restricting all visitors was in the person's best interest as they may have been less likely to contract the virus, but there is a wider issue around what an individual sees as being important to their best interests. I think if I had a few weeks to live, I would want to see my husband and children.

■ The fifth principle, which states that the least restrictive option should be used. Finally, if a decision is made (or an act done) on behalf of a person who does not have mental capacity, it should be the least restrictive option available and the person's rights and freedoms should be enabled, as far as possible. Stopping people seeing their loved ones is hugely restrictive. Care homes are people's homes, and people living there should be able to welcome family and friends as such.

The Law Society's guide *Identifying a deprivation of liberty: a practical guide – The care home setting* (2015) suggests that restricting visiting times in a care home may potentially have been a liberty-restricting measure where a Deprivation of Liberty Safeguard application should have been made.

The Human Rights Act 1998 sets out the fundamental rights and freedoms that everyone in the UK is entitled to. It incorporates the rights set out in the European Convention on Human Rights (ECHR) into domestic British law and remains applicable for people living in care homes. Article 8 of the Act protects people's right to respect for their private life and their family life. Guidance from the Equality and Human Rights Commission makes it explicit that family life includes the right to enjoy family relationships. This includes the right to live with your family and, where this is not possible, the right to regular contact.

The guidance suggests that there are situations when public authorities can interfere with your right to respect for private and family life but that this is only allowed where the authority can show that its action is lawful, necessary and proportionate in order to protect public safety and protect health.

It is clear that while a public authority can make decisions that interfere with people's human rights, care home staff may not do so.

The fundamental standards replaced the previous 'Essential Standards' and were intended to give people who use services (and those who provide them) a clearer picture of the standards that must be met. They were created from, and in line with, the Francis Report recommendations. The Fundamental Standards state that care and treatment must be appropriate and reflect service users' needs and preferences. Furthermore, care and treatment must only be provided with consent.

These standards underpin the regulations of the Health and Social Care Act 2008 (Regulated Activities) Regulations 2014:

- Regulation 10(2)(a) – Dignity and respect: People's relationships with their visitors, carer, friends, family or relevant other persons should be respected, and privacy maintained as far as reasonably practicable during visits.

- Regulation 9(3)(e) – Person-centred care: People using the service and/or those lawfully acting on their behalf must be given opportunities to manage as much of their care and treatment as possible. This has to be balanced against the need to consider the well-being of other people living in the home:

- Regulation 9(3)(b) – Person-centred care: "When planning how to meet a person's preferences, providers should take into account, and make provision for, any impact this may have on other people using the service."

It's not easy to weigh up all the requirements. Clearly this changed when the Coronavirus Act (2020) came into effect, but a few providers were choosing to act prior to this.

Perhaps there should have been more consideration as to how to manage visits to the homes rather than imposing isolation from family and friends on people before the law permitted it? It would be easier when the weather is better, and people can use gardens or go out for a walk. It may be that more consideration is going to be needed as we come out of full lockdown. Simply because a home-wide decision is easier, it doesn't mean it is lawful.

Sefton Hall, Dawlish

I am sure many will have seen this Devon care home on the BBC news. They closed to visitors as required by the Coronavirus Act, but were still very aware that families and residents were missing each other. They had the idea of recreating a drive-through fast food restaurant by offering a drive-through visiting day.

Putting the needs and wishes of people living at the home at the forefront of their planning, they set up the grounds with protection from the warm sun, distanced 'visitor stations' and time slots. This enabled families and residents to see their loved ones from the safety of their cars after eight weeks apart.

The television footage was very moving with people suddenly realising who they were seeing and bursting into huge smiles that reached from ear to ear. It must have been lovely for the staff too.

Consent
"No man is good enough to govern another man without the other's consent."
(Abraham Lincoln)

"For in reason, all government without the consent of the governed is the very definition of slavery."

(Jonathon Swift)

Key Messages

■ Consent is everyone's business.

■ Consent without full information is not consent.

■ Consent is a process not a form to sign nor a checklist.

■ Provider oversight of consent should consider the full process, not just completion of forms or risk assessments.

■ Staff need to understand the legal and professional frameworks for consent and know who can give consent.

■ Consent is a big issue; few things are more important. It is fundamental to good care and treatment. Every decision, every act of care, every sharing of information, however small, however important, should be made with full awareness and consideration of the need for informed consent.

■ Consent, in law, is voluntary agreement with an action proposed by another.

■ Consent is an act of reason; the person giving consent must be of sufficient mental capacity and be in possession of all essential information in order to give consent and must also be free of coercion or fraud.

Not everyone using health or social care services is able to give their consent. Those providing care and treatment must then act in accordance with the various pieces of legislation and guidance that support decision-making. There are anomalies and grey areas within the various pieces of legislation and professional guidance which can create confusion. It is important providers ensure that staff understand which specific guidance or laws relate to their services.

The guidance and laws used in this section related entirely to the UK – although the European Convention on Human Rights informs laws in all member states. The variation in laws around consent vary from country to country, even within Europe where, for example, the age at which you can consent to sex is 18 in Turkey compared to 14 years in Serbia, San Mario or many other nations.

There is also that hugely important word 'Informed': it must be *informed* consent. Informed means fully informed and able to understand the risks, potential benefits, alternative treatments and likely outcomes. Informed consent applies as much to care homes and GP practices as to hospitals. There is no use a care home saying, "Take this medicine Nelly, it will make you feel better" and not explaining what the medicine is actually for and accepting a refusal if someone doesn't want to take it (and has capacity).

It's quite hard to cite particularly good practice in relation to gaining informed consent. There is very good practice in many services but there are also times when what is obtained is not truly informed.

Montgomery v Lanarkshire Health Board (2015)

A woman was admitted to hospital for the delivery of her baby. There was a relatively high-risk (around 10%) of shoulder dystocia because of the mother's diabetes and her small size. In lay terms, a shoulder dystocia is an obstructed labour in which, after delivery of the head, the baby's shoulder gets caught above the mother's pubic bone and the baby isn't delivered without assistance. It is an emergency situation.

For this mother, there was a relatively low risk of a prolonged lack of oxygen from shoulder dystocia. She was not advised of the risks of vaginal delivery as opposed to Caesarean section. Unfortunately, the worst-case scenario happened, and her baby was born severely disabled.

The obstetrician's evidence was that she did not advise the mother of the increased possibility of shoulder dystocia because the risk of a serious problem for the baby was small. If the condition and potential for serious brain damage had been mentioned, most women would choose to have a Caesarean section. The judgment in this case was that a doctor's assessment of a patient's interests had outweighed the patient's wishes.

When the case reached the Supreme Court, the principal issue was whether the obstetrician's failure to warn the mother of the risk of shoulder dystocia was negligent.

Around this time there had been a change in the social, medical and legal landscape. People were now regarded as having autonomous rights and an ability to make choices for themselves. There was more access to medical information and patients were often better informed than previously. Expectations had changed. Professional guidance for doctors had also changed and there was greater emphasis on the concerns and choices of patients.

The government published their Human Rights and Democracy report in 2015 and the courts were increasingly conscious of the value of self-determination, particularly in cases involving issues of withdrawal of treatment. The Supreme Court ruled that:

"An adult person of sound mind is entitled to decide which, if any, of the available forms of treatment to undergo, and their consent must be obtained before treatment interfering with her bodily integrity is undertaken. The doctor is therefore under a duty to take reasonable care to ensure that the patient is aware of any material risks involved in any recommended treatment, and of any reasonable alternative or variant treatments. The test of materiality is whether, in the circumstances of the particular case, a reasonable person in the patient's position would be likely to attach significance to the risk, or the doctor is or should reasonably be aware that the particular patient would be likely to attach significance to it."

Whether a risk should be regarded as material depends on the patient's perspective rather than the view of the doctors. Healthcare professionals must share information fully and support people to make decisions, even if they do not think it is the best course of action.

In this case, the patient was found to have the right to be advised of the risk of shoulder dystocia and decide what risks she was prepared to run. The court accepted that she would have opted for a Caesarean section with proper advice. It awarded her damages of £5.25 million.

What happens when informed consent isn't obtained?

Report of the Independent Inquiry into the Issues raised by Paterson (February 2020)

The government report, published in February 2020, recounts the details of the investigation leading to the conviction of Ian Paterson, a surgeon in the West Midlands, who was found guilty of wounding with intent and imprisoned. He had harmed patients in his care. The scale of his malpractice shocked the country. At the time of his trial, Paterson was described as having breached his patients' trust and abused his power.

Most of the patients treated were women who had breast procedures. The term "cleavage sparing mastectomy" is mentioned in some of the patient accounts. This procedure has no definition and is not a recognised practice. As a woman facing breast surgery, how reassured would you feel by a surgeon who agreed to spare you your cleavage?

The patient stories are a litany of uninformed consent.

Patient 53

From the report:

"Patient 53 is deceased. Her husband and daughter told us of her experience. Patient 53 had a lump in her breast and was referred by her GP to Solihull Hospital as an NHS patient. Following a biopsy, Paterson told her she had cancer. He said patient 53 could have the lump removed but would need chemotherapy afterwards, or she could have a mastectomy, which had a higher chance of getting rid of all the cancer. Patient 53 chose to have a mastectomy and was operated on by Paterson.

Five years later, patient 53 became very ill and died. She had secondary liver cancer. Her family wonder if the secondary cancer was caused by Paterson leaving breast tissue behind following patient 53's mastectomy."

Patient 7

Patient 7 was initially seen by a colleague of Paterson's at an NHS hospital because she had breast lumps, before Paterson took over responsibility for her care. Following a scan, he told her that her lump was getting worse and that he needed to act. Patient 7 was reluctant to have surgery and asked whether there was an alternative course of action. Paterson told her that if she did not have an operation "it will start to deform your breast, very quickly". Paterson also refused patient 7's request for a second opinion and told her, "mine is the greatest opinion". He also told her that there was no time to be seen on the NHS as the lump was growing rapidly and therefore he had to see her as a private patient.

Patient 7 was seen at the private hospital in preparation for surgery but had no further test prior to her operation. On the day of the surgery, patient 7 was asked to sign a consent form for the operation while lying on the trolley. She was also asked to consent to a mastectomy if Paterson found during the operation that any cancer had progressed. Patient 7 had the lump in her breast removed, but afterwards noticed that Paterson had also removed tissue from a different area. When asked about this, his response was that he was able to remove the lump through a different route and argued that he left patient 7 with a "nice scar", which she disputed.

These are just two stories from many but are indicative of a total disregard for offering patients the opportunity to give informed consent. Perhaps one of the saddest reflections is that others knew but his charismatic personality meant they didn't challenge him.

While there are no doubts that Paterson's failings were much wider than not obtaining properly informed consent, the report acknowledges there were others involved who should also have challenged the lack of informed consent. Had they done so, fewer patients would have suffered harm.

Who should have raised issues around consent and where were the opportunities to protect patients?

Consent for procedures is often obtained by others on behalf of surgeons or doctors. In termination clinics, it is usual practice to have the drugs prescribed by someone working remotely, or for the surgeon to have not seen the patient prior to them being brought into the treatment room. In many private and NHS hospitals, nurses run pre-operative assessment clinics. In busy hospitals and departments, junior medical staff take consent before surgery, particularly for emergency surgery.

In every operating theatre, interventional radiology suite or surgical treatment room across all providers registered for surgical procedures, the World Health Organisation Five Steps to Safer Surgery should be in use routinely. If all five steps are used properly, many problems disappear and risks are mitigated. Avoidable harms should be avoided. For this section, there is an important part of the process that supports the team to ensure that valid consent has been obtained.

The guidance document, *World Health Organisation: Guidelines for Safe Surgery* (2009) offers a five-step process.

Step 1. Verification: This consists of verifying the correct patient, site and procedure at every stage from the time a decision is made to operate to the time the patient undergoes the operation. This should be done:

- *when the procedure is scheduled*
- *at the time of admission or entry to the operating theatre*
- *any time the responsibility for care of the patient is transferred to another person*
- *before the patient leaves the pre-operative area or enters the procedure or surgical room.*

The step is undertaken insofar as possible with the patient involved, awake and aware. Verification is done by labelling and identifying the patient and during the consent process; the site, laterality and procedure are confirmed by checking the patient's records and radiographs. This is an active process that must include all members of the team involved in the patient's care.

If only these steps had been followed fully when Paterson was operating...

Step three says:

Step 3. Time out:

The 'time out or 'surgical pause' is a brief pause before the incision to confirm the patient, the procedure and the site of operation. It is also an opportunity to ensure that the patient is correctly positioned and that any necessary implants or special equipment are available.

The Joint Commission stipulates that all team members be actively involved in this process. Any concerns or inconsistencies must be clarified at this stage. The checks during the 'time out' must be documented, potentially in the form of a checklist, but the Universal Protocol leaves the design and delivery to individual organisations.

The detail of the wording is the important bit; that *all team members* be actively involved in this process. This is key when considering consent. All team members, all involved health or social care professionals, should be assured that proper consent has been obtained; it is an active process. It is not adequate to 'think' that the person obtaining consent has sufficient knowledge of the procedure to ensure the person is fully informed of the risks, benefits and alternatives. It is unlikely that a healthcare assistant will have the depth of knowledge of a surgical procedure to be able to provide details of the levels of risk around surgical site infections or allergies to contrast dyes. They might be able to say there is a risk of an allergic reaction but not know what the frequency of such reactions is or what the potential consequences of anaphylaxis are. It's not good enough to say, 'It's not a big problem, few people react badly'.

One assumes that Paterson had a chaperone when he examined women and that leads to the question about why the chaperone didn't raise concerns about the consent process. In step one there were several people involved who should have checked that informed consent was obtained but clearly didn't do so effectively. The patients may not have known that 'cleavage sparing mastectomies' were not a thing, but the anaesthetist and theatre staff jolly well should have done. They also failed in the responsibilities to ensure consent was obtained.

In non-surgical settings, adult social care or a medical ward, for example, it's not informed consent around the use of bed rails if someone else has just suggested it would be safer and staff simply put them up telling the person, "they'll stop you falling out of bed". The bedrails restrict a person's liberty and come with risks of their own.

It may be worth noting that Paterson was still operating in 2011, well after the guidance from the World Health Organisation was issued.

Who can give consent in health and social care settings?

The answer to this question is more confusing than it might first appear and several pieces of legislation impact on the answer, depending on the circumstances. The first and most obvious answer is that any adult over 18 years of age who has capacity to understand what they are consenting to is the only person who can consent to care or treatment. That seems simple enough, but then questions pop up about people who may lack capacity due to conditions such as dementia, who are under 18, who are unconscious, who are prisoners, who are not making wise decisions, who are a bit confused sometimes and putting themselves at what we consider to be a risk of harm.

Can anyone be made to have treatment against their will? Can a spouse give consent? Can a parent of a severely disabled young adult? Can family give consent on behalf of an elderly relative? Can they insist something is kept from them? Can you insist on treatment against medical advice? Who consents to Do Not Attempt Cardiopulmonary Resuscitation Orders? Do you consent to a doctor not offering treatment?

Barts Health NHS Trust

The winner of the 2019 HSJ award for digitising patient services, Barts developed this initiative after a patient complaint in 2017. A Bengali-speaking patient developed a serious complication after an invasive procedure. They required surgery and did recover but complained that they had not understood that this was a recognised complication. It highlighted that he had not given informed consent, as required.

The investigation identified time constraints and language barriers as obstacles to ensuring patients fully understand what they are consenting to.

Animations describing the procedure, its benefits, risks and alternatives, in multiple languages was proposed as a possible digital solution. The vision was for animation-supported consent to become embedded routinely in the patient pathway, using an online platform to inform, empower and support shared decision-making before consent.

The trust launched a website that allowed patients to watch videos of their forthcoming procedure, in multiple languages, before consent. The animations described the procedure, its benefits, risks and alternatives.

Review of the initiative by the trust showed that the animations, in five languages, had been viewed over 8,000 times thereby saving about 660 hours of face-to-face explanation time. They had increased efficiency and standardised quality of information, meaning they had helped more than 50% of patients to understand the procedure. They were able to provide evidence that the project had led to reduced costs and enhanced patient experience. A win/win for staff, patients and the trust.

Millstream Surgery, Oxfordshire

This practice writes to every child when they reach 12 years of age, explaining how they can make appointments independently and confidentially, if necessary. At 16, all patients are given independent access to online appointment booking.

Mental Capacity Act (2005)

Perhaps the most important piece of legislation, or certainly the one most likely to impact on the most people, is the Mental Capacity Act (2005). The government publishes a Code of Practice and guidance, which can be found at www.gov.uk/government/publications/mental-capacity-act-code-of-practice and www.gov.uk/government/collections/mental-capacity-act-making-decisions

The full Act is available at www.legislation.gov.uk/ukpga/2005/9/section/1

The Mental Capacity Act (2005) came into force in England and Wales in 2007. The Act aims to empower and protect people who may not be able to make some decisions for themselves. It also allows people to plan ahead in case they are unable to make important decisions for themselves in the future.

It applies to anyone over 16 years of age who is unable to make decisions for themselves because of illness, injury or a disability, whether that be a permanent or temporary condition. It is applicable in all health and social care settings in England and Wales.

In Scotland it differs, with the Adults with Incapacity (Scotland) Act (2000), which sets out in law a range of options to help people aged 16 or over who lack the capacity to make some or all decisions for themselves. It allows other people to make decisions on their behalf.

There is no equivalent law in Northern Ireland at the moment, but the professional guidance from the General Medical Council and Nursing and Midwifery Councils apply.

Here are the key principles.

A person must be assumed to have capacity unless it is established that he lacks capacity

I remember my mother being admitted when she fractured her neck of femur and needed surgery. She was a 92-year-old who was deaf and had little vision; her sight was restricted to seeing blurry shades of grey. Many staff spoke to her with the assumption she also lacked capacity. Nothing could have been further from the truth. When she eventually became exasperated with people asking us what she'd like to drink, or whether we thought she was in pain, she said (quite loudly) while looking at me, "Tell that scruffy man in the green pyjamas that he is very rude and that if he has a question he might do better if he bothers to ask me." The consultant had the good grace to look slightly embarrassed and changed his practice. The assembled ward round giggled behind him.

How many hospitals insist on all people over 70 having a capacity assessment as part of their pre-operative assessment? They shouldn't routinely assess people, of course. The assumption is that people have capacity.

A person is not to be treated as unable to decide unless all practicable steps to help him to do so have been taken without success

Just as a person whose first language is Sylheti may need an interpreter, so a deaf person may need a BSL interpreter and a person with a learning disability might need Easy Read information or the support of a Makaton signer. My mother was perfectly able to make her own decisions if someone helped her put her hearing aids in, so that she could hear the question. Far more people can understand things if they are put in everyday language rather than jargon. Simple words are good for everyone. It might mean changing the time of asking the question, it might mean ensuring someone is pain free before asking something. It might just mean explaining something in a way that is familiar to the person.

If someone asked whether you wanted fish for tea, there would be a number of different views as to what this meant. My mother-in-law would think I was offering smoked salmon sandwiches and scones, someone else might think they were being asked whether the nanny was cooking the children fish pie for their early evening nursery meal, others might think it was a trip to the 'chippie' to get cod and a pea fritter.

It is the professional's job to help people understand. Many people being asked whether they have 'passed a motion' might be utterly confused and they might not be able to decide whether they needed 'anything to help'. It might be better to ask a younger child if they have done a poo or a rough sleeper whether they have crapped today.

I was reflecting on some examples of good practice and could only come up with a couple of specific examples where I have got it wrong – no consent per se and not in a health or social care setting but around ensuring I had provided the right support to enable people to understand. Both are children, but the situation makes the point well, I think.

Sonia

Sonia was a 14-year-old child who had a learning disability and language processing disorder. She had arrived at the residential special school I was working at because her father felt he was a little overprotective and wanted to allow her to broaden her horizons. He felt that, as a single father, there were activities he couldn't support Sonia to take part in. Sonia settled quickly and loved having female company; she liked dancing, swimming and choir, she started experimenting with make-up (not always successfully). Each weekend she ran to her father when he arrived to collect her and told him all about her week. She began to learn to cook, to sew, to do chores and became much more independent. It was a joy to see her growing into an increasingly confident and capable young woman. We thought we were doing really well as a team supporting this personal growth.

Over the summer term, I led a series of camps and residential trips so that many of the children could experience new things, try new activities and see the wider world. Younger ones started off camping in the school's extensive grounds, and the complexity and challenge grew for each year group. Sonia's housemother arranged for us to go to Jersey. She had good contacts and a very persuasive manner, which found us free accommodation and several meals out. Off we set in our yellow minibus for a fantastic few days in the Channel Islands. We did fun things, and everything went well with trips to the zoo, barbecues, a smart restaurant, giant cabbages and much more. The weather was glorious and so we decided to visit St Brelades Bay, which has the most beautiful, safe beach; it was crowded but we managed to find a suitable patch to mark out our territory as the girls started getting ready to swim, paddle or sunbathe.

We heard Rachael, another pupil, shriek, "Sonia, what the f**** are you doing?" Which rather caught our attention. On turning around, we saw a 14-year-old girl standing stark naked in the middle of a crowded beach attracting an excessive amount of unwanted attention. One of the staff members threw a picnic rug over her and helped her change without further exposure. We explained what the problem was, and the poor child just looked confused. The rest of the day passed without problem and we all settled down to enjoy jumping the waves.

Later, when the girls were getting ready for bed, we asked ourselves how it had happened, Sonia had been swimming several times a week at the school and occasionally at local leisure centres. What we came to realise was that when she was at school or at a leisure centre, we either used communal changing areas so we could supervise properly or help those who needed help, or we used individual cubicles in a changing village. In the communal area nobody was bothered about anyone else stripping off. It was entirely female and the girls all shared rooms. Sonia had arrived into a culture where everyone was comfortable with each other and adapted well to the freedom and body-confidence that offered. Had we been more thoughtful, had we understood and prepared her, she was perfectly capable of adapting behaviours to different settings, as long as she knew the rules.

We had failed her and compromised her dignity by not allowing her the opportunity to understand fully that there were different expectations in different settings.

Peter

Peter was also a teenager with speech and language processing difficulties, being educated in a different special school.

My children were young, and I was only doing the odd bit of part-time lecturing. This meant that, when my husband asked whether I'd consider teaching a few lessons, I was able to say yes. The school was finding it a challenge to recruit qualified teachers and they had Ofsted looming. I had adult teaching qualifications and could do a few useful things, so became a supply instructor. One of my key responsibilities was for teaching food technology, supported by an excellent teaching assistant.

The lesson was one of the first where I taught Peter. It was intended to start the children understanding about safety when cooking and this particular lesson was around the safe use of sharp knives. It was very simple, just preparing a fruit salad. The objective was, after all, to get the children to handle the knives safely and not about creating a showstopper.

I'd explained carefully, shown how to hold a knife, how to put a knife down away from the edge of the table, how to chop on a board, and then they were able to make their fruit salads under supervision. It was going really well, although the odd strawberry may not have made it into the bowls. We wandered among the dozen or so children, helping where necessary. As Peter was one of the more able pupils, he probably got less attention than those who found the physical task of holding a knife correctly, or remembering the instructions in the correct order, more challenging. I'd done pictorial instructions as a flow chart for everyone to follow and had laid out the process on a spare table so they could see what to do when.

When I did get around to Peter, I could see he had done really well and had a bowl of bright coloured berries and soft fruit. He'd made his own syrup, as an extension task for the more able children. I stood and chatted as he picked up a banana and began to slice it, as instructed. Once it was chopped and in with all the other fruit, he looked and me and asked, "When do I peel it, Miss?"

Clearly I hadn't paid sufficient attention because we then had to spend our afternoon break picking out slices of banana and doing the job with better instructions from me. Peter proudly handed over his creation to his housemother to have for his supper but was scathing of me, "Mrs Salt, didn't know you had to peel bananas".

Again, not consent, but an example where giving the right information and enabling someone capable of understanding the opportunity to do so would have allowed Peter to deliver a perfect outcome for himself.

A person is not to be treated as unable to decide merely because he makes an unwise decision

There are two pieces of legislation that can appear to conflict and which staff in health and social care services need to have a good working understanding of: the Care Act (2014) and the Mental Capacity Act (2005). The MCA code of practice offers guidance but unfortunately changes the wording used and is not the same as the Act itself.

The Code says: "People have the right to make decisions that others might think are unwise". Taken alone, this could leave staff thinking that people had an absolute right and that there should be no interference.

The second sentence clarifies it further: "A person who makes a decision that others think is unwise should not automatically be labelled as lacking the capacity to make a decision". That key word 'automatically' is critical when interpreting the guidance.

The Act is about protecting people who are unable to make decisions, whether wise or unwise. It is not about the right to make decisions more generally if someone has capacity. It provides guidance on recognising a possible lack of capacity and helps staff understand how they may decide for the person while remaining within the law.

Our right to make whatever decision we wish, provided it is not prohibited or otherwise legally overridden, is not given to us by the Mental Capacity Act (2005) but is a fundamental right for adults.

The Care Act (2014) sets out the powers and duties regarding care and support, with the general duty to promote well-being. For health and social care staff this can seemingly create a conflict with the staff not unreasonably wanting to protect people from harm and reduce risks. That's not a bad thing unless in so doing they remove people's rights to make their own informed decisions.

In healthcare settings, patients rarely disagree with the advice of the medical team; they may question a planned treatment and be given more information, but an outright refusal to be treated is rare. When it happens, the medical team may well think this calls into question their capacity to understand and retain information; after all, the medical team hold the expertise. What the medical team cannot have is the patient's knowledge of the things that are important to them and the factors that impact on their decisions. They can try to explore this and answer more questions or provide further information, but in the end the patient's right to make what they consider an unwise choice is paramount.

There is ample case law that shows the courts will uphold the right of people with capacity to make unwise decisions about their care or treatment. They are worth a read to gain a better understanding of how courts react to cases where capacity is disputed.

LB Hillingdon V Stephen Neary 2011 EWHC 1377

Stephen was a 21-year old man who had autism and severe learning disabilities. He needed ongoing care at all times and lived with his father.

When his father needed respite care, the Local Authority found a residential placement for Stephen for what Mr Neary believed would be a few days until his own health needs had been addressed. It resulted in a 12-month legal battle to allow Stephen to return home.

The court found that Stephen had been unlawfully deprived of his liberty.

CC v KK [2012] EWHC 2136 (COP)

KK was placed in a care home and restricted using a local authority Deprivation of Liberty Safeguards Standard Authorisation. KK was found to have mental capacity by the judge in the face of several professional views that she lacked capacity. When living at home, KK frequently became distressed when alone and used her care-line device to contact call centre staff for reassurance.

She appeared in court and convinced the judge of her understanding of the situation because she was clear about the possible consequences of a return home. Staff were criticised for assessing her mental capacity in relation to risks about a return home based on two opposing options – at home unsupported or in residential care.

The judge made it clear that KK should have been given information about the full range of alternatives, the risks and benefits of each, to enable them to make their decisions. The option of living at home with a full support package was not offered.

An act done, or decision made, under this Act for or on behalf of a person who lacks capacity must be done, or made, in his best interests

Where a person lacks capacity and there is no Lasting Power of Attorney, decisions must be made in the person's best interest. The decision and influencing factors should be recorded by the health and social care staff involved.

Lasting Power of Attorney

A Lasting Power of Attorney (LPA) is someone appointed and registered by the donor (the person the LPA is acting for) who can make decisions relating to the donor's health and care, if they lose capacity. Simply being next-of-kin does not mean someone can offer consent or make decisions on behalf of someone else. Health and social care staff accepting decisions and consent from someone who has accepted the LPA (often a family member) should ask to see the registration documents. If the LPA isn't registered with the Office of the Public Guardian while the donor retains capacity, then it is not valid.

An LPA for health and welfare can be used to make decisions on, for example, where the donor should live, their day-to-day care (for example, diet and dress), who the donor should have contact with, whether to give or refuse consent to medical treatment

Deputy

If someone lacks capacity and has not registered an LPA to act on their behalf, then a close relative, spouse or partner can apply to become a Deputy to the Court of Protection. If agreed, this confers the rights to make decisions and offer or withhold consent on behalf of the person it relates to.

The court will usually only appoint a personal welfare deputy if there's doubt as to whether decisions will be made in someone's best interests, if there is a family dispute about care, or if someone needs to be appointed to make decisions about a specific issue over time, for example where someone will live.

Without an LPA or Deputy, it falls to the involved professionals, in consultation with close family, spouses or partners, to decide in the best interests of that person. Case law examples show us how the courts consider capacity and the rights of people to self-determination.

Aintree University Hospitals NHS Foundation Trust (Respondent) v James (Appellant) [2013] UKSC 67

This case concerned how doctors and courts should decide when it is in the best interests of a patient, who lacks the capacity to decide for himself, to be given or not to be given life sustaining treatment.

After Mr James developed complications from a chronic lung problem, he was admitted to the critical care unit because he needed to be ventilated. In the following months he suffered some severe setbacks and his condition fluctuated. A deterioration in his neurological state meant he was thought to lack capacity to make decisions about his ongoing medical treatment. He did, however, seem to recognise his wife and family and his friends.

The trust applied to the Court of Protection for a declaration that it would be in the patient's best interests for certain treatments to be withheld in the event of a further deterioration. These were treatments such as cardiopulmonary resuscitation. The family took a different view from the clinicians, believing that, while they accepted that he would never recover his previous quality of life, they believed that he gained pleasure from his present quality of life and would wish it to continue.

The Mental Capacity Act Code of Practice suggests that it may occasionally be in the best interests of a patient not to give life-sustaining treatment "where treatment is futile, overly burdensome to the patient or where there is no prospect of recovery", even if this may result in the person's death.

The trial judge interpreted these words as inapplicable to treatments which would enable Mr James to resume a quality of life which he would regard as worthwhile: they did not have to return him to full health. Three months later, the ruling was overturned. Sadly, Mr James' condition had deteriorated further. The new declaration decided that futility was to be judged by the improvement or lack of improvement which the treatment would bring to the general health of the patient. It was ruled that 'recovery' meant recovery of a state of health which would avert an ever-present prospect of death.

The discussion around why the rulings were made says:

"The starting point is the strong presumption that it is in a person's best interests to stay alive.

In considering the best interests of a particular patient at a particular time, decision-makers must look at his welfare in the widest sense, not just medical but social and psychological; they must consider the nature of the medical treatment in question, what it involves and its prospects of success.

They must consider what the outcome of that treatment for the patient is likely to be; they must try and put themselves in the place of the individual patient and ask what his attitude is or would be likely to be; and they must consult others who are looking after him or interested in his welfare."

The Supreme Court Summary stated that, "The judge was right to consider whether the proposed treatments would be futile in the sense of being ineffective or being of no benefit to the patient. He was right to weigh the burdens of treatment against the benefits of a continued existence, and give great weight to Mr James' family life, which was 'of the closest and most meaningful kind'."

He was right to be cautious in circumstances which were fluctuating. A treatment may bring some benefit to a patient even if it has no effect upon the underlying disease or disability. It was not futile if it enabled a patient to resume a quality of life which the patient would regard as worthwhile.

Most of us will never be called upon to make such difficult decisions where the family disagree very strongly with the professional views, but all settings should consider and record how best interest decisions, such as imposing a Do Not Attempt Cardio-Pulmonary Resuscitation order on younger people with learning disabilities or not treating a potentially reversable condition in an elderly person, have been made.

Before the act is done, or the decision is made, regard must be had to whether the purpose for which it is needed can be as effectively achieved in a way that is less restrictive of the person's rights and freedom of action

I'm sure there are many examples of very good practice which will come to me later. I need to clear my head of one of the worst practices I have seen around least restrictive options, an example that we looked at earlier in the context of the Hellomynameis campaign. It was long before the Mental Capacity Act (2005) came into force and before the Care Quality Commission existed, but even at the time, it was pretty poor consideration of people's capacity to make decisions balanced with achieving the least restrictive option and maintaining people's safety.

The provider had three care homes that they called 'hotels for aged gentlefolk'. They were very clear that they weren't care homes despite accommodating people with complex care needs and many with quite advanced dementia. The provider assured us they only provided 'discreet care'. They were unable to define discreet care, but it became evident what they meant was unsafe or absent care, to maintain the notion that the person was coping just fine with hidden support.

Certainly, the provider often used the least restrictive option. They used to send a very confused resident out alone around the streets of Brighton with a little card in their pocket, so that he could be returned home easily when he got lost. Apparently, the local police often brought him back and had some concerns about his inability to crossroads safely, which the provider dismissed, claiming they did not understand older folk.

They handed out very smart umbrellas as walking aids, so the guests weren't embarrassed by having to use a walking frame. They didn't subject guests to intrusive assessments, or interventions, for skin integrity or nutritional status.

The unfortunate result of this lack of risk assessments was that one person was left sitting in the same domestic reclining chair for two years, as they were unable to sleep in the single divan that was offered in place of an adjustable bed. They were unable to transfer to another chair or to leave the room as they were too heavy for staff to lift and the guest house didn't believe in hoists.

They came to our attention because the local hospital had informed us that a resident had fallen and impaled their eye on something, necessitating surgical removal of their eye.

Clearly, this isn't what the Act intends. It is not a carte blanche to avoid any protective restrictions. It is about allowing people to have the maximum control they can within the limits of their capacity at the time and balancing their rights to make as many of the decisions that impact upon them against other risks.

Deprivation of Liberty Safeguards

Sometimes, caring for a person who lacks capacity to make important decisions for themselves involves reducing their independence or restricting their freedoms. Those people living or being cared for in a hospital or care home, may have their routine and everyday choices decided for them, and they may not be allowed to leave.

In some cases, this may amount to a 'deprivation of liberty'. This is not always a bad thing; sometimes it is essential to ensure the person remains safe, but it should only happen if it is in the person's best interests. It is not acceptable to restrict someone's liberty because it is easier for staff, or because someone wants to do something others think isn't a good idea.

The Mental Capacity Act (2005) includes the Deprivation of Liberty Safeguards (DoLS) – a set of checks that aims to make sure that any care or environment that restricts a person's freedoms is both appropriate and in their best interests. If a care home or hospital plans to deprive a person of their liberty, they must get permission. To do this, they must follow strict processes called the Deprivation of Liberty Safeguards, which are usually managed by the local authority.

By far the highest number of applications for authorisations under the Deprivation of Liberty Safeguards are made by care homes, but that doesn't mean that they are irrelevant for other services. The Deprivation of Liberty Safeguards framework applies to care homes and hospitals in England and Wales, and not to other settings.

A Deprivation of Liberty does not just mean a locked door. It is normal for services to lock external doors as a security measure; telling someone they are not permitted to go outside, however, is likely to be a deprivation of their liberty. Most people with dementia living in care homes and hospitals will receive care that falls under the definition of a Deprivation of Liberty and that isn't about poor care; it's about providing safe care while ensuring their right to make decisions are maintained, as far as possible.

In care homes, staff and providers may want to consider whether they offer maximum freedom and support people's liberty. They need to be able to demonstrate that the correct processes have been followed where they have decided to deprive somebody of their liberty. The following should be given consideration.

Being continuously supervised and controlled

If people are subject to continuous close supervision and control, it may well be considered a deprivation of their liberty. Staff in care homes and hospitals need to provide ongoing observation and may have established routines around mealtimes. The time lights are dimmed, or the time people are made to get up in the morning. It may constitute a deprivation of their liberty of they have not consented to one-to-one supervision while on a hospital ward or in a care home. Hopefully the days of care home residents being up, dressed and having breakfast before the night staff have finished their shift are long past, and enforcing such a regime would clearly be depriving someone of the choice to stay in bed and sleep because they'd had a disturbed night.

Continuous surveillance and control might include the use of technology such as sensors or CCTV to protect people. While this might well offer physical protection, it might also deprive them of their liberty. This could apply to pressure sensors or bedrails, where someone is unable to get out of bed or stand up and walk around safely. If someone has capacity to understand they might fall or they have designated someone to have lasting power of attorney, then consent should be sought for using technology that might be considered as constraining them.

Not being free to leave

If a person is not free to leave the home, ward, hospital or unit where they are being cared for then they may be deprived of their liberty. Even if they haven't asked to leave (but the answer would be no if they did) then they are being deprived of their liberty. It generally applies to people who lack capacity but can also be used as a control measure for others who have capacity. A day surgical unit that asks everyone on the list to arrive by 7am and then expects them to change into a gown and dressing gown and to sit around for five or more hours watching daytime television isn't depriving anyone of their liberty unless they say, when asked, "No, you aren't allowed to go off the unit, sorry". Then you probably are depriving someone of their liberty. Better to give them the correct information, explain that they are second on the list and may be going to theatre in the next hour, or to say, "Yes do, we have a pager that you can take so we can contact you if you need to come back before midday".

If it's an elderly person in a care home who wants to go for a walk, unless you have applied for, or have, an authorised Deprivation of Liberty Safeguards, you are breaching the legislation if you stop them. Similarly, a blanket rule that residents must have an escort to go out into the community or may only go on planned activities, is a restriction that is not permissible if a person with capacity has neither given consent or a Deprivation of Liberty safeguard has not been considered for someone without capacity. People with capacity are entitled to come and go as they please, to spend all their savings on taxi fares to go to the station and watch trains and to eat six ice creams a day, if that is what they want to do. If staff believe that they are not able to make that decision safely (as opposed to wisely), they need to make a best interest decision in consultation with the person and their family and apply for a Deprivation of Liberty Safeguards authorisation.

Providers and staff need to be mindful that some families are very protective, very risk averse, and may want to restrict a much-loved family member's liberty because they don't want them to make potentially unwise choices. The family view cannot ever overrule the rights of a person who has capacity or who can be supported to make their own decisions. Two daughters may feel their mum is far too wobbly on her feet and might fall if she walks out to buy her own knitting supplies, but if their mother wants to do it, they have no right to stop her. They can provide as much wool and knitting patterns as they like, they can negotiate with her and tell her their anxieties, but they cannot legally stop her and any staff listening to the family, rather than their resident, is making a very unwise decision.

Restricted opportunities for access to fresh air and activities

This may be considered a deprivation of someone's liberty – even if it is due to staff shortages.

As an aside, it can also mean an increased risk of vitamin D deficiency, which brings its own problems. Supplements may address the vitamin deficiency but won't address the loss of liberty. Being outdoors is significant benefit in maintaining good mental and physical health. It is sad that so many people living in residential accommodation rarely feel the wind in their hair or the rain on their faces. They lose touch with the seasons and their world contracts further. It's much sadder if this is because someone else feels the outdoors is a dangerous place, with too many risks to manage.

One of my greatest pleasures is year-round swimming outdoors, preferably in rivers or the sea. I am well-padded, so the cold isn't a huge issue and we don't use wetsuits, although my husband has invested in neoprene gloves for winter dips. I'm now too old to worry about what others think, which brings a new freedom that I would be loath to lose. Over the years we have very happy memories of shrieking and giggling like teenagers when plunging into the River Dart, the pools at the end of the Newlands Valley or crashing into waves in Ventnor. I can't imagine a time when it would no longer be appropriate, but I can imagine a time when my children might think they knew better and try to limit us. They will do so not because they want to make us unhappy, but because they want us to be immortal, to stay safe, to be protected. Meanwhile, we would very much like to live until we die and not sit in the corner watching television programmes that are not of our choosing. We shall swim as long as we can drive or walk to a beach or river.

I know this is likely to happen as I regularly chat with an 87-year-old woman who swims in the sea every day, come wind, sun, rain or snow. Her daughter is also a keen swimmer but has concerns about her mother being on her own when she swims and about her falling on the slippery rocks that she walks over to reach the sea. Her mother has not yet succumbed to the pressure to stop and has no intention of doing so just yet. The daughter recognises her mother has a right to live her life as she wishes and she accepts there may be some degree of risk which her mother is prepared to accept. The Deprivation of Liberty Safeguards doesn't apply as she remains in her own home, but the idea that we should be supported to make our own decisions, as far as is possible, is valid in all settings. This silver haired woman's insistence that she wants to take the risk affords her social contact, improved physical and mental health, and makes her a much-respected and visible part of her local community.

Elizabeth and Phillip

Our local 'village elders', who live in the next village to us, walk across the Downs each day. This helps them maintain core stability, muscle tone, cardiopulmonary capacity and mental health. The two nonagenarians do a three-mile, circular walk in all weathers and throughout the year. Sometimes chatting happily to each other and sometimes scowling at each other, as they walk ten feet apart. Phillip is a little forgetful but can make polite conversation about most subjects. The family are concerned about their well-being and ability to continue to live in a rambling and isolated, Victorian farmhouse with an oil-fuelled Aga and open fires.

The family want them to move to a smaller property in Bristol, near where they live. They tell them they can walk in the park and it will be easier to get to the shops, and that they'll be able to see their grandchildren more often.

Phillip is unwilling to move and loves the Downs. He wants to be near his friends and to sail on a neighbour's boat, sometimes. He wants to grow raspberries and cucumbers, as he has always done. He doesn't want to be dependent (although that time is perhaps approaching). He certainly doesn't want to live in a city flat without a garden. Elizabeth might be easier to persuade, but she has friends locally and likes her yoga class, where everyone is over 70. She enjoys painting in the garden and watching the nesting birds. She looks forward to church on Sundays with coffee afterwards, in a tiny Saxon church, where the entire congregation could fit into a minibus and where coffee is served with or without powdered milk.

They have adapted as they have aged. They have sold their own yacht and Phillip now only goes to sea as a guest. They have a freezer full of ready meals that just need warming up. They have employed cleaners and a gardener to mow the lawns. They aren't yet ready to compromise further, but it is clear that decision-making is getting more challenging and they are feeling pressurised into doing something neither of them wants. They love their children and don't want to upset them. The children love their parents and want to keep them safe.

I rather suspect that if they were given options and helped to come to an agreement, it might be much easier for all concerned, but it is not our place to become overly involved. I can drop round scones to have with a cup of tea in the garden, I can take them fish and chips occasionally, but the decisions and discussions are between them and their families at this point. Perhaps if a bungalow in the nearby harbourside village was suggested rather than a move to a big city, they might admit that caring for a seven-bedroomed house set in an acre of garden was getting a bit much. Perhaps if a daily housekeeper was suggested, with a promise of more time to paint or garden, they might accept it as something helpful. I suspect there are middle paths – which everyone would be fairly happy with and which Elizabeth and Phillip could be persuaded to consent to. They could still go to yoga and sailing. They could have a garden. They could have a 'daily'. They could be supported to make their own decision that the time had come to accept more help.

Of course, they are not subject to Deprivation of Liberty Safeguards, but the principles of the Mental Capacity Act still apply and they shouldn't be forced to move against their will.

The key messages I would want to offer are:

■ People may be helped to make what others consider 'sensible' decisions, with some compromise and options that are not entirely binary. Life is rarely black and white.

■ Pressurising someone to consent rather negates the idea of consent.

Mental Health Act (1983)

An adult may be detained in a hospital if that person has one of the mental disorders listed in Mental Health Act (1983). Both psychiatric hospitals and most acute hospitals are registered to detain people under the Act. Detention should not be the first choice; it is a significant reduction in someone's liberty. Doctors and Approved Mental Health Professionals must always think about alternatives that do not involve the person being held in hospital.

People can be detained if:

■ They are suffering from a mental disorder that requires medical treatment in hospital.

■ They need to be in hospital for their own health and safety or to protect other people.

■ The medical treatment that they need is only available in the hospital.

Before someone can be detained there needs to be an assessment. An application to detain someone against their will must be made by a doctor, nurse or social worker specialising in mental illness. An application for detention can also be made by the person's closest relative. In addition, two doctors must confirm in writing that the detention is valid.

Someone who lacks capacity to consent to remain in hospital may be treated as an informal (voluntary) patient but only if their care does not deprive them of their liberty. Someone wanting to leave who is at risk of harm or who is a risk to others must either be detained under the Mental Health Act (1983) or an application must be made for a Deprivation of Liberty Safeguards approval.

The Mental Health Act Code of Practice says that a threat of detention must not be used to force someone into hospital as an informal patient. If someone is thought to need hospital treatment and is not wanting to consent, they retain the right to refuse admission unless they are sufficiently unwell to be detained under the Mental Health Act (often referred to as sectioned). Consent obtained through coercion or threat of sanction is not valid consent.

Imagine a patient who is staying on a voluntary basis at a specialist unit for people with eating disorders doesn't want to join in with art therapy. It would be entirely wrong to suggest that if they didn't participate they risked being sectioned. Detention is not about compliance with treatment. If someone lacks capacity for whatever reason, then the Mental Capacity Act (2005) should be used, where appropriate. Just disagreeing with the need for admission is not proof of a lack of capacity.

Where someone is assessed as lacking capacity to consent to hospital treatment, the least restrictive option should be used, in line with the Mental Capacity Act (2005).

In 2018-19, 49,988 new detentions under the Mental Health Act were recorded; the actual figure is likely to be higher as some providers didn't submit data. The demographics make for interesting discussion and show significant differences between different groups. For example, the rates of detention for 'black or black British' people were over four times those of the white people. Community treatment orders for males were higher than the rate for females. Individual practitioners and services might want to reflect on their own rates of detention and whether there is equity across various demographic groups.

Patients detained under the Mental Health Act (1983), unsurprisingly, have rights built into the Act. There are strict limits on the length of time they can be detained. The duration of the permissible detention depends on which section of the Act is used:

- Under Section 2, the person is admitted for an assessment and necessary treatment. They can be detained up to 28 days.
- Under Section 3, the person is admitted for immediate treatment and can be detained for up to six months.
- Under Section 4, the person may be admitted as an emergency and detained for up to 72 hours.

Patients held under the Mental Health Act (1983) can ask for a review of the situation by another doctor to decide whether the detention is appropriate. They can also appeal to an independent mental health review tribunal to assess whether they should be kept in hospital.

The police also have powers under the Mental Health Act. Section 136 of the Act allows the police to take someone to a place of safety or keep them in a place of safety. It is most often used in public places to remove someone who is behaving in a way that suggests they are at serious risk of harming themselves or others.

It can't be used to remove someone from their home. They must discuss the situation with a healthcare professional before acting.

R v. Canons Park Mental Health Review Tribunal, Ex Parte A

England's High Court of Justice, Queen's Bench Division, rejected the decision of a mental health tribunal to detain an involuntary patient for treatment. Her refusal of treatment basically made her untreatable and negated the legal ground for commitment.

The patient had been detained in a psychiatric hospital for depression with an impulsive personality. About seven months later, she applied to be released.

Before the tribunal ruling, her condition was reclassified to 'psychopathic disorder'. The law entitles those patients classified as psychopaths or mentally impaired, but not those patients classified as mentally ill or severely mentally impaired, to be released from involuntary commitment unless a criminal offense is committed.

The court determined that under the provisions of the Mental Health Act (1983) and the European Human Rights Convention, the tribunal ruled that the patient was entitled to be released.

The key message is that under the Act there are situations where people's liberty may be restricted lawfully, and people may be treated without consent. There are protective measures built into the Act, but individual healthcare professionals and provider organisations have a responsibility to ensure that the person's rights are upheld, and any restrictions are minimised as far as is possible.

The Mental Health Act (1983) Code of Practice and children]

There are numerous pieces of legislation that impact on the care of children with mental health problems. In addition to the Mental Health Act (1983), health and social care workers with responsibility for the care of children and those in hospital should be conversant with other relevant legislation. Healthcare professionals in other settings should also be aware of the wider legislative framework.

The pertinent other pieces of legislation include the Children Acts (1989) and (2004), the Mental Capacity Act (2005) for those over 16 years of age and the Human Rights Act (1998). They should also be aware of the United Nations Convention on the Rights of the Child.

That's quite a big ask, and while they should understand the principles and key messages, I am not suggesting they need to be able to quote the legislation verbatim.

The best interests of the child or young person must always be a significant consideration. This is enshrined in law: Section 1 of the Children Act (CA) sets out three general principles, the first of which is the paramountcy principle that states very simply that the welfare of the child is paramount.

The law about admission to hospital and treatment for mental health problems of children aged 16 and 17 differs from that of children under 16. In both cases, whether they are competent or have capacity to make decisions about any admission is an essential consideration. Children who are competent or have capacity can be admitted to hospital for treatment for mental health problems as a voluntary patient if they offer their consent. Parental consent is not necessary (although the active involvement of parents should be encouraged).

Where a child is not competent or lacks capacity, then the consent of someone with Parental Responsibility may be accepted and the child accommodated as an informal patient. In cases where a child cannot be admitted informally and the criteria for detention under the Mental Health Act are not met, the High Court may authorise the admission by way of a section 8 order under the Children Act (1989). Whether the court is prepared to assist will depend on the facts of the particular case.

Consent by children

Aside from the Mental Health Act and consideration of detention, particular consideration is required when anyone is seeking consent for the medical treatment of a child. The professional bodies offer advice but there are complexities that each provider and each healthcare professional should understand.

Whether a child has capacity to consent depends on the individual's ability to understand and weigh up options, and to consider risks and benefits and longer-term consequences. At 16, a child can be usually be presumed to have the capacity to consent to medical treatment. A child under 16 may have the capacity to consent, depending on their ability to understand what is involved. Wherever possible, a child under 16 should be encouraged to involve their parents in making decisions about care and treatment. That's usually pretty straightforward in a child attending an independent hospital to have their tonsils removed. It's a bit more complicated in some other types of services.

If a child under 16 is to be offered treatment then the healthcare professional providing the treatment must assess whether the child is capable of understanding what they are agreeing to or refusing, with regard to the complexity of the decision being made. A child who has the capacity to consent to something simple, like stitches in a bad cut, may not necessarily have the capacity to consent to more complex treatment which may have a long-lasting impact.

If a child lacks the ability to consent, then parental consent should be obtained and a decision should be made in the best interest of the child.

Where a child does have capacity, they should be encouraged to involve their parent's in the decision-making process. The child's decision should usually be respected but it might be best practice to involve others such as an independent advocate or a named or designated doctor or nurse, if their involvement would help children make their decision.

In most of the UK, the position when a child refuses treatment that the parents or doctors feel is in their best interest is very complex. The professional body advice is to seek legal support on the individual circumstances.

Gillick v West Norfolk & Wisbeck Area Health Authority

This landmark case saw Victoria Gillick, a mother with five daughters under the age of 16, seek a declaration that it would be unlawful for a doctor to prescribe contraceptives to girls under 16 without the knowledge or consent of their parent. As a result, the term 'Gillick Competence' is widely used to describe a child under 16 years of age who has been assessed as competent to give consent to the medical treatment being offered.

In 1983 the judgement from this case laid out the criteria for establishing whether a child under 16 has the capacity to consent to treatment. It was determined that children under 16 can consent if they have sufficient understanding and intelligence to fully understand what is involved in a proposed treatment, including its purpose, nature, likely effects and risks, chances of success and the availability of other options. If a child passes the Gillick test, he or she is considered 'Gillick competent' to consent to that medical treatment or intervention. A child may have the capacity to consent to some treatments but not others. The understanding required for different interventions will vary, and capacity can sometimes vary, if a child is very unwell or has certain mental health conditions. Each individual decision requires assessment of Gillick competence. Best practice would be that this assessment is recorded along with the measures taken to encourage the child to inform their parent.

The Fraser guidelines were sanctioned by the House of Lords following the ruling in the Gillick case. They were originally only related to the prescription of contraception but, since a case in 2006, they are now applicable to all sexual health services including termination of pregnancy. The House of Lords sanctioned the provision of sexual health advice and treatment for a child under 16 years of age, as long as:

- He/she has sufficient maturity and intelligence to understand the nature and implications of the proposed treatment.
- He/she cannot be persuaded to tell her parents or to allow the doctor to tell them.
- He/she is very likely to begin or continue having sexual intercourse with or without contraceptive treatment.
- His/her physical or mental health is likely to suffer unless he/she received the advice or treatment.
- The advice or treatment is in the young person's best interests.

The Tavistock and Portman NHS Foundation Trust

This trust offers a range of mental health assessments and treatments to patients and, by their very nature, a patient's active participation is vital to the process. It recognises that consent is a fundamental principle of the work of the trust.

The trust consent policy and guidance goes beyond the level offered by most services and shows an understanding of their patients and the need for gaining consent prior to commencing treatment. Much of their work would not be feasible if the patient did not want to participate.

They have developed an Opt-In policy for assessment of young people over 16 years of age which states:

"It is the trust's usual practice to write to young people, who have not self-referred, asking them to opt-In and confirm that they would like to be seen here. The Adolescent Department then gives a deadline of one week for the young person to make contact. If no response is received after the first week, a reminder letter is sent with a copy to the referrer and a further week given to await contact.

"To minimise the waiting time, the young person has a choice of contacting the Adolescent Department, Referrals Coordinator by telephone or by returning the Opt-In form which is enclosed with the original letter and prompt letters. If there is no further response after the second letter, the case is closed on the system and the referrer is written to advising them of the outcome."

This is very clear as to how they ensure that children between 16 and 18 years of age are consenting with an option to refuse treatment.

They also offer clarity on a child's right to consent:

"For children under 16, under the law clinicians may assess patients and determine whether they have sufficient understanding of what is to be offered, both its risks and benefits, and alternatives to treatment, and if a patient has sufficient understanding then they can consent to treatment.

For under 16s who are deemed competent, it is recommended practice in the Adolescent Directorate for parents of children under 16 to be seen at least once during the course of assessment. This is usually discussed with the young person."

The full professional guidance is considered with an active encouragement about parental involvement for each child.

The service ensures that consent from children is only accepted after an assessment of their competence, in line with the professional guidance on seeking consent from children:

"Judgments about competence can only be made on a case-by-case basis. As Rutter (1999) points out '…there is no universally acceptable level of competence that applies to an individual child. Rather, the question is of a child's competence in a particular context, for a particular type of decision, given particular circumstances'. When there is genuine doubt over competence it may be useful to get a second clinical opinion (something that is always required where Section 58 of the Mental Health Act 1983 pertains). In any event, clinicians must make a full record of the basis for any judgment about competence. The criteria are derived from Re C and it will be important to indicate whether the young person was not competent because he or she: 'is unable to take in and retain the information material to the decision especially as to the likely consequences of having, or not having treatment'; or 'is unable to believe the information'; or 'is unable to weigh the information in the balance as part of a process of arriving at the decision'. (Chapter 15 of the Mental Health Act 1983 Code of Practice 1999)."

I wonder how many services working with children are as proactive in ensuring compliance with the full guidance around consent by children under 16. If you see children, do you record the basis on which you have decided that they are competent to consent?

Are they caring?

Key messages

- A compassionate culture is essential to improving and sustaining performance across organisations.
- Compassion is not an optional 'add-on'; it is a requirement of professional and regulatory standards.
- Compassion and kindness are about responding to personal preferences rather than imposing one's own view of what caring means.
- Feedback is a vital tool to build a caring culture.
- You cannot care for people using services if you are not kind and compassionate towards your staff and each other.

"I have come to realise more and more that the greatest disease and the greatest suffering is to be unwanted, unloved, uncared for, to be shunned by everybody, to be just nobody."

(St Teresa of Calcutta)

> From the Care Quality Commission key lines of enquiry, prompts and ratings characteristics for healthcare services:
>
> "By caring, we mean that the service involves and treats people with compassion, kindness, dignity and respect."

My understanding is that the word 'care' has multiple sources but has a strong connection to the Latin words 'cura', meaning pains, concern, treatment and charge, and the word 'curo', meaning manage, trouble, take care, pay attention. In Old English it is close to the word 'carian' meaning to be anxious or solicitous, to grieve, feel concern or interest. The world over and throughout history, caring has been an important word which has varied little in meaning.

Caring is not an optional extra, it is the foundation on which health and social care is based. The Code for Nurses and Midwives starts out by setting a standard that registrants will treat people with kindness, respect and compassion. The General Medical Council guidance, *Good Medical Practice*, states that good doctors work in partnership with patients and respect their rights to privacy and dignity. They treat each patient as an individual. The Code of Conduct for Healthcare Support Workers and Adult Social Care Workers in England requires care workers to promote and uphold the privacy, dignity, rights, health and well-being of people who use health and care services and their carers.

I make no apologies for the length of this section; it is absolutely vital to get it right and while all the key questions (or 'domains', in CQC-speak) are weighted equally when aggregating ratings, without having a truly kind and compassionate service it will be very difficult to achieve high ratings in other areas.

Caring is often the domain of the regulatory framework that is perceived as the best understood and the area that staff feel is a real strength. It is also the domain where it is hardest to provide evidence and to pin down exactly what it is that makes a member of staff, a team, or a service, exceptional. We all think we know what caring means but ask staff to describe why they think they are exceptional, and the answers are often woolly at best. I cannot quantify how often I have asked the question about what makes them believe they are providing outstanding care or what makes them special. All too often staff (including quite senior staff) will say things like, "We are just a really nice team", "Everyone is really kind", "Oh, we're lovely. We all work together and get along really well". That's good, but it's hardly aspirational or particularly moving.

In order to build on the vague claims of niceness and grow it towards genuine caring and compassion for all, it is fairly essential for the individuals, teams and leaders, to reflect on where their experiences were founded and what they understand caring and compassion to look like. It can vary a surprising amount in practice. It isn't about imposing one's own view of kindness onto others.

True compassion comes from an underpinning respect and recognition that we are all equal and that individuals have a right to want or need something different to others. Corporate expectations of 'niceness' and caring can never be truly outstanding because it is just that – corporate. Truly exceptional care has to be based on the needs and wishes of individuals. It is also about the response of individual staff members who are sufficiently confident in the culture to step outside the norms. It is personal and responsive. It recognises and is comfortable with difference. It never imposes.

It is almost impossible for providers to be rated as 'Outstanding' for caring if they are not building a culture of kindness, tolerance and compassion towards their staff and each other.

One only needs to read any of the volumes of the Francis Report, published in early 2013, in response to serious and long-standing concerns with the Mid Staffordshire NHS Foundation Trust to see that had building a caring and empowered culture taken precedence over the control of targets, asset stripping and redundancies, then the very sad report might never had needed writing. Had the trust focused on building positivity, compassion and a shared responsibility among its staff groups, then patient care would almost undoubtedly have been much better. One of the key themes that was identified as part of the report section on culture was that:

"Aspects of a negative culture have emerged at all levels of the NHS system. These included:

- a lack of consideration of risks to patients, defensiveness, looking inwards not outwards
- secrecy, misplaced assumptions of trust, acceptance of poor standards and, above all, a failure to put the patient first in everything done.
- The emergence of such attitudes in otherwise caring and conscientious people may be a mechanism to cope with immense difficulties and challenges thrown up by their working lives."

As early as 2001/2002, the NHS staff survey results for the trust showed that staff felt that the target driven culture and control of finance took precedence over staff morale. The Barry Report in August 2005 reported an aggressive, inappropriate and inefficient management style that reflected a systems failure. In May and July 2006, the trust had asked for £1m pounds to support staff redundancies.

By 2008 the trust was in the lowest (worst) 20% for the national inpatient survey and the Healthcare Commission had written to the board with concerns about basic nursing care.

With a culture that suspended staff for raising concerns, where there was a lack of support from managers and an executive that didn't mention staff well-being or patient care as a priority, is it any wonder that staff felt demoralised and demotivated? The impact is very well known, sadly. Had the focus been on supporting the staff, building trust, recognising and rewarding good practice and creating shared responsibility, would the outcomes have been different? I rather suspect so.

Following the Winterbourne View scandal, Steve Scown, the Chief Executive of Dimensions, an organisation which provides care for people with learning disabilities and autism, including challenging behaviour and complex needs, writing in *The Guardian* said:

"Many care workers supporting vulnerable people have been in the sector for a long time. But things have changed. We are working hard to transform our whole organisation to deliver personalised support that gives the people being supported choice and control over that support.

We recognise and reward good practice and measure performance against our values. These include having ambition for the people we support and working in partnership with them and their families and having the courage to do the right thing in the face of adversity."

He recognised that the culture of the organisation and the way staff are trained and supported is key to how services are provided.

I think now is a good time to share my experiences of being cared for, which demonstrate well the difference between genuinely caring and emotionally intelligent staff, who went the extra mile, and one who thought (incorrectly) that they were compassion personified and perfected. Reflecting on these linked personal experiences helped me understand and define excellence in caring. Far from being the regulator's voice, these are a patient's voice.

Many years ago I 'found a lump'. I knew immediately that it was almost definitely a breast cancer and would have been surprised if I had been told it was anything else. I was referred to a one-stop clinic and seen by a consultant who initially told me not to worry as there were hundreds of possible causes for lumps and most were benign. I know this was meant to be reassuring but clearly when I was sent from there for a core biopsy the likelihood of a cancer increased. I was left wondering how experienced this consultant was if they didn't have a rather good idea – given that I knew myself.

One returns in the afternoon for a discussion about next steps and initial diagnosis – my understanding was confirmed when everyone else at the clinic went in ahead of me and had a five-minute slot. Eventually I was called back into the room to see a consultant who had a Macmillan breast care nurse specialist with her. They had their soft and kind faces on, but to say I was unreceptive to this approach was an understatement. The surgeon told me that she'd known at once what it was – at least that bit was reassuring about her knowledge base. When they asked whether I had any questions I asked why I had been lied to and mentioned that I was considering changing hospitals because I wanted a team I could trust and who were prepared to be a partner in care, rather than treat me like a child. The entire day had felt dishonest. I probably wasn't, in truth, being particularly objective or considering their perspective of wanting to be gentle in the breaking of bad news. At one point the surgeon had to leave the room while the clinical nurse specialist looked awkwardly at me before fetching them back to arrange a follow-up appointment. I left feeling more upset about the earlier dishonesty than the idea of surgery.

You're probably thinking this is an example of staff who felt they were being caring and got it wrong. Far from it.

The next appointment transformed my opinion. I was expecting a frostiness and distant but competent care. I got an apology, an explanation that on reflection they had understood my point and that they understood that not everyone wants a head on one side and a touch of the forearm. I was even more impressed when the surgeon opened their notebook and handed me some printouts of the prognostic indicator tool used to determine the preferred treatment plan and comparative survival outcomes, the minutes of the MDT and a research article on wide local excision (lumpectomy) and axillary clearance compared to mastectomy. She had my attention, my respect and my co-operation at this point. That process of reflection and considering things from the patient's perspective had resulted in a definite improvement in how I experienced care.

She went on to prove her exceptional surgical skills as well as her ability to learn and adapt, to put the needs of the patient first. On the day of surgery, she'd told me to bring my lowest cut bra and was careful to make sure the scar was in the right direction to be covered by it. I was woken from surgery by her shaking my big toe to rouse me sufficiently to tell me the details of the procedure. A few weeks later she came in early following a phone call, with no prior appointment, just so I could see her about a new second lump, before I started chemotherapy.

The excellent breast care nurse also adapted her approach and became far more pragmatic – which I genuinely appreciated. On my move from recovery to the ward I was placed in a bay opposite a patient who was both incredibly nosey and incredibly insensitive. In hindsight, it was quite funny but at the time I was less tolerant. This other patient came behind the curtains as I was getting changed from a gown into my own clothes. She told me not to worry she had seen it all before. She then said, "Cancer, is it?" I made a non-committal grunt and asked her to leave. She ignored me, sat on my bed and said, "It's terribly sad that Jade Goody dying of cancer, isn't it? She was no age at all". I conceded it was indeed sad but pointed out it was cervical cancer rather than breast cancer and that nowadays most women survive breast cancer, thankfully. To this day I ask myself why I engaged with her. She barely caught her breath before telling me, "That woman in the South Pole, she died from breast cancer, didn't she and she was a doctor… And Wendy Richards off 'Are you being served?' She had a really long and painful battle before she died, didn't she?"

My husband rang the breast care nurse specialist who swung into action, arrived on the ward, packed up my belongings and moved me to a single room immediately. She was sensible enough to take the risk and discuss my situation with my husband rather than telling him that she could only do something if I raised concerns personally. I shall be forever grateful to her.

Luckily, I remember more about Roger Federer taking the world Grand Slam record with his 15th title than my post-operative recovery. That is in no small part to a Ghanaian night nurse called Sisi. I was struggling a little with nausea and the heat – it was an extremely hot July. The hospital had kept the short stay ward open and there were very few patients over the weekend. On her second night Sisi brought me some homemade African ginger cake, which she claimed was a miracle cure for sickness. I'm not sure whether it was that or the anti-emetics, but something worked. As another powerful example of caring she somehow managed to chill the sheets. She arrived each evening with clean sheets that had been put in a plastic bag in a fridge somewhere. She also found ice cubes and filled a hot water bottle with iced water and crushed ice. The bed after she'd made it was heavenly. Unforgettable. Not expensive – ice is cheap, after all, but it made a huge difference.

These were truly compassionate staff who put the patient first, who were confident enough in themselves and their organisation to step outside of usual practice and who were willing to reflect, adapt and learn.

Opposing this comes the story of someone who thought they knew how to be a caring professional. I have told it with a degree of amusement at supper parties ever since.

Shortly after I had finished chemotherapy and radiotherapy, I needed to have a routine blood test unconnected to the cancer treatment. For convenience, I went to a local community hospital that had a phlebotomy clinic. It was pouring down and when I entered the reception area the place was deserted. I saw a couple of chairs with hideous crocheted cushions, so moved one and awaited some sign that the building was in use. About 15 minutes later, a woman in a white coat appeared and said, "Where's your form?" I passed her the blood test request form, which she scrutinised before telling me I was sitting in the wrong place, was dripping water on the floor and shouldn't have moved the cushions. In my best compliant patient mode, I moved to the seat she was pointing to only to be told off again. Apparently, it was too late to sit down as she would take my blood before even having a cup of coffee to get herself going.

I followed her into a room of curling laminated posters and overfilled shelves. "Sit down, Treessa, and roll up your arm, sweetheart," she said. I tried to explain it was Mrs. Salt or Terri, but she explained very clearly that Terri was a boy's name and she much preferred Treessa. I tried to say my name, even in full, was never Treessa, but she wasn't having any of it. She was even more upset about my choice of arm.

"Not that one," she barked. I explained that I had no lymph nodes on the right arm, and it is better to use the left. "I'll decide which vein to use," she said, "It's nonsense about lymph nodes and infections, they're all over your body, so it doesn't matter if some have been removed". I was quite insistent, and she clearly thought I was just being difficult. She poked around trying to find a usable vein with limited success so took a breather to chat to me while tapping my elbow crease furiously.

"Breast cancer is it?" she said. I was a bit bemused as although this diagnosis was on the form, it was entirely irrelevant to the tests that I was there for. I made a non-committal grunt, as is my want when I don't want to engage but don't want a battle. She then went on to say in her most empathetic, head-tilted and reassuring voice, "You can't tell which one is the falsie you know". I explained that they were, in fact, both my own but regardless, that wasn't what I was here to discuss. She wouldn't let go and became more and more offensive while thinking she was being kind and reassuring. "It's so good these days you can get ones you can swim in and everything… Did all your hair come out then? That's hard, isn't it? Did you have it all cut off for the Little Princess Trust? Some people fight so bravely…" On and on she went. Her voice got more and more patronising with a "Bless you, poppet" after every sentence.

I said I wouldn't have a plaster thank you, as I was allergic to them, but she insisted that despite them bringing me out in a blistering rash, she knew best and was the professional here. She stuck a plaster on and that is the point I finally exploded and told her that my opinion of her was not especially high, explaining with barely suppressed rage, that I had found her anything but professional. She simply didn't understand. She looked hurt momentarily, put her head on one side, nodded slowly then grabbed my hand, stroked it and said, "I'd be angry too, if I had cancer, Treesa. Bless you, Poppet".

I'm sure she thought she was being compassionate and supportive but failed to understand being genuinely kind is not imposing your own view of compassion on others.

Evidence and growing kindness

As mentioned already, most of us know what kindness looks like but sometimes it's hard to put it into words (or to evidence in CQC-speak). In the chapter on evidence or opinion, I talk about the 'Book of Good' introduced by Sussex Community NHS Foundation Trust. I know several other organisations have used a similar cheap and effective means of recording good practice. There are other examples, but a particularly lovely one comes from the town where my Godmother lives in Clonakilty, County Cork, Ireland.

Gaelscoil Mhichíl Uí Choileáin

This is a co-educational, multi-denominational primary school serving the town of Clonakilty and the surrounding areas. For the past three years they have stopped giving out homework in December and asked each child to complete a daily act of kindness. The children then record their activities in their own Kindness Diary. The acts can be any level of kindness and might include helping unload the dishwasher, making a Christmas card for an elderly neighbour or sharing your sweets. It can be playing with someone who is often left out of playground games or making a parent a cup of tea (assuming the child is old enough).

If children or staff notice any acts of kindness during the school day, they are encouraged to write about it and post it in the school 'kindness bucket'. At the end of term, the kindness is celebrated and shared. Such a simple way to give a clear message that being nice is good for everyone and something organisations should be proud of. It isn't a huge leap to see how this could be used in all manner of regulated organisations and how people using services, visitors and other staff, could be encouraged to identify good practice in compassionate care.

I quite like social media and I think it's potentially another useful means of spreading a positive culture and good news. It can be used at the simplest level to show what organisations are doing for the staff, residents, families and the outside world. It can also be a repository of evidence and used to remind staff about happy stories and the times that they have gone 'over and above'. Many organisations are now using social media platforms to gather feedback too.

Castle Keep Care Home, Hull

Castle Keep is registered to provide personal and nursing care. It is a single storey, purpose-built home. The home is divided into two parts, Willow and Nightingale. Both support people who are living with complex dementia care needs. They are currently rated 'Good' overall.

They posted a lovely picture of their home just before Christmas showing a carefully crafted false fireplace and chimney made from cardboard boxes and whatever else such temporary structures are made from. The staff had created this huge masterpiece because one person living at the home was very upset that there was no fireplace to hang stockings from and nowhere for Father Christmas to appear from. I suspect the staff enjoyed making it as much as the resident enjoyed hanging their stocking. It felt like such a normal activity – decorating a home for Christmas. What made it special was that the decoration was how the resident wanted it not how the staff felt it should look. A huge 'red brick' fireplace was slightly incongruous in a modern bungalow but that didn't matter; it was about truly considering what was important. Tasteful decorations weren't given priority over an elderly person's preferences.

Another example picked up from social media shows how the simple things make a big difference.

Burcot Grange, Bromsgrove

Burcot Grange is registered to provide accommodation and personal care for up to 40 older people, including people living with dementia. People's bedrooms were en suite and some people had a 'suite' that included a lounge and kitchenette. It is currently rated as 'Outstanding'.

The provider posted a picture of an incredibly happy and proud group of staff holding a huge banner that showed the world they were 'Outstanding'. It made me look at the report, which said:

"They told us about a couple who were staying at the care home for respite care. In the middle of the night one person could not sleep. Different mattresses were tried but not successful and the person wanted to go home. The solution to this was that the registered manager and the person's relative drove to the person's home to get their own mattress. The respite stay went ahead, which gave the couple the time they needed to recuperate."

Another relative said that their family member, Maud, loved a bath. Even though there was a bath in their own room, staff took their relative to Burcot Lodge next door (the provider's other home). This relative said, "In the Lodge, there's a lovely big deep bath. The staff take Maud and staff put music on and light candles. It's the highlight of her week."

The registered manager apparently reiterated that this was 'everyday' practice. That is why they were given the 'Outstanding' rating – because a truly personalised and considerate attitude from staff meant people felt cosseted, they felt they mattered. It can't even be a one off to impress the inspection team if you want the rating. In fact, wanting the rating should never really be the driving force at all.

Is it worth the extra effort? I imagine the staff at Burcot Grange go home and tell their partners that it was a lovely day at work and that Maud was so happy to have her candlelit bath. Even from the written report I can feel the gentleness and humanity offered to Maud. I know the relatives will feel they can trust staff, so aren't constantly 'checking up on them' or hiding cameras to catch them out. I just know Maud will be protected from harm and there will be fewer minor injuries and less pressure damage. I suspect Maud will sleep and eat better, and be more engaged with the world around her. Definitely worth it for everyone involved.

You don't have to be in an outstanding organisation to be caring

Being kind as an individual member of staff, leader, peer, surgeon, carer, pharmacist, dentist or receptionist is an easy first step towards supporting your organisation's journey towards an 'Outstanding' rating. It might seem a long way off, it might seem an unattainable goal, but it really isn't. If most members of staff are committed to kindness and thoughtfulness towards others, the rating would likely follow; those who didn't commit would be pulled into the cultural norm by peer pressure and role modelling. If all staff decided to perform one act of exceptional kindness a day, what a lovely organisation it would be. If, however, staff decide it's just about getting through the next shift, then it isn't going to be pleasant for anyone.

Let's consider the example of babies, they don't generally move directly from sitting unsupported to running in a single move. It takes persistence and practice. It needs the support of parents that allow a little risk-taking and that encourage standing and walking as intermediate steps. It needs that baby to have the inner drive to move from its bottom. Luckily most do – just as most staff in health and social care settings want to be kind and provide compassionate care. Even in the services that are struggling, which are perhaps rated the lowest, that have poor reputations, that are going through challenging times, there are times one can still see or feel the embers of a burning passion for providing compassionate care.

It is those embers that must be fanned, and a tiny flame elicited to spread the warmth across the organisation. Good practice, kind care must be recognised, valued and rewarded. Staff need the kindness from each other and their leaders just as much as the people using the service. More perhaps, because the way they are treated, the way they feel about their work, will be mirrored and magnified in how they treat the most vulnerable.

The difficulty of waiting for an inspection team to arrive before showing that kindness is that we are very good at spotting shortfalls in care, very good at noticing staff talking over patients or not making eye contact. We are less good at seeing the evidence that supports an 'Outstanding' rating for caring – we ask staff and get vague answers that assert things like, "We're nice and a good team". We rely on NHS Friends and Family results or local surveys and feedback from service users and their relatives. We ask staff to give us examples.

If a caring culture isn't embedded, then that isn't going to come out in the data. If organisations don't themselves recognise and reward compassionate behaviours, then how can a team visiting for one or two days be expected to see it? You need it to be the norm that staff are kind to each other, to visitors, and to people using services.

A kind and compassionate culture will also underpin and build on performance in all other domains. Empathetic staff who understand that it's unpleasant and unkind to leave a patient unable to see properly and who take the trouble to clean their glasses and ensure they are worn, will likely see that the extra time taken to do that small, caring task will show as improved patient outcomes. This might be a reduction in falls, a greater engagement with others, possibly improved continence because they are more confident in taking themselves to the lavatory; there might also be financial benefits through a reduced length of stay.

A kind staff group would not leave someone without appropriate analgesia. They would not be too busy to support a new mother with breastfeeding her pre-term baby. They would not tell a student they should have rung at eight o'clock if they wanted an appointment when they couldn't swallow anything due to tonsillitis. Yes, it's hard to find the time, but only until you realise that finding the time often reduces the overall time to provide high-quality care both for individual services and across regions.

My granny used to say, "Look after the pennies and the pounds will look after themselves". I believe that this is true of good care too; take care of the seemingly small things and some of the bigger problems might not even occur.

Isle of Wight NHS Trust and Earl Mountbatten Hospice

It would be fair to say that the Island trust has faced significant challenges – it was placed in special measures in 2017 by NHS Improvement. The trust moved from an 'Inadequate' rating overall to a 'Requires Improvement' rating in June 2019. There is more to do, and some services remain in need of significant cultural changes.

End of Life care across the trust had improved to a 'Good' rating. The narrative in the report says, "Staff went the extra mile providing personalised compassionate care and considered patients well-being. They ensured patients had basic food supplies when they dropped them off and they drove one patient home along the seafront, as they said they had not seen the sea for a long time."

This is the perfect example of fanning the embers of kindness that were there all along but were rather hidden under an overwhelming cultural greyness. The report from 2017 (that was the one that saw the trust go into Special Measures) saw kindness and compassion in end of life care. The mortuary staff clearly understood the need for thoughtfulness, personalised care and compassion, but something stopped this spreading across the trust.

Luckily, the current leaders at the trust seem to have a better understanding that recognising, valuing and sharing good practice is a far more effective tool to bring about change than any KPI.

The trust has begun working with the local hospice, which is rated 'Outstanding' for caring. Earl Mountbatten Hospice report is a lovely read that talks about personalised care, dignity and respect. Sharing the work of the hospice and the way staff 'go the extra mile' has clearly had an impact and will continue to do so. The impact is, and will continue to be, far more than using the same model of syringe drivers to reduce errors. End of Life care is spread across the entire trust and is everyone's business; good practice and a positive staff attitude here is likely to promote similar improvements in other areas of the trust.

Kindness is also cyclical. The kinder you are as a member of staff or a team, the better the feedback, and that makes you feel good about what you are doing. When you feel good about your work, you usually approach people at work more positively. Being told you are exceptionally kind and that the junior doctor on call is really grateful for the cup of coffee and biscuit as they haven't managed a break is far more likely to see you repeat the kindness. The junior doctor who is feeling frazzled but nurtured is more likely to find the energy to smile and be gentle with the frightened parents in the emergency department. Those parents worrying about meningitis are more likely to be reassured by a calm and gentle doctor telling them it's chicken pox and more likely to tell someone the doctor was lovely. The feedback comes back to the doctor who feels good, remembers the mug of coffee and takes some homemade flapjacks for the ward staff. The ward staff feel valued, smile and are happier. They smile at their patients and the ward atmosphere is nicer, so patients are happier and feel more cared for. Everyone wins.

The latest report for the Isle of Wight NHS trust in June 2019 rated the Medicine core service as 'Inadequate', overall. There is one sentence in the report that says, "Staff did not always treat patients with compassion and kindness, respect their privacy and dignity, take account of individual needs". Not something I imagine anyone would want to read about the care they were providing, regardless of the type of service. Even when this is the verdict overall there are glowing embers where individual staff do show they care. There remain pockets of compassion and staff who still find it within them to show kindness.

About two years ago, there was a consultant rheumatologist at the Newport hospital who was caring for a man with an end stage life-limiting condition. The man was relatively young at 58 years and fully competent. He had always enjoyed a tot of a single malt whiskey as a nightcap each evening, until he was admitted. His family had brought a bottle in and asked whether the staff could pour him a glass each day. The decision was that no, they couldn't 'allow' this as it might aggravate his condition, might pose a potential risk of falls or he might drink too much. He couldn't have it in his locker because someone else might drink it by mistake. It might be stolen. Every possible barrier and excuse were put in place, until the family spoke with the rheumatologist and asked again whether it was possible. The rheumatologist tried to persuade the ward staff that it was a good idea and a small pleasure for a man that was dying, albeit not imminently. The ward staff continued to find reasons why not, so the rheumatologist decided to prescribe it on the patients medicine chart and agreed with the chief pharmacist that the family could bring in an unopened bottle and that the pharmacy staff would decant it into a medicine bottle with a proper label so that the nursing staff could administer it as a daily dose and at other times, on request.

If the consultant rheumatologist and the pharmacist could find a way around the system and work in the patient's best interest and wishes, it should be possible to build on that kindness through staff supervision, team meetings, sharing in newsletters and hospital awards.

Ty Gwyn Residential Care Home

Ty Gwyn Residential Care Home is a residential care home near Leicester that was providing personal care to eight older people with learning disabilities at the time of an inspection in May 2019. It was rated as 'Good' overall and 'Good' for caring.

What the report says was that, "People gave lovely feedback about the caring approach of the staff at the home. One person said, 'The staff are very kind and will help you in any way they can'. Another person said, 'The staff are very nice, I like being at home here'."

Staff were friendly, encouraging and supportive to people. One member of staff said, "This has always been like a family home. We've got so much passion for the people here."

The narrative shows a very caring staff group with lovely relationships that were valued by both staff, families and residents. Why haven't they been rated 'Outstanding'? I would suggest that is for the staff team to reflect on. It is the managers task to lead the staff team towards the next level. Clearly, with committed and appreciated staff, that step isn't insurmountable. They might just need support to recognise excellence and find a way of recording it.

What improvements can they make? How can they better demonstrate what they are doing? How can they collect and act on feedback to improve the residents' lives? Are they forgetting to collate evidence of caring practice simply because it's part of their everyday practice?

Caring when it's hard to care

Providing health and social care isn't always easy. Some of the most vulnerable people that pass through the doors of regulated services, in need of care, treatment, support or reassurance, are often quite hard to work with. How a staff group or individual staff respond to the complex needs of people whose distress or lack of cognition causes unwanted behaviours is often humbling.

I understand completely that the relentless challenges staff face in their work can cause compassion fatigue among staff. Their peers don't step in to provide support, to encourage them to see the person and recognise the behaviours as either a pathological lack of ability to engage positively or because of something in the situation creating distress, rather than a personal attack. Their leaders may be fretting about ticking boxes to show that the paracetamol cupboard temperature has been checked daily or that there are green stickers on cleaned commodes and getting cross when those ticks are missing. Sometimes priorities get skewed and the demands of a regulation, rather than the needs of the individuals receiving care, becomes the driving force. Nothing should be done simply because it appeases a regulator. Everything should focus on the needs of the people using the service. If that is not understood, an 'Outstanding' rating will continue to escape the most well-ordered services with a whole host of checklists.

We'll talk about the financial and personal cost of pressure damage elsewhere, but a kind staff group who understand the discomfort of sitting in one position, unable to move independently, will be more likely to support the person to a comfortable position than a member of staff who thinks it's necessary because a chart needs filling in. They'll be more likely to see a reduction in pressure damage simply because they can empathise.

What support is there? Again, I think it is for the provider and staff team to determine the best ways of managing situations. The provider and leaders need to listen to their staff and accept good ideas. An additional member of staff to provide one-to-one care may be expensive but it's a whole lot less expensive than staff members 'burning out' and going off on long-term sick leave. It's much cheaper than someone taking an overdose in a lavatory in the emergency department. It's much cheaper than the closure of a care home because staff working under intense pressure have snapped and lashed out.

I was challenged quite recently about the language I accepted in a report that I was quality assuring. I had let the term 'challenging behaviour' (when written about people living with dementia) pass through without comment. A member of the panel pointed out the people weren't trying to challenge. They had no capacity to manage their own behaviours and that they were showing their distress, fear and anxiety in the only way they could. They suggested the report be amended to say distressed behaviour rather than challenging behaviour. It is so much easier to be kind to a distressed person than a person who is challenging. It hopefully brings out the nurturing and compassion rather than challenging behaviour which is often 'managed'. The staff member was right, and I have now changed my language and check all reports that pass through my hands to ensure we are looking from a patient perspective.

Hampshire Hospitals NHS Foundation Trust

Winchester is a beautiful, historic city which was recently ranked third in The Halifax Quality of Life survey, moving up from ninth position. People living in this part of Hampshire are healthier, better paid, better educated and have plenty of luscious green surroundings, along with a river that's good for children to swim and paddle in and an easy commute to London. A fantastic place to raise a family, if you are a young accountant married to a university lecturer. A bit harder to be poor though.

A couple of years ago, a 13-year-old girl was brought to the accident and emergency department at the hospital. On arrival, she was clearly in a very volatile and distressed state and exhibiting the sort of unpleasant behaviour that onlookers 'sniff and tut' at. She was admitted to the children's ward as her father wasn't coping and she was considered to be at risk. She wasn't generally well received. Paediatric nurses, on the whole, like working with beautiful bald babies that smell of vanilla and doe-eyed, curly haired, pre-school children with a wheeze. Loud, violent, swearing 13-year-olds aren't necessarily their dream patients.

This poor child had certainly been through a lot and it was no wonder she was acting out in a fairly dramatic way. She had been living in a different county with her mother until her mother became pregnant with a new partner and she found herself being hurt because she was no longer wanted. She ran away and somehow managed to get to Winchester to find her father: a journey of about 200 miles. She found him, miraculously, but he was homeless and living in temporary accommodation above a pub. There was a kettle in the corner, as the only means of cooking, and a shared lavatory. There was no bath or shower.

She had been with her father for a month at the time of admission. Despite having a child protection plan she had dropped off the face of the earth. Dad didn't have a GP. She didn't go to school. Her father tried but couldn't cook and they were living off instant noodles and value-range baked beans heated by the can being placed on the radiator, which came on for a limited time each evening. They were just about surviving until the father got his new girlfriend pregnant. The girlfriend was also in the pub accommodation and was clear that she didn't want the child around, so the child started hanging out downstairs with the dope smokers and the alcoholics. Still no concerns were raised because she was under the radar. She started acting badly and having major tantrums, but her father didn't seek help, he was too scared he'd get into trouble. At the inevitable point when it all imploded and the child had started to self-destruct, all he could do was call an ambulance and have her taken to the local hospital.

On arrival to the ward, the local safeguarding team were able to confirm a child protection plan had been in place and she was admitted as a place of safety. She was filthy – not grubby, filthy. Her clothes were soaked, and she was cold; this was winter. She had long, matted, tangled hair that was crawling with head lice. She had severe infected eczema on her face, neck and arms. She had a swollen face and very sore eyes. She just looked incredibly unappealing and terribly sad.

The ward was full of beautiful babies with bronchiolitis and toddlers with chesty coughs. Amongst them came this 13-year-old girl, hurling things around and shouting abuse very loudly. The nurses' instinct was to protect the little ones, the cuties. Of course, they mainly had parents who could protect them just fine. The one in most need of protection was the scary one they struggled to manage. She was put in a side room and the door closed as she was 'destroying the room'. Staff were not unreasonably scared of entering and disturbing her further since she had calmed and was curled up in a desolate ball of dejection in a corner.

This was a very frightened child whose 'trashing the room' was symbolic rather than significant. She had emptied the paper towels and ripped them to shreds, emptied the bin and thrown the mattress on the floor. There was lots of noise.

At a ward round shortly after the admission, a junior doctor, a GP trainee, asked whether they had tried talking to her and was met with looks of horror at the very idea. "No, you'll get hurt if you try that," was the consensus. The staff had taken her shoes away because, "She might kick someone". She hadn't hurt anyone, but it was assumed she would. The junior doctor felt that if you tell someone they are bad, they are likely to be bad, so decided to go in and talk. Fortunately, the doctor had a good understanding of teenagers in distress.

The doctor said "You're making lots of noise. What do you want me to hear?" which was ignored, and the child carried on screeching. The doctor talked about her eczema being sore and said they needed to make it better. Then asked what the child liked doing.

It turned out she liked colouring, so the doctor sent the other staff (who were acting like bodyguards) away and sat and coloured with the girl. The nurses had assumed she was 'too old' for colouring.

When the doctor asked what the girl wanted, she was able to say, in no particular order:

- A home
- A school
- Parents who love me
- To be normal

The doctor acknowledged they were reasonable things to want and that the child was in a horrible situation, not of her own making. They said they couldn't promise to make everything better, but they could stop her skin hurting and they could get rid of the nits and sort her hair out. They also said they could help sort out somewhere better to live and find a school.

The doctor said they couldn't make her parents love her but explained that they probably did, and that they just weren't coping very well as adults.

In return, the girl had to understand this was a children's ward and that there were lots of very sick babies and frightened parents. The doctor apologised that she hadn't been looked after very well so far but said the ward was really busy. Her screaming and throwing things made it harder for everyone.

They 'pinkie promised'.

While the doctor sorted the administration and started the referrals processes, they asked a healthcare assistant to take their personal debit card to a nearby supermarket to buy some nice shampoo, the largest bottle of hair conditioner they had, a hairbrush and some bobbles and some pretty pyjamas along with the largest chocolate bar that they sold. She also gave the healthcare assistant a prescription for some headlice lotion, as the hospital pharmacy was closed.

When the staff member returned with the goodies, she and the doctor bathed the child while she watched television on the doctor's laptop and ate chocolate. Every tangle was persuaded out. The nits were treated, and the child then slathered with cream for the eczema before dressing in her new PJs and having her hair French plaited. She then sat in the playroom with the little ones, colouring and chatting like the bright, engaged and happy child she deserved to be.

Liaison with the local authority meant she returned to new accommodation with her father five days later, but it broke down within an hour and she was readmitted. A rapid response and staff who knew and accepted her more readily saw her move to a stable foster placement within a couple of days.

Caring isn't hard. It isn't expensive. It was thoughtfulness, empathy, shampoo, chocolate and nit lotion. It changed the whole experience (and potentially the life) of a distressed and neglected child. It saved staff stress, saved costs and improved the experience for other patients. All it took was seeing the vulnerability through the behaviour and responding to it.

Another example from the same hospital involved a 53-year-old man, let's call him Mick, with motor neurone disease. Motor neurone disease is a rare condition that progressively damages parts of the nervous system. This leads to muscle weakness, often with visible wasting. It is often life shortening and can leave people with limited control over their bodies.

Mick was initially admitted with pneumonia which was treated but as his condition was progressing rapidly it was agreed he was no longer able to live independently at home and needed round-the-clock nursing care. He was an intelligent, professional photographer and was absolutely clear he did not want to be placed in an elderly care home. Trying to find an appropriate placement that he could accept proved incredibly challenging and so he remained in the hospital for some considerable time. On a good day he was able to lift a spoon to his mouth, but the number of 'good days' decreased as he languished in hospital. The level and type of care he needed was usually found in homes for people living with dementia, but his cognitive functioning, his thought processes remained intact.

As delays in finding appropriate placement persisted, Mick developed another episode of pneumonia and some significant pressure damage. Every time he became unwell, the care planning process was stopped until he was medically well enough for discharge. Then the assessment had to begin all over again. He was still in hospital nearly a year later but had been medically fit for four months. Four or five months being well enough for discharge but with nowhere to go. He was cared for in bed for most of this time and became depressed to the point where he decided to go on hunger strike. His perspective was that he would eat once a home had been found for him that wasn't a hospital.

A junior doctor working on the ward where he was an outlier had begun to get to know and understand him. On a quiet weekend afternoon, two junior doctors asked him about the degree to which he was prepared to take risks to overcome the misery of being stuck in bed all day. He had full capacity and wanted more than anything to see outside the ward and feel fresh air. He said he dreamed of the sun on his face, but rain would do. The two core trainee doctors borrowed a wheelchair from the outpatient department and hoisted Mick into it. Not all the ward nurses were supportive but didn't actually stop them. They found several pillows to wedge Mick in reasonably securely, and a safety belt to prevent him tipping out too easily. With Mick wrapped up warmly in blankets, they headed out around the hospital. Mick wanted to go outside so they ventured into the garden and got stuck. Luckily, a passing porter helped them back onto the path from the grass. This was the first time anyone had heard Mick laugh in months. The two young doctors then told him it was their break time and they wanted coffee, so they took him to the on-site coffee shop. They told Mick he could sit and watch them drink coffee or join them, but they'd been working all day and needed a snack. Mick said he couldn't as he had no money, but they assured him they would be able to afford to pay. He chose a hot chocolate and a cheese and ham toastie. He fed himself for the first time in several months and declared it delicious. He talked about the sadness of not being able to look at his photographs. The doctors said they could apply for a grant for an adapted laptop and find someone to help upload his photos – which they did. His whole demeanour changed because a couple of young doctors didn't get too preoccupied with risk and cared enough to find a solution. They saw the person, not the problem.

Sadly, Mick developed pneumonia again and never was able to leave the hospital. How much more important did that hot chocolate and 'toastie' become?

Specialist services

While all services should be capable of demonstrating compassion towards people who use them and actively involve people in care, providing evidence of this can be a challenge. This might be because they are working with very small cohorts or the circumstances in which care needs to be provided make showing the compassion more difficult. Much easier for an inspection team to see kind care on a maternity unit than in an operating theatre, for example. Much easier to be a kind GP practice than a prison healthcare service.

Critical care can be a place where it's relatively easy to provide excellent care and where staff have plenty of opportunity to show compassion, but where it isn't always easy for inspection teams to see that excellence. It tends to be a reasonably contained service with patients who are generally unable to be anything but compliant and relatives who are effusively grateful for all the staff do. That possibly means the bar is set higher though. It's normal to see staff supporting and working with patients and relatives in a kind and gentle way. How do they go above and beyond? How do they show outstanding care?

It's quite hard without any preparation. Most intensive care units in district general hospitals have quite small units with just a few beds. The number of beds range from those with fewer than ten beds, such as South Tyneside NHS Foundation Trust, which has just six, and Northern Devon Healthcare NHS Trust with eight beds; to the largest teaching and specialist trusts such as the Royal Brompton and Harefield NHS Foundation Trust with 102 beds or Leeds Teaching Hospitals NHS Trust with 106. Inspection teams may see just a handful of patients or relatives throughout the inspection visit. How do they decide whether the compassionate approach is truly outstanding?

Worthing Hospital and St Richard's Hospital

When we inspected Worthing Hospital and its sister site, St Richard's Hospital, in 2019, the trust had already prepared. They had thought ahead and printed off a few copies of a booklet they called *Always going above and beyond*. It contained brief vignettes of where staff had 'gone the extra mile'. Where the care went from what one might expect of critical care staff to the exceptional. Obviously, this couldn't all take place while we were on the units but was a series of patient stories, collated over the preceding year or so. It was used to provide evidence for the inspection team, but more importantly it was used as a tool to remind staff of the work they were doing and to celebrate excellence. It was also useful to us as a tool to guide conversations so that staff were able to tell us about the individual patients and the way they had been cared for. It allowed us to check out the validity of the claims; to feel the investment that staff had made.

Examples of the vignettes included a story about staff arranging a funeral for the spouse of a long-term patient in the hospital chapel and supporting their ventilated patient to attend. It was the discussion with staff that this led to, rather than the few written sentences, that demonstrated so perfectly the attitude and level of compassion among the staff group and unit leaders.

We often joke that to be rated 'Outstanding' for caring we need there to be a wedding, a birthday and a tale about a pet. Within the vignette booklet was the story about a ventilated patient's dogs.

The hospital already had Pets as Therapy dogs visiting wards regularly. Pets as Therapy is a national charity who provide visits of volunteers with their behaviourally assessed animals. They provide a visiting service in hospitals, hospices, nursing and care homes, special needs schools and a variety of other venues across the UK.

This patient was very unwell and ventilated via a tracheostomy and was feeling very miserable; he was missing his own dogs. The staff on the unit couldn't admit unknown dogs to the hospital, so arranged for the patient to be taken outside into the grounds, where the patient's family had brought his dogs to visit him. We were told his recovery and mood improved from that visit and his recovery was significantly enhanced by seeing his pets.

The Applegarth

The Applegarth is the registered name for the Humankind arm of North Yorkshire Horizons. They provide community substance misuse support for adults in North Yorkshire. Feedback from clients and carers during the inspection was universally positive about staff treatment of clients.

Clients said that staff went the extra mile and that the support they received had exceeded their expectations. Clients told the inspection team that the 'hubs' were safe and welcoming, and that staff approached them with kindness, empathy and with no judgement. Clients who used the service said that they had been "treated as a whole person, not just... substance use". It had made them feel normal. One person said that the service had "saved them". Clients noted that there were added benefits from having staff members in the team with lived experience, as they felt it provided hope as well as an extra level of understanding.

Staff recognised and respected the totality of clients' needs. They sought to meet clients' social and emotional needs, as well as their physical ones. One of the recovery plans we reviewed detailed how staff had assisted a client in de-cluttering their home and sorting through their possessions, to improve their welfare and that of their family. The Skipton hub had distributed homelessness kits, including sleeping bags, tents, warm clothing and toiletries, to provide to clients in need. The service also had a separate fund that clients could request the use of to improve their quality of life. Prior to the most recent inspection a client had been granted the funds to decorate their home and buy their children new bedding.

Northumberland, Tyne and Wear NHS Foundation Trust

Northumberland, Tyne and Wear NHS Foundation Trust is one of the largest mental health and learning disability trusts in England.

The report for the acute wards for adults of work age and psychiatric intensive care units said:

"The occupational therapy department which covered the four wards at Hopewood Park (Beckfield, Longview, Springrise and Shoredrift) had introduced a 'social inclusion programme' that was designed to support patients to access services and activities in the community. Examples of activities included a gardening project at a local church and modelmaking as part of preparation for Sunderland's 2018 Tall

Ships Race. The social inclusion programme was celebrated in a national magazine, as an example of work which both improved patient well-being and reduced the social stigma of mental ill-health."

Registering the Right Support

Since the BBC Panorama programme in 2011, which exposed the abuse of people at Winterbourne View hospital, there has been increased scrutiny of how the health and social care needs of people with a learning disability are being met.

The Care Quality Commission have committed to taking a firmer approach to the registration for providers who support people with a learning disability and/or autism in 'A fresh start for registration'. In October 2016, we published the state of health and adult social care in England 2015/1612 in which we identified concerns that providers were continuing to apply to register residential services that were not consistent with the new service model for people with a learning disability

The Moorings, Poole

The Moorings is a residential care home which can support up to six people.

The service has been developed and designed in line with the principles and values that underpin Registering the Right Support and other best practice guidance. This ensures that people who use the service can live as full a life as possible and achieve the best possible outcomes. The principles reflect the need for people with learning disabilities and/or autism to live meaningful lives that include control, choice, and independence.

This is one of those inspection reports that one can read and almost *feel* how good the service is. It would be hard to deny that this was an exceptionally caring service – despite caring for a group of people with complex needs. The report says:

"Staff regularly went above and beyond for people and genuinely cared for them. For example, one staff member was so committed to making sure they were there to support one person (who had an extreme fear of health settings) during planned surgery, that they made alternative family and childcare arrangements so that they could be there. Two staff members had worked with the person over a prolonged period to be able to get them calm enough to agree to go to the hospital. Another staff member wrote to us about when the person was admitted to hospital as an emergency, 'My colleague slept on the hospital floor and the registered manager sat in a chair from the afternoon till 3pm the next day to ensure the person was safe and because they genuinely care for them. There aren't many managers that would do that. I am unbelievably proud to say I work with such genuinely caring people as it's not a job with a staff team and service users. It's a family.

"Staff had an in-depth knowledge of the people. Staff were fully familiar with people's likes and preferences including the music they liked to listen and sing along to, creating a truly person-centred environment and using this detailed knowledge to make people comfortable and reduce any anxiety or distress. We observed staff singing along with a person about what they were going to listen to when they went out in the car and finding videos of a specific TV show they liked to watch on a tablet computer."

The latter paragraph is something that is so important, yet so overlooked. It's about seeing people as individuals and respecting their preferences. So often I have gone into care homes or even hospital wards and heard loud pop music or heavy metal blasting out. Music is good if it's what people want. Often, staff turning on Iron Maiden at maximum volume suggests they aren't fully cognisant or are uncaring of their patients' or residents' wishes. Obviously, if there is one service user and they actually want Metallica 18 hours a day, that's a different thing.

> From the Care Quality Commission key lines of enquiry, prompts and ratings characteristics for healthcare services:
>
> *There is a strong, visible person-centered culture. Staff are highly motivated and inspired to offer care that is kind and promotes people's dignity. Relationships between people who use the service, those close to them and staff are strong, caring, respectful and supportive. These relationships are highly valued by staff and promoted by leaders.*
>
> *Staff recognise and respect the totality of people's needs. They always take people's personal, cultural, social and religious needs into account, and find innovative ways to meet them.*
>
> *People's emotional and social needs are seen as being as important as their physical needs.*

The importance of touch

I guess, because I am first and foremost a paediatric nurse who has spent most of my adult life working and living with children in a multitude of settings, I am very aware of the power of touch. It's extremely hard to resist picking up and cuddling a crying toddler who is holding their arms up to you after their mother has had to go home to care for her other children. I take great pleasure in holding tiny babies and rediscovering anew the magic of their tiny hands and button noses. I've held children with special needs who were frightened by their own loss of control. I have cradled dying children who were waiting for their parents to arrive from their hospital accommodation. It feels almost second nature.

Unfortunately, as a nation we have perhaps become a tad paranoid about touch – a huge pity when touch can be such a powerful tool to show empathy and compassion. Obviously, the touch must be wanted and accepted by the recipient. Obviously, there are limits, but is it wrong to gently bounce a toddler and sing 'the wheels on the bus' to distract or calm them (even if you are a GP or a midwife)? Is it wrong to sit stroking the hair of an elderly and very distressed woman who has just had a stroke and doesn't know where they are?

I suspect, as health or social care professionals, we should invert the question and ask ourselves what it must feel like to be 'an untouchable', to never feel the warmth or comfort of a hug. I'm not suggesting every dentist receptionist should embrace every patient that walks through the door, but I am suggesting we should consider compassionate touch as a human right. It cannot be a compulsory thing and people's personal space and preferences should be respected (staff and service users' alike), but I'd find it pretty sad if healthcare professionals could not recognise body language or other cues that suggested someone was or was not comfortable with the level of touch being offered. I would suggest that in the very best organisational cultures you often see staff touching each other, too – the hug to say, 'Good Luck' for an interview; the touch of an arm to say, 'I understand how hard that was'; the touch to say, 'I have no words to help with the pain of your bereavement, but I do care'.

Should you kiss patients? Now that's an interesting question, isn't it? Instinct says probably not, but instincts can be wrong. I remember an inspection of an accident and emergency department where several elderly people had been held on trolleys in the corridor for a few hours. Staff were conspicuous by their absence. There were three of us and it felt very natural to sit around and chat to a few of the patients, to see how long before anyone came to check on them. One very elderly woman was particularly taken with one of the inspectors on our team. He was sweet with her and sang her a few old favourites and talked about his cat. She then proclaimed very loudly that he was, "Lovely and that she wanted to kiss him". He initially laughed it off, but she was quite persistent. In the end, he said, "Oh go on then, just a peck on the cheek". She flung her stick-like arms around his neck and planted a huge, wet, slobbery, kiss on his cheek. She then laughed and declared it was, "The best kiss all year". She continued smiling to herself. Was that acceptable? It brought pleasure to her and harmed nobody. There was no risk attached to it. It wasn't a safeguarding issue. It was a kind and gentle interaction between a healthcare professional and a patient.

If you've sat through the night with someone you've cared for over many months, but who is now unwell and very frightened or tired and have held their hand for most of the night, is it so very wrong to gently kiss the back of their hand as they finally drift towards sleep?

I certainly used to kiss babies and little ones when I worked in clinical care; I still do, given half a chance. Blowing raspberries on feet often brings incomparable joy to both parties – but only with small children and in certain settings. Context is everything. Well considered, individual and personalised care is key to responding to a need with a hug or a kiss.

There is science behind the need to encourage health and social care practitioners to touch. Research suggests that it probably has far greater impact than merely feeling nice. Human beings are highly social creatures who often touch each other during social interactions. Although the physiologic effects of touch are not understood fully, it appears to sustain social bonds and to increase co-operative behaviours. Oxytocin is a hormone known to facilitate social bonding, and touch affects oxytocin release. A study by Morhenn *et al* (2012) showed that massage increases oxytocin levels. They suggest that their findings may help explain the mechanisms through which social connections reduce morbidity and mortality.

- Oxytocin promotes trust and attachment between individuals. However, oxytocin has a more complex role than solely enhancing prosocial behaviours. There is consensus that oxytocin modulates fear and anxiety.
- Oxytocin produces antidepressant-like effects and a deficit of it may be involved in the pathophysiology of depression in humans.
- Levels of oxytocin increased when there was food sharing. This comparatively higher level of oxytocin after food sharing parallels the increased level of oxytocin in nursing mothers, sharing nutrients with their kin.
- Trust is increased by oxytocin. Disclosure of emotional events is a sign of trust in humans. When recounting a negative event, humans who receive intranasal oxytocin share more emotional details and stories with more emotional significance.
- There is improved wound healing: oxytocin is also thought to modulate inflammation by decreasing certain cytokines. Thus, the increased release in oxytocin following positive social interactions has the potential to improve wound healing.

Touching costs nothing.

Stonebridge Nursing Home, Redditch

Stonebridge Nursing Home is a residential care home for up to 52 adults. The home has four wings, each with its own lounge and outside gardens, with bedrooms on two floors. Three wings provide care for people living with advanced dementia and one wing specialises in providing care to people living with long-term mental health conditions. Certainly not always the easiest people to care for.

The report is a joy to read but there are a few notable sentences that stand out and help the reader understand why this service was rated as 'Outstanding' for the caring key question. Below is an excerpt from the inspection report:

"There was a culture of fostering kind and supportive relationships between people and staff living at the home. Staff and management were fully committed to ensuring people received the best possible care in a loving and compassionate way.

"Staff were highly motivated and passionate about the care they provided to people living in the home. Staff acted professionally, although we saw they were not afraid to show love and affection, for example by hugging people, when people needed it, with their consent. Their passion was echoed by the provider and management team, who described people and staff as 'Family'. One person told us, 'It's the friendliness and caring shown, not just for me but for my family as well'."

Beechcroft Green Nursing Home, Gosport

Beechcroft Green Nursing home is one of a group provided by Contemplation Homes Limited. It is currently rated as 'Good' by the Commission.

The report says, "Our observations of staff interactions with people showed that people were treated with kindness, compassion, dignity and respect. Staff recognised when people may be becoming anxious and spent time with them offering reassurance. People were clearly relaxed and comfortable in the company of staff."

That paragraph reads quite nicely but is probably a bit succinct for others to learn much from. That's not the inspection team's shortcoming – there is a move towards shorter, easier to read reports and this one published in October 2019 is well written.

I know the home well because my already deaf and blind, 94-year-old mother was moved to their care after she suffered a major stroke and was not expected to live very long. She is very frail, unable to communicate much and spends most of her time in another world. The stroke left her with advanced dementia. She is immobile and more or less cut off from the world because of her condition. When people approach her or try to provide care, she can become very distressed and consequently lashes out, scratching, spitting and hitting staff who are trying to help her. She isn't always easy to care for. I describe this to enable people to understand the effectiveness of compassionate touch rather than as a judgement on her distressed behaviour.

The staff are kind and pleasant but there are two who stand out as truly empathetic and compassionate. They are two of the home's senior registered nurses. Whenever I visit and they are on duty they come to talk to me about how my mother has been. Last week it was about a small wound under her eye that looked slightly infected.

While the nurse was talking to me about not knowing how it had happened, she held my mother's hand and stroked it very gently. She continued to provide the reassurance and human contact through that seemingly insignificant touch.

It isn't insignificant, of course. I don't know whether the nurse even registered that she was doing it; it was just a normal everyday occurrence. It wasn't contrived for my benefit; she didn't use it as a formal part of any risk assessment or care plan. It was simply nursing at its best. A subconscious reaction to distress in another person. I suspect she wasn't thinking about oxytocin and dopamine release, she just intuitively knew touching calmed a distressed, elderly person who was unable to communicate in any other way.

The impact of Coronavirus is likely to reduce how often those most likely to benefit from being touched are actually touched. Social distancing is going to see people withdrawing from each other. I'm not sure what the answer is – massage sessions maybe? Pets certainly add scope for affectionate touching.

The power of music

"Joy, sorrow, tears, lamentation, laughter… to all these music gives voice, but in such a way that we are transported from the world of unrest to a world of peace, and see reality in a new way, as if we were sitting by a mountain lake and contemplating hills and woods and clouds in the tranquil and fathomless water."

Albert Schweitzer

Sometimes music reaches people in a special way and can be an excellent response to distress, to fear, to sadness, to anger or simply to bring pleasure. Most people have pieces of music that ignite cherished memories or make them smile as soon as the introduction is played. Who cannot still sing the words of Band-Aid's, 'Do They Know It's Christmas?', a single song that had the power to raise £8 million to help address the Ethiopian famine.

Why is it so vital in health and social care?

We all know that music should be an integral part of early child rearing. Research undertaken by a team of researchers in the 1990s showed that exposure to music from early childhood onwards helps children to speak more clearly, develop a larger vocabulary, and strengthen social and emotional skills. When dancing and moving to music, children develop better motor skills whereas singing along to a song helps them to practice their singing voice. In general, exposure to music supports children in their development process to learn the sound of tones and words.

Interestingly, further research also indicates that parents develop a stronger bond to their children when they enjoy music together. This way music is not only a tool that contributes to the growth and development of a child, but it also helps the family to spend quality time and have fun. Is the same true in health and social care settings? I rather suspect it is.

"The essence of good dementia care is human connection, and music lets us do that"
Lucy Frost, Dementia Specialist Nurse and Nurse Consultant, Sussex Community NHS Trust.

Music therapy can help to manage and reduce agitation, isolation, depression and anxiety in people with dementia. The Alzheimer's Society suggests that, "Music therapy has the power to improve the lives of some of the most vulnerable people in our communities." Research has shown that music therapy can significantly improve and support the mood, alertness and engagement of people with dementia. As a result, music therapy sessions can often reduce the use of medication. It can also help people who may find it difficult to communicate verbally, whether due to a physical or cognitive disability, emotional distress or mental illness.

In their 2018 report entitled *What would life be – without a song or dance, what are we?*, Bamford and Bowell say that: "Music can provide a true lifeline for those both with and without dementia by promoting social connection, restoring a sense of self and bringing joy even in the most challenging of times. The ability to connect to music is an innate aspect of being human; having a diagnosis of dementia need not undermine this."

Music is not just a useful tool for people living with dementia.

A research article written by Wilson *et al* was published in the *Journal of applied Arts and Health* in 2014. This article presented a one-year evaluation of the Open Arts studio at Hadleigh Old Fire Station (HOFS) in Essex, England, which had been established to provide opportunities for mental health service users to carry out artmaking independently with professional support. The report said, "Participatory arts projects are thought to increase mental well-being and social inclusion for people with mental health difficulties. Members' comments indicated increased social support, confidence, motivation and mental well-being, in addition to decreased social isolation."

Research published in *Journal of Intellectual Disabilities* by Pavlicevic *et al* in 2014, said that, "Long-term shared therapeutic musicking provides young adults with ongoing opportunities for experiencing confidence and self-esteem, with feelings of shared acceptance and success, and also provides young adults and their families with opportunities for developing and sustaining friendships. In addition, families experienced meeting other parents and carers in the communal reception area as supportive and countering their isolation."

Why then are health and social care environments not full of joyful music? I don't mean that Bing Crosby or Val Doonican should be piped on a loop in every care home. And I certainly don't mean that patients recovering from surgery in a day care unit should be subject to the latest top ten, playing loudly for the staff.

Chestnut Tree House, Arundel

Chestnut Tree House is a children's hospice in West Sussex. I know the service well and have visited many times over the years since it was built. On one inspection, carried out while working for the previous regulator, there was a young child being cared for in the Stars Suite (accommodation designed specifically to care for a child and their family after the child's death). I spent some time talking with the bereaved parents in the child's bedroom, having been invited in by them. They talked to me about their daughter, who was dressed in the sweetest Beatrix Potter pyjamas. They said that they really appreciated the support from the hospice staff in helping them prepare to say goodbye to little Rosie.

The mother told me that they had a routine at home where Rosie had her bath and put on her pyjamas each evening. The mother said she then usually took Rosie outside to sing 'Twinkle, Twinkle, Little Star' to her, find the special star and say goodnight to her grandmother, who had died the previous year. It had become a habit they continued, despite Rosie becoming so ill.

After Rosie had been brought to the Stars Suite to rest before her funeral, the staff helped the parents continue their family routine. They had helped move Rosie outside each evening and supported her mother to hold her. The parents tried to sing 'Twinkle, Twinkle' but couldn't manage it. The staff took over and sung the nursery rhyme for them; sometimes the parents had joined in and sometimes they couldn't. The parents were able to say that the singing together had really helped them feel a bond with the staff who they hadn't met prior to bringing Rosie to the Stars Suite. It helped staff to build a positive relationship and opened communication in the most difficult of circumstances.

Wellbeing teams – Greater Manchester

Wellbeing teams – Greater Manchester is a domiciliary care agency. It provides personal care and support to people living in their own houses and flats. It provides a service to adults including supporting people with a diagnosis of dementia. Their staff understood the value of music in providing care that went beyond the essential.

Their report showed that, "Workers were encouraged to offer 'spa experiences' for other personal care tasks such as showering or applying creams". A worker told us, "If you're showering someone, you're doing it anyway, but people enjoy it more if there's music playing, and they feel they are being pampered and feel they are having a massage rather than having cream put on". The registered manager told us, "We want to think about how we can elevate the visit. All workers have a data allowance on their phones, and we expect them to use it to put music on if the person wants it."

The Wishing Well (Music in Healthcare) is an organisation that works in partnership with several NHS trusts and charities across the South East, bringing live interactive Music for Wellbeing into hospitals and hospices. Their musicians work closely with healthcare staff to make sure that our approach is right for each person. I was fortunate to see two of their musicians at work.

More information can be found at: http://wishingwellmusic.org.uk/our-team

East Surrey Hospital

This was one of my favourite moments on inspection in the past couple of years. It was a well-led inspection, focusing on leadership at all levels of the trust. There was enough space within the timetable to allow the team to visit wards and departments, to get a feel for how well the hospital was managed and led. An Admiral Nurse invited me to come and see the work the trust was doing to improve the care of patients living with dementia.

Admiral Nurses provide the specialist dementia support that families need. They work alongside people with dementia, and their families: giving them one-to-one support, expert guidance and practical solutions. Their dementia expertise helps families to live more positively with dementia and to face the challenges with more confidence and less fear.

We went onto an elderly care ward about an hour or so after lunch had finished. It was very quiet, almost silent, with most patients appearing to be enjoying an afternoon nap. One or two visitors were starting to arrive and spoke quietly with the staff at the nurses' station or sat by their relatives.

The Admiral Nurse consultant told me that there was to be music. I groaned inwardly, expecting a sort of loud, vintage, karaoke session. I put on my 'How lovely' face and continued down the ward beside him. Still quiet. I was beginning to wonder whether he'd got the wrong ward. He guided me into a bay of about six elderly women, most of whom were beginning to wake up and call out. One person, Violet, was still dozing in her bed, her hands rapidly twiddling her blanket.

She'd been admitted during the previous night and had been very unsettled and frightened, apparently.

There were two women standing close by her. One had a violin and one a bag of other instruments. They gathered around her and then the violinist started playing at a volume akin to a whisper. Not much response. Very quietly, the other woman started singing, 'I'm forever blowing bubbles'. Violet's eyes remained tightly shut but her jaw moved, almost imperceptibly, in time to the music. Then, as they increased the volume very slightly, her lips started mouthing the words. No sound, no drama, almost as if she were singing it to herself as she worked at something; her lip movements became more recognisable, her fingers twitched less rapidly and moved in time to the music.

Violet's two daughters arrived towards the end of the song, clearly anxious and keen to see how their mother was. At the end of the song, Violet opened her eyes, looked at the musicians with a huge smile and said, "That was beautiful". Her daughter cried and later said her mother had not engaged meaningfully with anyone for a few months prior to this.

Using feedback

From the Care Quality Commission key lines of enquiry, prompts and ratings characteristics for healthcare services.

Feedback from people who use the service, those who are close to them and stakeholders is continually positive about the way staff treat people. People think that staff go the extra mile and their care and support exceeds their expectations.

The use of feedback from people who use services, those close to them and other people visiting the service is a prerequisite for an 'Outstanding' rating. That is not why providers should collect and analyse feedback though. Providers and individual health and social care professionals should collect feedback as a means of assessing and monitoring how well their service is meeting people's expectations and needs. Tools for supporting feedback are available through statutory instruments such as the NHS Friends and Family test but that probably isn't sufficient to gain a true understanding of how people perceive your service or what improvements people might like to see. Feedback needs to be built into every conversation, ideally.

Staff need to get used to asking for feedback, not necessarily formal recordings online or a written analysis of the service, just an ordinary conversation. It's not difficult for a GP to ask, "Has that been helpful? Is there anything else I can help you with today?" It's easy for a consultant on a ward round to ask whether the patient understands and is happy with the treatment plan. It's quite usual for an independent hospital matron to walk around the hospital to talk to patients about their experience.

What's as important as collecting the data is understanding it. What's as important as asking people to tell you about the service is listening to and hearing what they have to say. It's very, very easy to hear the positives and dismiss any negatives, but we learn so much more from the less positive comments. Culturally you need to build on good practice. You want to understand what people tell you is good and use that to improve further, but if you ignore the things you don't want to hear your journey towards being 'Outstanding' will take much longer.

There are a multitude of ways to gather feedback, from direct conversations to suggestion boxes or residents' meetings. If you don't gather and respond to feedback you are more likely to find you must use valuable resources addressing formal complaints. The NHS Friends and Family test is a comparative indicator tool, but it doesn't tell us (or you) everything. Results aren't delivered in real time; they aren't contextualised, and they don't provide the detail necessary to drive specific improvements. It's also limited to the services that treat NHS patients.

> The NHS Friends and Family Test (FFT) was created to help service providers and commissioners understand whether their patients are happy with the service provided, or where improvements are needed. It is a quick and anonymous way to give your views after receiving care or treatment across the NHS.
>
> Since its launch in 2013, around 70 million pieces of patient feedback have been submitted. The FFT is in use across most NHS services, including community care, hospitals, mental health services, maternity services, GP and dental practices, emergency care, patient transport and more.
>
> There is updated guidance from April 2020 for providers about the Friends and Family Test on the NHS England and NHS Improvement website.

West Midlands Ambulance Service University NHS Foundation Trust

The trust's primary role is to respond to emergency 999 calls, 24-hours a day, 365 days a year. 999 calls are received in one of two emergency operation centres. In addition, the trust provides a patient transport service employing 400 staff, a Hazardous Area Response Team of 49 staff, and provides clinical teams to three air ambulances. Air ambulance services in the region are provided by the Midlands Air Ambulance Charity. Paramedics and doctors on the service are funded by the charity but are provided by the trust. They are rated as 'Outstanding'.

The report is clear that the rating was given for staff who 'went the extra mile'. Porters employed by the trust but working on site at NHS hospitals supported patients who were arriving at the hospital or awaiting collection. They sat with distressed patients to provide emotional support. The porters also sat on vehicles with patients where more than one patient was being collected. The ambulance liaison assistants and porters told us of occasions when they had waited after their work hours with patients when transport was delayed, and a department was shutting, for example hospital outpatient departments.

If they were assessed purely on the feedback from the NHS Friends and Family Test alone, I suspect the rating would be different.

The evidence around the Friends and Family Test for this service showed that, from April 2018 to March 2019, the trust scored better than the England average for recommending the trust as a place to receive care with regards to its see and treat activity for five out of the eight months where data was available. However, for Patient Transport Services (non-emergency transfers) the trust scored worse than the England average for recommending the trust as a place to receive care. How then could they be rated 'Outstanding' after inspection? The response rate was very low, with less than 0.1% of eligible patients responding. Trust data for February 2018 was suppressed as less than five responses were received.

This is why context and an understanding of the data is so important. If less than one tenth of patients completed the survey, that means the results are not necessarily representative of the majority of people using the service. People who have a poor experience are more likely to share their views and write reviews than those who have a positive experience. A study of buying habits and customer service in retail completed by Dimensions Research and sponsored by ZenDesk, showed that respondents who suffered a bad interaction were 50% more likely to share it on social media than those who had good experiences, and 52% more likely to share it on an online review site. If these figures transfer approximately to the Friends and Family Test, as one might imagine they would, then it's clear that such a low figure might not offer a fair reflection of what people thought of the service.

So, what can you do about it? An ambulance service might struggle to get large numbers filling in an online or paper form when they've just been provided with a short journey to an appointment; many people who are eligible for patient transport are not able to fill out forms. The new guidance suggests that patients should be able to provide feedback at any point during their care and treatment. The guidance says that providers should ensure that all patients can give feedback if they want to. They should take proactive steps to allow people to give feedback whatever their communication needs. This will be considered under the Caring domain as part of the inspection framework for all eligible providers.

It makes sense (and is a requirement of NHS England and NHS Improvement) to actively promote the Friends and Family Test, in order that results are reliable. If your service is generally 'Good' or better, it's nice for staff to see that recognised. It reassures future service users that they will be well cared for. A positive score of 96% of people recommending the service is far more valid if 52% of people using the service have completed the survey. The guidance says that parents, carers, volunteers or staff can give help to those who need it to give feedback. It cautions providers to be careful that the feedback represents the views of the patient, not the staff, relative or provider themselves. Some trusts have designated staff or volunteers who visit patients and talk to them about their experiences. They may speak to people in the outpatient department, on the wards, in day surgery units or any other part of the hospital and record their views as part of the Friends and Family Test. Some community trusts phone people and ask for their views. In general, people appreciate being asked for feedback and like that someone has bothered to ask.

Milner House, Leatherhead

Milner House is a nursing home that provides care to older people, people with physical disabilities and complex medical needs, which for some includes living with dementia. They were rated as 'Good' following an inspection in October 2019.

The Caring section of the report is a nice read; it says:

"People were treated with kindness and compassion. We observed a special interaction between one person and a member of staff in which they shared a joke and the staff member stroked the person's hair. Afterwards the person said to us, 'We are always like that. Staff are so friendly; you can have a proper chat and laugh with them.' People's relatives and friends echoed that Milner House was a welcoming place to be. One visitor told us, 'There is such a family atmosphere here. I would like to live here when I need care in the future'."

The reason this service is included here is because of the way they used feedback. One woman, Elsie, had been a volunteer at a centre for disabled riders when they were a little younger. She had worked at the centre for over 20 years and missed seeing horses regularly. Milner House had a Wishing Tree initiative where people could make a wish (also known as provide feedback); Elsie's wish was to be with horses again. Unfortunately her physical ill health meant she could not be taken to visit the centre, but the staff arranged for the centre to come to her and she was visited by a large piebald cob pony called Daisy.

Imperial College Healthcare NHS Trust

Horses must be the new dogs…

I had the privilege of inspecting Imperial College Healthcare NHS Trust and was humbled by the commitment to excellence that many of their staff showed. I was invited onto wards to see for myself the care that the staff in a focus group of about 150 staff were so proud of. The staff were providing care in buildings that were no longer really fit for purpose. There were environmental challenges to overcome to ensure that patients continued to receive compassionate care, as the buildings crumbled around them.

A patient in the intensive care unit received a special equine visitor when his wife fed back how important the horse was to him. The patient had been in both St Mary's Hospital and the Hammersmith Hospital intensive care units for about four months. Previously he had competed in dressage for many years with this same horse, 'The Footsy'. Complex arrangements were made (this was in central London) and 'The Footsy' was brought to the hospital with another companion horse to keep him calm on the journey. The patient was accompanied by a clinical team who enabled him to go outside and see his beloved horse. His wife reported that the patient was, "So much perkier, brighter and alert since he heard his horse was coming to visit. It's been fantastic."

Was it worth it? Again, I imagine the staff went home that day with photos of the horses to show their children and remembered exactly why they do the jobs they do. I suspect they were smiling at each other and feeling like a cohesive team. My guess (but there is no direct evidence around visiting horses to support this) is that this patient's recovery was enhanced, and his length of stay may well have been shortened. There is a good research basis for saying that social isolation and disengagement from usual social activities has a significant negative impact on patient recovery and experience in intensive care units. Animals, for many, are part of their families and a lack of contact can feel like a bereavement.

Harveys Gang

Harveys Gang is possibly one of the best examples I have seen of patient feedback and most effective ways of ensuring that a patient understood and was involved in their own care and treatment.

Harvey Buster Baldwin was a six-year-old who became very unwell with acute myeloid leukaemia. He spent many weeks in hospital and developed a curiosity about the vacuum system that transported his blood to the pathology laboratories. This interest in pathology was fed back to the staff. Children's ward staff spoke with pathology staff and a visit was arranged under the supervision of Malcolm Robinson, the Harveys Gang chair. Harvey was given his own white lab coat with a badge that said he was a trainee biomedical scientist. He understood where his blood ended up and why testing sometimes took a long time. He and his parents felt fully involved in his care.

Very sadly, Harvey died a year later but he left an enduring legacy. Worthing Hospital received the world's first Ortho-vision blood grouping machine, which was named in memory of Harvey (and which had his picture on), and Harveys Gang grew and grew. Today it offers young patients across the world the opportunity to understand more fully what happens to their blood or other samples and why. It has reached as far as Tasmania, the USA, Norway, the UAE and many other areas of the UK.

All because a little boy asked, and the staff listened.

St Barnabas Hospice

Another example of people asking and staff listening without judging comes from 'the old' St Barnabas Hospice in Worthing. A group of patients were asked by day hospice staff about activities they would like, to help with service planning and to ensure people felt involved and able to make decisions about how care was provided. Somehow the conversation turned to funerals and understanding what the stage after dying was like. A few patients said they were curious and wanted to know what happened after the curtains at a crematorium were drawn during the funeral service. Rather than dismissing the suggestion as entirely inappropriate, unpleasant or possibly too upsetting, the staff member leading the group suggested the staff might need a little time to think about and come to terms with the idea. It was suggested that the patients who were saying they would like such an activity might want to take a little time to consider whether they really did want this or whether they had just 'gone with the group'.

In the following few days, the chaplain spoke with each person who had declared an interest. They were told what they might experience. They were offered the opportunity of seeing photographs instead. Staff were given the opportunity to explore how they felt about supporting such a visit. Then it was made to happen. A group of about ten hospice patients went to visit a crematorium and see behind the screens. They had the opportunity to ask any questions they wanted and to have honest answers. It was, apparently, a good afternoon out.

I do wonder if sometimes how we respond to specific requests is more about our own fears and anxieties or perceptions about what is right than the wishes of the people we aim to serve. Sometimes it is necessary to listen with an open mind, knowing it is OK to take a little while to consider a request and for people to be offered the chance to rescind their request at any point.

Are they responsive?

Key messages:

- The best service in the world isn't much use to people if they can't gain access.
- Services should be planned around what people need and want.
- Personalised care involves taking risks sometimes.
- Ensuring equality for all should underpin every consideration and decision.
- Good care and treatment are about what people using services want and need, not what staff think they should want.

"No society can legitimately call itself civilized if a sick person is denied medical aid because of lack of means."

Aneurin Bevan

> By responsive, we mean that services meet people's needs.
>
> Services are tailored to meet the needs of individual people and are delivered in a way to ensure flexibility, choice and continuity of care.

In the responsive domain, the Commission considers several aspects of access to care and how well providers and staff meet individual needs.

My background in paediatrics perhaps confers an advantage in seeing that meeting individual needs is not hard. Personalising care does not make it more difficult for staff – it makes for happier more co-operative patients, fewer complaints and a much nicer work environment. As ever, good care costs less. That is not to say you should necessarily redecorate your GP waiting room in sunshine yellow when you know Mrs Jones is due to attend for her leg ulcer dressing because she thinks it's a more cheerful colour than the current beige. Beige can be drab and quite depressing on a wet winter's day though. Perhaps it might be worth asking the people that are sitting there most regularly before you next redecorate? There is no 'perhaps you should' when the place being redecorated is someone's home.

The responsive domain is about how easy it is for people to access services. For NHS trusts, are there enough appointments, and at the right times, to meet demand? For a GP practice, can people get through to the telephone triage system or can they get help quickly in an emergency. For sexual health services, can people see someone without needing to take time off work or school? Can mothers with pre-school children bring their babies with them?

If you are a tertiary centre in, say, London, can patients access all the testing and clinics they need on a single visit? Are there sufficient cardiology technicians to allow the testing to be prior to the patients' appointment with the consultant cardiologist? Or do they have to travel to London on several days for different tests at their own expense or use patient transport services? How does this impact on their ability to work?

How easy is it for people to get to the service? Is there parking on site or close by for women who have just undergone a surgical termination of pregnancy? Are there sufficient disabled parking bays for a child development centre or a pulmonary rehabilitation gym? If it's a specialist service that serves a large catchment, how easy is it to arrive by public transport?

South Central Ambulance Service NHS Foundation Trust

In common with many NHS healthcare providers, there is an ever-increasing demand placed on the ambulance services. South Coast Ambulance Service provides a non-emergency patient transport service which provides transport across Buckinghamshire, Berkshire, Hampshire, Oxfordshire, Surrey and Sussex.

They transport people who are unable to use public or other transport due to their medical condition, and this includes those who are:

- attending hospital outpatient clinics
- being admitted to or discharged from hospital wards
- needing life-saving treatments such as radiotherapy, chemotherapy, renal dialysis or DVT treatment.

The service leaders understand that attending hospital can be a challenging time in a patient's life. They have a Patient Charter that explains the patient's rights and responsibilities when using the patient transport services.

In order to meet the commitment of the charter, the service uses volunteer car drivers. They actively recruit local people who like driving and who like meeting new people. Volunteers use their own cars for patients who experience difficulties travelling to their appointments but are offered a mileage allowance, ongoing professional support, uniform and equipment. All are subject to full recruitment checks and all now complete a training programme.

In areas where there is high demand but a shortage of drivers, the local ambulance crews and team leaders have worked with several local voluntary organisations to recruit and train more drivers. The response to a personal approach has been such that the station staff thought they probably saved the equivalent of two staff for three days a week. It meant the employed crews could focus on people with more complex needs. It also meant the person being transported received support from someone who had a little more time to stop and chat. For the organisation, it meant they were more likely to meet their targets and staff in contact centres were less likely to have to deal with calls about delayed crews. A simple win, win.

Many large hospitals now have volunteers at the entrance who help people trying to find their way around. They give directions and are a friendly face to be greeted by (that first impression is important). In a few places it is taken further, and volunteers will happily walk people to their destination, meaning they don't get lost and delay outpatient clinics.

I've not seen any in a hospital yet, but a few commercial car parks have people on bicycles showing people to the vacant spaces. We went to one in Liverpool near the Hilton hotel where we were at a conference. Gunwharf Quays shopping village in Portsmouth has little green and red indicator lights above spaces to show the vacant ones. It's so nice to be able to drive straight into a space.

Car parking comes up as an issue at virtually every hospital inspection. It's not going to be the same for smaller services where there is less rapid movement and high demand, but in trusts it's an issue. So much so that on one recent inspection I was told it was the highest clinical risk. I suspect the person answering hadn't really understood what was meant by clinical risk but clearly felt that car parking was one of the biggest problems that they faced – it even made the television news.

I wonder whether trusts with multi-stories could use volunteers from a local college or sixth form to direct people to spaces: it could even count towards their Duke of Edinburgh's Gold award. Maybe the fitting of the light system would be cost effective. I wonder how many clinics have been delayed due to car parking issues? How many meetings missed? How many staff late for their shifts?

Certainly, I have been extremely late for meetings due to parking and I recall once getting stuck in a multi-storey in a south coast city hospital for about an hour trying to park.

Stanley Medical Group: Clifford Road

Stanley Medical Group is a large practice providing care and treatment to patients of all ages, based on a Personal Medical Services contract agreement for general practice. The practice is part of the NHS North Durham Clinical Commissioning Group (CCG). The practice offered a 'Commuter's Clinic' on a Tuesday evening until 7:15pm and a Thursday morning from 7:30am for working patients who could not attend during normal opening hours.

From January 2016 the practice was part of a pilot scheme to identify patients who were at high-risk of diabetes, whose needs would not have otherwise been reviewed. From the beginning of the pilot to 19 October 2016, the practice identified 575 patients with impaired glucose regulation. Less than 8% were subsequently confirmed as diabetic. The remaining 92% were included in the practices recall for a review, under the long-term condition review process. Patients were also engaged in the prevention of onset for diabetes and offered diabetes education via the local Diabetes Prevention Program. The pilot scheme will be rolled out across other practices in the North Durham area.

The practice had supported health advisers to run monthly 'Walk away from diabetes' at the practice for those patients identified as pre-diabetic as part of a local scheme.

Berkshire Healthcare NHS Foundation Trust

Berkshire Healthcare NHS Foundation Trust was formed in 2001 and gained foundation trust status in 2007. The trust provides specialist mental health, community health and specialist learning disability services to a population of around 900,000 people within Berkshire. The trust also provides out-of-hours GP services across the county. The trust operates from just under 100 sites across the county, including community hospitals, Prospect Park Hospital, clinics and GP practices. Staff from Berkshire Healthcare NHS Foundation Trust also provide healthcare and therapy to people in their own homes. The trust currently manages 369 inpatient beds across 12 locations, has an annual income of £245 million and employs 4,400 staff members.

Mental health services are at best stretched. There is an increasing demand and resources are precious. A hospital inpatient ward for adults with mental health problems is not necessarily the best place for them to be treated and get well.

The trust mental health service was running a pilot project aimed at reviewing patients who had three or more admissions to the crisis service within the last 12 months. Themes resulting from this audit had shown the need for improved safety plans and improved goal setting from community mental health teams. The project had been running for the past nine months and had resulted in a 28% reduction in admissions for patients who met these criteria. The team were in the process of obtaining patient/carer feedback on their experience of being within the project.

Hollinwood Medical Practice, Oldham

This GP practice is run by Hope Citadel Healthcare Community Interest Company. Hope Citadel Healthcare is a not-for-profit community interest company, who have been commissioned by local CCG's to provide NHS services to the local population where the practices are located. They say of themselves, "We are not your typical GP practice and our aim is to do healthcare a bit differently. It's what we call Whole Person Healthcare."

Whole person healthcare looks at people in their wider setting, as whole people. There is an understanding that good health is not just related to clinical matters but that it is affected by many complex factors such as social, economic, community issues, beliefs, family circumstances and employment. While recognising that people's healthcare needs are complex, there is also an understanding and commitment to addressing needs that place increased demand on GP services. Some of the initiatives they support or offer reduce the burden on the appointments system and reduce costs for the NHS overall. People were given someone to turn to that wasn't necessarily a GP.

Their 2018 report says:

"The provider employs focused care practitioners, and one was based in the practice, GPs referred patients to the focused care practitioner if their physical health needs were being addressed but they required more holistic help. Members of the team encouraged and motivated patients, helping with issues such as housing, debt, benefits and asylum applications and appeals, social isolation, attending appointments within secondary care and encouraging the uptake of health screening. We saw evidence of detailed care planning for these patients, and cases were regularly reviewed by the focused care worker and GPs. The focused care worker had on average 35 active cases seeing patients on a regular basis, but also provided emergency contact in-between appointments. We were provided with many examples of the positive impact the work had on patients and their families lives and data provided by the practice highlighted just some of the outcomes, for example in 2017, 12 patients attended for smear test who had previously refused, six homeless patients were rehoused, five supported through the Asylum process, successful reduced the reliance on emergency services with four patients and they supported 84 patients to receive appropriate benefits."

The practice was instrumental in setting up various social and support groups that supported the needs of the local population, focusing on those most vulnerable and or socially isolated. Some of these were organised and run by the practice and others were hosted by the practice in partnership with other health and social care providers.

The practice hosted a 'Thriving Communities' programme in partnership with the local authority which supported people back into work. The practice also supported initiatives such as adult learner's week. The practice was aware of the higher than average child poverty and poor health outcomes for children within the local area, and so were partnering with the local authority to deliver a new group 'Healthy Gems' – a health education programme targeting families with children under five years of age.

London North West University Healthcare NHS Trust and Infinity Health

The joint winners of the 2019 HSJ Award for Driving Efficiency Through Technology, Infinity Health is a team of clinicians, designers and software developers that worked with London North West University Healthcare NHS Trust to improve workflow and communication challenges and transform the way healthcare professionals co-ordinated their activity and shared critical information. London North West University Healthcare NHS Trust is a large provider with more than 8,000 staff serving a population of over one million people.

The Infinity ePortering solution was implemented in the emergency department at Northwick Park Hospital in 2018 and is used to co-ordinate over 100,000 transfer requests per year. Using the system, staff can request a collection or patient transfer using secure mobile devices and porters can accept and share their activity in real-time. It was a significant improvement for the clinical, operational and facilities teams. The average time to complete a request has been reduced by six minutes, which translates to a saving of over 10,000 hours of staff and patients' time each year. It also brought about improved efficiency and patient experience and transformed staff experience.

Meeting individual needs

"The most thoroughly and relentlessly damned, banned, excluded, condemned, forbidden, ostracised, ignored, suppressed, repressed, robbed, brutalized and defamed of all 'Damned Things' is the individual human being.

The social engineers, statisticians, psychologists, sociologists, market researchers, landlords, bureaucrats, captains of industry, bankers, governors, commissars, kings and presidents are perpetually forcing this 'Damned Thing' into carefully prepared blueprints and perpetually irritated that the 'Damned Thing' will not fit into the slot assigned it.

The theologians call it a sinner and try to reform it. The governor calls it a criminal and tries to punish it. The psychologist calls it a neurotic and tries to cure it. Still, the 'Damned Thing' will not fit into their slots."

Robert Anton Wilson

What do we call people who don't fit into our notion of what a patient, service user or resident should be like?

When we talk of pathways, do we forget that each person experiences the pathway in a different way, and some may have challenges to moving along the pathway? Are we willing to step outside the box and allow care to be personalised, or do we fear that allowing individuality will make the job of providing care and treatment harder?

I'll start with a story fairly similar to the one about Emma in the introduction. It shows the ongoing need to allow considered risk in order to personalise care and improve the experience of people using services. It's slightly more current, so shows that the underlying message about balancing personal fulfilment against risk never really changes. The best leaders, the best services are courageous, but not foolhardy.

Callum

Callum had been known to us since he was a small child. He had a progressive neurological disorder and was referred to the special school my husband was the Head of early in his career. When he started in the primary department, Callum could walk (albeit with a bit of a wobble) and could speak quite clearly; his struggles were just beginning but his parents wanted him settled and in familiar surroundings as his disease progressed. He was an absolute delight, gave everything his best and loved most sports.

As the school expanded, a new sports hall and swimming pool were built. Callum had grown into a 14-year-old who was reliant on a wheelchair and whose speech had become much harder to understand.

Everyone was excited about the new facilities and all classes were offered swimming lessons. It was a beautiful pool; our own children developed their swimming abilities by using it regularly. Callum's class were going for their first swimming lesson since the pool had been upgraded. Everyone changed and gathered on the poolside. The more able-bodied laughed, jumped, climbed, or edged into the warm water, watched by several staff including my husband. Callum was still sitting in the wheelchair in his swimming trunks and towel: He was unable to stand at this stage of his disease. All too late and very sadly, the assembled staff realised that there was no hoist in the pool area; most of the children were physically able and it hadn't been considered in the commissioning. The Equality Act 2010 was still a little way off.

Callum tried so hard to be brave about his disappointment. He was known to be a good swimmer and loved the water and was a frequent visitor to the local sports centre. Toby decided the level of disappointment was not acceptable and spoke with Callum who, whilst having some difficulty with clear speech, didn't lack the ability to make decisions. He grinned widely and pinched his nose in response to the question, "Do you want to dive in from your chair?" The reactions from staff were mixed apparently, but one jumped in the water, in their shorts, ready to act if necessary. Toby pushed Callum to the water's edge and tipped the chair over the side so that Callum could dive in with more enthusiasm than technical skill. He surfaced laughing whilst the staff breathed a sigh of relief and joined in the laughter. He swam for the rest of the lesson and every lesson thereafter. The school invested in a tracking hoist system to allow more children to access the pool and then offered it at the weekends to a local support group for families with disabled children.

I am not suggesting that schools simply throw children into swimming pools without any consideration of risk. There was consideration and mitigation with adults in the water ready to act, a knowledge of the individual and their swimming capabilities and plenty of adult helpers watching carefully. He was old enough to make decisions and understood what he wanted to do. The decision to take the risk was his to make.

Mavis

Mavis had been a patient in an acute hospital for far too long when I met her. She was mildly confused and physically about as well as she was going to be, but not able to manage at home. She was what used to be termed rather unkindly a 'bed blocker'. Mavis was very happy in her corner bed in a bay with five other women of similar age. I went onto the ward, introduced myself, said I'd like to speak to a few patients and enquired which bay had people well enough for a chat. The doctor sitting at the nurses' station said the ladies in Bay 3 always liked to talk. A strange look was exchanged between the ward sister and the Director of Nursing, who was guiding me around. The sister muttered something about checking they were all up and washed before rushing away, which seemed odd given it was just after lunch. The Director of Nursing seemed to be wanting some inane conversation about the new whiteboards (it was a long time ago). I walked towards Bay 3 with the Director of Nursing trying to distract me at every step; I'm not daft, I can smell a rat well enough. Something was going on.

I found Bay 3 and said hello to the five smiling elderly women who were all chattering away except the patient in Bed 3, in the corner by the window. She seemed a little distressed; there were three staff, including the ward sister lined up against the wall trying to calm her. Again, it seemed odd they were calming her from the other side of the bed to where she was sitting, with the curtain pulled part way across the window, on a lovely sunny day. I was curious.

I introduced myself and Mavis told me her name then said they had taken Sammy away. They had stolen his lunch and he would be hungry. She missed Sammy and was worried he was dead. The three staff and the Director of Nursing all looked uncomfortable, squirming almost. They hadn't moved from the wall. I raised my eyebrows and jumped in, "What is going on that you aren't telling me? Who is Sammy?"

Another exchange of looks, a slightly embarrassed glance at me and the curtains were drawn back. "There's Sammy", said Mavis, beaming.

"I'll get his lunch" said the ward sister, reappearing with half a tuna sandwich cut into small pieces. I watched as the healthcare assistant and ward sister helped Mavis walk around the bed to the window where a seagull was frantically tapping on the glass, awaiting his lunch. They opened the window and Mavis fed the seagull very happily. She then returned to her chair and told me what a lovely place it was, how they even let her keep Sammy and helped her look after him.

As I walked out, the Director of Nursing and ward sister began apologising and saying they knew they shouldn't because of the infection control risk but it made such a difference to Mavis who had been quite depressed before Sammy appeared. They told me they resisted any attempt to move Mavis from her corner bed because of Sammy. I asked them to quantify the risk, but they couldn't. I couldn't either but I could see the positive impact the somewhat unorthodox use of hospital tuna sandwiches had. It was a lovely example of staff putting the needs and wishes of someone they were caring for at the heart of their decision-making. I was just sad that the staff thought I might have objected to them making a very elderly patient happy.

Pathways for Care

This is not from a CQC report but ably demonstrates how a commitment to equality and consideration of individual wishes – also known as seeing the individual – helps staff provide excellent care and brings great benefits to service users and staff alike. It is shared with a name change but with the young woman's consent.

Ana

Ana is a young woman who lives in her own flat with 24hr background support and one-to-one support in the community. She has autism and sometimes struggles with accepting her diagnosis, which causes her to have low self-esteem and anxiety (which sometimes result in behaviours which challenge staff). A functional assessment was completed to help identify the triggers to the behaviours she was exhibiting and to develop a positive behaviour support plan to help staff provide consistent and proactive support. In order to ensure staff fully understood the plan and how Ana wanted to be supported, a staff workshop was facilitated by the specialist practitioner.

Ana often found it difficult to manage her emotions and stress, which could result in self-harm. Due to this, the clinical nurse specialist spent a number of one-to-one sessions with Ana, to discuss the feelings she was having and what triggered them. This meant that coping strategies and interventions could be developed as an alternative to self-harming. As a result of the work a Wellness Recovery Action Plan was put together for Ana to refer to daily and for staff to have an additional toolbox to use to provide proactive and personalised support.

Ana was awarded a certificate of achievement for not self-harming for three months – a huge achievement. Her support staff met with her regularly to set goals as part of her person-centred plan. In the past year Ana had achieved a number of goals, including a parachute jump, walking over the O2 Dome in London, and she completed the Duke of Edinburgh gold award which was presented to her at Buckingham Palace. Ana has also just been to London on the train independently to meet friends, which was a real achievement for her. She is now planning more activities and trips independently!

As regards the parachute jump and walking over the O2 Dome – the risk assessment and management process was, with support, led by her. Her family and social worker were all involved. Prior to her move to our service she lived in a residential college who had stated that such activities were too risky to be engaged in, something that Ana found difficult to accept. She is highly motivated to embrace life and experience new things.

The staff accompanied her to training exercises for the parachute jump and to the event on the day in order to provide emotional support. They did not, however, make the jump with her – something that she was OK about. She has said that she would like to do it again with a member of staff, and there are a few volunteers for this, so it looks as though this is going to happen.

The walk over the O2 Dome was a far more energetic affair and involved being tethered to a safety line. No training was required for this and on the day she was joined by her mother and the Pathways for Care Operations Director. They apparently all had a great time.

I am told that little staff preparation was required as positive risk-taking and a focus on wrapping services around people's individual needs, choices and aspirations is an integral part of the culture of the service. I would debate that and suggest a continuous and constant review of the service they provide, a shared team commitment towards risk and enabling people to live a full life coupled with a shared staff and management understanding of risk required quite significant preparation.

How much nicer for staff to enable and support achievement than to write someone off as not being capable of the achievement?

Moston Grange Nursing Home, Manchester

Since 2016, all organisations that provide publicly funded adult social care are legally required to follow the Accessible Information Standard (AIS). The standard was introduced to make sure people are given information in a way they can understand. The standard applies to all people with a disability, impairment or sensory loss and, in some circumstances, to their carers.

The report for this home, which caters for people with complex needs including dementia, says:

"Ensuring information was provided to people in an accessible way was a fundamental aspect of the 'whole service' approach to providing person-centred support. The home had well-established technical solutions in place which included accessing dedicated computer packages that created a wide range of signs, symbols and visual prompts that could be utilised for people who could not access written communication.

"Multi-sensory communication equipment had been purchased and introduced for people who were unable to access verbal communication and we saw this had been used to good effect. Promoting the use of touch as a calming/soothing method of communication for people in distress was also widely used by staff across the home.

"A number of staff were highly proficient and experienced in the use of British Sign Language, and a number of staff were able to communicate with people whose first language was not English."

This is another example of an 'Outstanding' rated service where the rating awarded is about attitude rather than expenditure. The report recognises that staff understood the importance of touch and effective communication.

Its lovely that some of the staff had bothered to learn British Sign Language to allow them to understand and respond to people's needs and preferences. It's not a hugely difficult or expensive thing and must make life much nicer for both the people using the service and the staff. A quick search of the internet shows numerous videos that can be used to learn the sign language. Use your search engine and type in British Sign Language video. It's really not hard. Maybe do a session as part of your staff meetings? Maybe have it playing on a Raspberry Pi computer in the staff room. Have the leaders learn it first as a very good use of role modelling.

British Sign Language (BSL) is a sign language that is the first or preferred language of many deaf people in the UK. There are 125,000 deaf adults in the UK who use BSL, plus an estimated 20,000 children. Which means there are few services where staff do not come into contact with BSL users. Staff learning BSL would certainly help in GP surgeries, polyclinics, acute and community hospitals, care homes, scanning centres, sexual health services and mental health services. It might even help deaf staff integrate and feel supported by their colleagues.

I was at a trust inspection fairly recently and was approached by a learning and development manager who was deaf. She talked to me at some length about the difficulties deaf women faced during labour and how her choices had been limited because her deafness was considered a risk that required a consultant-led delivery. She talked about not being offered an interpreter as BSL wasn't considered a 'proper language'. She spoke about antenatal checks being difficult because the midwife was looking down at her growing bump and not at her face so she couldn't lip read. It did chime and made me think that I had never asked about interpreters for the deaf despite always asking about interpreters.

Defence and National Rehabilitation Centre, Stamford Hall

Facilities and premises are innovative and meet the needs of a range of people who use the service.

Technology is used innovatively to ensure that people have timely access to treatment, support and care.

The Defence Medical Rehabilitation Centre, Stanford Hall, is run by the Ministry of Defence but has strong links and sponsorship from Nottingham University Hospital Trust, Loughborough University and University Hospitals Birmingham NHS Foundation Trust. Its patients are serving members of the armed forces, but it is envisaged that it will also benefit civilians who have suffered traumatic injury. It isn't a regulated service but does provide insight into excellence.

It combines technology with proven therapy. It has buildings and spaces specially designed to aid assessment and healing processes and deliver the specific functions of rehabilitation medicine. It has impressive facilities including gyms, a range of swimming and hydrotherapy pools, a gait lab and all the elements essential for its clinical purpose. That purpose includes rehabilitation of the most seriously injured members of the armed forces but also, importantly, returning those who have been injured in the course of training, sport and road accidents to work.

The design of the building and the architecture have been carefully thought through to match very precisely the clinical needs of patients and best rehab practice. The space includes carefully crafted courtyards which serve a clinical purpose as well as being pleasing in their own right, social spaces, places for relaxation and doing all of those things that serving members of the armed forces would associate with their ship, regiment or air station. It has the feel of a military establishment, but patients know immediately that it is somewhat different. Unlike most medical buildings put up today, it recognises the role that architecture plays, alongside medicine and technology, in creating the right environment to help in the successful rehabilitation of patients.

It puts the patient first, both in the choice of its site and landscape as well as the innovative approach and the attention to detail that the programmes offer to injured military personnel.

It is clear that the planning of the service meets some of the characteristics of an 'Outstanding' service despite not being subject to the hospital's inspection framework. It goes further though, and it is the attention to detail and personalised care that really marks it out as exceptional.

Will

People's individual needs and preferences are central to the delivery of tailored services. The services are flexible, provide informed choice and ensure continuity of care.

Will is a young man of 26 years of age. He is a corporal in the army. Unfortunately, he suffered a head injury whilst taking part in competitive sport and needed surgery that involved removing a bone flap from his skull. He was at the centre for rehabilitation after discharge from the acute hospital where he was treated. To reduce the risk of further injury to his brain, which was only protected by his scalp, he was advised to wear a protective helmet during the day. It was a pretty standard white helmet with wide chin straps; very clearly worn for medical reasons. Will didn't like wearing it despite the persuasion and reasoning by the staff.

Realising Will's determination and sense of self was of huge benefit in his rehabilitation programme, the staff found an alternative. They asked the Defence Medical Centre Benevolent Fund to pay for a specially adapted baseball style cap with a peak and logo from a sports team that Will supported. The cap did not need a chin strap but clipped on at the back of his neck. When worn underneath a 'hoodie' it looked remarkably similar to outfits that many image-conscious young men chose to wear.

With his new helmet Will was more prepared to face the outside world and venture out on activities and visits as part of his rehabilitation programme. How he looked was vitally important to him and the staff recognised that this had an impact on his recovery.

Concord Medical Centre

Concord Medical Centre is situated within the Bristol, North Somerset and South Gloucestershire Clinical Commissioning Group (CCG) and provides services to about 14,500 patients.

> There are innovative approaches to providing integrated person-centered pathways of care that involve other service providers, particularly for people with multiple and complex needs.

The practice had invested in a scanner to test patients with suspected osteoporosis. It offered a free assessment for its own patients and a private service for those from other practices. This meant local patients received their diagnosis more quickly and without needing to attend hospital. In one year, the practice had provided 213 patient scans, including 136 for the local hospital to help reduce patient waiting times.

The practice had developed a joint service with the local oncology centre to provide in-house treatment for their own patients and patients from other practices in the community. The practice has the facilities to see up to 20 patients per day and offer a specialist treatment suite and community garden to support emotional well-being. The treatment provided at the practice includes chemotherapy, osteoporosis infusion treatment, biological monoclonal antibodies, blood tests, PICC line care, electrolyte replacement, venesections for polycythaemia and immunoglobulin infusions.

Greenside Court, Rotherham

Greenside Court in Rotherham is a nursing care home for adults with complex needs. It is currently rated 'Outstanding' overall.

The very best services recognise that they can't do everything in isolation. Sharing knowledge and working in partnership to improve services is always going to make for better outcomes for people using services. I'm not sure I'd want to go to a nightclub anymore, but I'm delighted to see providers taking risks to broaden people's horizons rather than keeping people safe, in cotton wool coverings.

Their report says: "The service was taking part in an exploratory study, with Leeds University. This study helped the provider have a better understanding of how people with disabilities maintain and make sense of the changes in their sexual, intimate and relationship needs, whilst living in a complex care setting. This had enabled the provider in the development of training, policy and practice. People who had taken part in the study had shared the learning with others and had been empowered to try new activities, such as visiting a nightclub. They were said to have achieved a sense of well-being, felt valued and listened to, and been able to develop and maintain relationships."

Cumbria, Northumberland, Tyne and Wear NHS Foundation Trust

This trust provides a range of mental health, learning disability and neurological care services across the north of England.

A little while ago the BBC shared a film about how the team on Marsden Ward in Sunderland had created 'Little Boxes of Love' for carers of people with dementia. These boxes included a candle, chocolates and love heart sweets, a photo frame and tissues. Included were cards with kind, inspirational words. They were created to let the carers know they were being thought about and that the staff understood the challenges they faced.

Follow this link to get the printable PDF: https://bit.ly/30LseDy

Sometimes excellence in the responsive domain is about personalising the care of families as much as the care of the people using services. The families of people living with dementia should be very much part of the team. They hold the key to staff knowing who the person hiding inside the patient with dementia is. They can share familiar music, touch, photos of past memories and the person's earlier life.

Similar boxes have been used by numerous services working with patients who are dying with a Coronavirus infection and the idea is readily transferred to other settings. There is nothing stopping any GP service sending a card of condolence or a child mental health inpatient unit sending regular updates to families that live far away.

Michael and James

Michael is a 28-year-old man who raises money for the critical unit at Western Sussex Hospitals NHS Foundation Trust by running marathons. He is an ex-patient who was diagnosed with Guillain–Barre syndrome, which affected his nerves and left him paralysed.

James was a young man I helped care for many years ago at the Hospital for Sick Children Great Ormond Street. He was 14 when he was admitted and also had

Guillain–Barre syndrome. Before their diagnosis both young men were healthy and active. James was a rugby player, as I recall.

Michael had been in the intensive care unit and was very weak. His mood was also affected and despite daily physiotherapy, speech and language therapy, occupational therapy and input from the medical team, his progress was slow. The team thought about how to help and considered hydrotherapy as possibly something that might be beneficial. They had never taken an intensive care patient for hydrotherapy previously and there were risks because Michael breathed through a tracheostomy.

It's that bit about thinking outside the box and being prepared to take a few risks to offer truly personalised and exceptional care. It would have been easier to leave Michael on the unit, recovering slowly and accepting that a young man was likely to feel a bit down if they were paralysed. The team decided that the risks and additional effort were worth taking. Within a few days they had researched and planned how to transfer a high-risk patient from the intensive care unit to the hydrotherapy pool. They thought carefully about safety. They risk assessed and developed guidelines. They held practice 'dry-runs'. The whole team was involved.

The sessions in the pool helped improve Michael's strength and mobility and as a consequence his mood also improved and allowed him to drive himself to an even better recovery. He returned to full fitness such that he could run marathons.

Risk has its benefits for all – the patient and their family.

James's needs were a bit different. He was a child and his parents were ever-present at his bedside. He'd been too ill to be anything but compliant in the critical care unit: his parents were simply grateful to have him alive. After he began the long process towards recovery, he was moved out of the critical care unit to the respiratory ward (because he was stepping down from ventilation and his chest muscles remained weakened). He was an absolute delight to spend time with, brave, intelligent, determined. Inspirational even.

Unfortunately, weeks of tiny steps felt like forever and he did become a bit despondent for two reasons. One was because he was a talented violinist who felt he'd never be able to play again and the other was his seemingly incurable athlete's foot. His feet itched like mad and he couldn't even scratch them.

It was arranged for him to have a visit from Sir Yehudi Menuhin to talk about his violin. Sir Yehudi turned up without any fuss and slipped quietly in James's cubicle with just a nod to the assembled staff who were pretending they were doing something close by. There was chatter and laughter. Then, there was the most beautiful, soul wrenching sound imaginable and the ward fell silent. Even the toddlers stopped to listen. It was entirely mesmerising. I'm not often moved to tears, and rarely by music, but I don't think there was a dry eye on the ward. It was simply beautiful.

Talking later, apparently Sir Yehudi had not pulled any punches with James. He told him that the struggle was necessary if he wanted to play. He explained how he had practiced daily since the age of four and that most people have a gift, but only if it is cherished and grown. That, he said, required hard work and determination through the darkest and hardest of days. James listened and then beat Sir Yehudi at chess.

Sir Yehudi returned several times to see James and play for him. He brought with him the most expensive violin in the world which is currently valued at over $16 million and trusted James to hold it. His input gave James a new sense of purpose; he wanted to show Sir Yehudi what he had achieved since his last visit. Slowly and steadily he progressed and eventually walked out of the ward.

His athlete's foot was treated by resorting to a very old-fashioned method of soaking his feet in Potassium Permanganate solution. He had pink feet but didn't mind because the twice daily foot spa's, where he had a soak and then we used a hairdryer to ensure his feet were fully dry, was a nice bit of pampering. Plus, his feet stopped itching. I suspect we carried on the foot spa's after the fungus was cleared but it was a nice time to talk.

"The violin, through the serene clarity of its song, helps to keep our bearings in the storm, as a light in the night, a compass in the tempest, it shows us a way to a haven of sincerity and respect."
Sir Yehudi Menuhin

Berkshire Healthcare NHS Foundation Trust
Some providers are making excellent use of social media and online services to provide support for patients and families in innovative ways. Often it is as important to support the families as much as the patients.

This trust has developed an online network for parents and carers of children with social communication difficulties or Attention Deficit Hyperactivity Disorder (ADHD) with access given by invitation only: The Young SHaRON (Support, Hope and Resources Online Network) online forums for service users and carers. The resource allows parents to post questions and comments, it is monitored and moderated by the clinical team. It also encourages peer support and guidance from other parents.

The service has a well-established carers group that runs weekly in both east and west Berkshire. It is facilitated by the services carers' lead who displays a genuine passion for the role. The group runs for two hours and is well attended with many carers returning regularly. There is a four-week rolling structure that covers: mental health services and diagnosis; helping relatives in crisis; and helping relatives in recovery. The final week has a question and answer forum with a panel of senior managers and medical staff from the service. The group aims to be supportive within a relaxed, and sometimes humorous, atmosphere.

Luther Street Practice, Oxfordshire

Luther Street is an urban service offering primary healthcare to people who are homeless including residents of five hostels. This clearly demonstrates a practice that has thought about the demographics of their local population and developed services accordingly. It's that thinking that is necessary. It's no use taking a good idea and thinking it will make you 'Outstanding' if you simply replicate it. You might want to take a good idea and think how it might work in your community or how you might adapt the idea for different groups.

"The practice had a clear ethos to improve the health of people who are vulnerable and those in excluded groups. Patients were very positive about the care and treatment they received, and we saw many aspects of outstanding care. All patients received a comprehensive health check on first registering with the practice, this helped to identify health and social care needs early. Appointments were for a minimum of 20 minutes to accommodate the more complex needs of patients. Volunteers supported patients by encouraging those who might not want to attend. All staff were involved in planning care and treatment at daily team meetings, ensuring a co-ordinated approach to meeting patients' care and treatment needs.

"The services included on-site podiatry and dentistry, which helped people access these services and staff visited homeless patients in remote locations to deliver care.

"An award-winning patient participation group involved homeless patients through surveys, and the feedback helped to change the way services were delivered."

Cuckoo Lane Practice, Hanwell

The report for this London based practice shows that good ideas have a multi-faceted positive impact and reinforce the premise that good care results in lower costs. The financial impact from both the examples given below means savings for the practice as well as savings for the wider NHS. Patients coming to the surgery is cheaper than home visits. Patients not missing appointments means less cost. Patients being supported to remain well in their homes with continuity of oversight and early intervention means fewer admissions. The King's Fund suggests that 70% of hospital inpatient bed days are for the elderly with continuity of primary care being shown to make a significant difference to that figure.

More importantly, it is much better for patients and staff. An elderly person who is supported to attend the surgery is less isolated because they have social contact from the support worker. Isolation is a huge issue with many elderly people developing depression and a decline in physical and mental health as a result of that isolation. If they have a regular review by the same GP or practice nurse and they are brought to the surgery by a trained volunteer or support worker, they are less likely to develop depression. If they don't develop depression, they are more likely to eat and drink to stay healthy. They may well be walking to the car with all the benefits which every step they take brings.

The practice report says:

"An example of integrated care for older people is that an Age UK support worker attended the practice three days a week, to support older patients who live on their own. The practice also provided transport to improve access for those patients who are housebound or find it difficult to get to the surgery. Patients reported satisfaction and liked being able to attend the surgery. This improves socialisation and reduced the amount of home visits by 20 during its first month.

"The practice took part in the 'shifting settings of care' program which supported patients with mental illness transitioning from secondary care to primary care to ensure a safe discharge process. A mental health worker, employed by the secondary care trust, would attend the practice every two weeks to meet with people recently discharged from hospital. The support offered was holistic which included information and advice about housing, income, social and general health. One impact being 19 patients who would have previously received care in secondary care settings in the past are now receiving their support and treatment in their GP surgery.

"The GPs also had access to a consultant psychiatrists help line at Ealing hospital where they would discuss concerns such as medication swaps and co-morbidities. Patients who experienced poor mental health were kept on a register and invited for annual reviews with extended appointments. Reception staff we spoke with were aware of signs to recognise for patients in crisis and to have them urgently assessed by a GP if they presented at the practice. The practice scored 100% for their Quality and Outcomes Framework (QOF) target for dementia."

Beech Hall, Leeds

Beech Hall is a residential care home providing personal care for up to 64 people aged 65 and over, many of whom live with dementia. The home consists of purpose-built accommodation spread across three floors. Two of these floors have been specially adapted to meet the needs of people living with dementia.

In the most recent inspection, the home scored an 'Outstanding' rating for the caring, responsive and well-led domains. It is a lovely read. The consideration of how to allow people to choose their activities and a little 'thinking outside the box' means that people are encouraged and supported to participate and enjoy activities and to stay mobile. That Silent Disco sounds like huge fun but it underpins falls prevention and pressure damage prevention. It helps people retain core stability without even realising it. Activities provided by staff who are genuinely interested in those activities has to be better than sitting around the dining table for yet another round of bingo delivered by a care support worker who is thinking about the silent disco they are going to at the weekend. I suspect the staff also enjoyed the silent disco; it certainly makes their job easier if more people are enjoying themselves and retaining their mobility.

"There was an exceptional range of activities available to people which enhanced people's quality of life, tailored to the needs of people living with dementia. Each of the three floors had its own individualised programme of activities based on people's preferences. People were able to access activities in any area of the home, giving them a large choice. During the inspection, a Silent Disco visited the home, with people happily dancing and singing.

"Each staff member was empowered to plan and deliver their own activities based on their strengths and interests leading to a highly creative approach to activities. This led to a great variety of activities delivered with passion and confidence by staff, including shopping trips, trips to the zoo, dancing, sewing, baking and growing vegetables. Throughout the inspection we saw people receiving an extremely high level of stimulation and interaction from staff."

The London Nightingale Hospital

One could, I suppose, argue that the Nightingale and Seacole hospitals set up as a response to the Coronavirus pandemic was the NHS at its most responsive. Certainly, they are a powerful example of the commitment from healthcare professionals and other key workers across the country to ensuring they continue to serve and meet the needs of their local population. They have seen an unprecedented coming together of staff from all sectors, sharing the planning and the execution of a significant increase in intensive care capacity nationwide.

Indeed, one of my team returned to the 'frontline' and went off to work at the London Nightingale. Others volunteered, but Emma actually got to don her scrubs and started working shifts. She has since returned to work in the Commission and shared a lovely story of how, despite the surroundings, staff still managed to humanise the care people received.

The NHS Nightingale hospital had a family liaison team who contacted the patient's family within six hours of admission and then daily. As part of the admission conversation, the family liaison team completed a poster which was laminated and stuck onto the wall of the patient's bed space. From this information, staff found out the patient, their work, their likes and dislikes and who is important to them. One patient lived with his wife and three sons, and he was a Muslim. The poster showed a request from the family to play an Islamic prayer on YouTube five times a day, in accordance with Salat, second Pillar of Islam, the requirement for all Muslims to pray five times every day. The Nightingale team were able to do so by using one of the portable computers at the patient's bedside. The patient seemed to respond well to hearing the prayer and was more alert, but calm and peaceful.

Accident and Emergency Department, Portsmouth Hospitals NHS Trust

There is a CQC report published in February 2019 which states, "There were occasions when the privacy and dignity of patients was not protected". As I may have mentioned before, even where there are some concerns about services, many people still received good care.

In 2019 a close friend, Edward, was referred to the trust for a prostate biopsy. Unfortunately, he haemorrhaged at home a day afterwards and was admitted via the accident and emergency department. He was seen quickly and cared for in a side room, because he were very embarrassed about the need for frequent trips to a lavatory and a very messy appearance. This was someone who was usually dressed in a suit and in charge of a large organisation; he was not used to feeling vulnerable or being less than perfectly groomed.

The team at the hospital were very respectful and thoughtful when Edward suggested going home rather than being transferred to a ward overnight. He had a wedding anniversary trip to Paris booked for the next day and intended to be on the Eurostar, as planned. Instead of transferring to a ward (his main concern was a shared bay and being left languishing rather than being pro-actively managed) the team and emergency department consultant, Simon, allowed him to remain in 'his' side room in the department.

The urologist was also accommodating and thoughtful, working to the timeline of the trip. He suggested deferring to the afternoon to see whether everything had settled sufficient to make travelling out of the country a safe enough option. Working with the patient rather than sticking rigidly to usual practice meant the patient did not discharge himself and agreed to remain overnight for observation.

The emergency department consultant arrived early the next morning carrying a large Americano with cold milk; he knew that the patient had refused the department instant coffee and was stubborn enough to continue to do so. The urologist also made sure, as promised, that he saw Edward before his morning list started and signed him off as fit for discharge and travel, dependent on normal blood test results, without needing to be seen again.

The emergency department reviewed the blood results and waved the patient on his way in time to drive to Ashford to catch the train a little later than intended, but still allowing three days in Paris. His padlock showing 25 years of marriage was hung on the Pont de l'Archevêché (Bridge of Love) because the staff had 'gone the extra mile'.

Personalised care is not usually expensive or complex. Often, people generally just want quite simple things. What raises care to the level of excellence is staff knowing that they can support and deliver personalised care and then deciding to do so. Personalised care is not about what staff or managers think people want but understanding and asking what is important to the people using the service. It's about listening and understanding what is important to people. Nothing more.

St Mary's Hospital, Newport, Isle of Wight

Making information accessible and ensuring the needs of patients and their families are met is important in an accident and emergency department. People coming into an emergency department are often frightened and uncertain. They don't want to bother staff who are terribly busy, so they sit fretting and worrying about little things.

St Mary's was a bit ahead of the field in providing basic information in a very accessible way. They introduced wipe-clean information boards in each of the cubicles in their major's area of the department ahead of most other trusts. I'm not sure everywhere else yet provides the same level of information in such an easy to see way. The boards show which colour uniform is worn by whom and who you may see in the department. It also gives the location of drinks vending machines and the café, along with where the cash point is and the phone number of local taxi firms.

End of life care

"Death is not the opposite of life, but a part of it."

Haruki Murakami

"Death is a challenge. It tells us not to waste time. It tells us to tell each other right now that we love each other."

Leo Buscaglia

Can there be any aspect of care or treatment that is more important to get right? I think it's the Royal Surrey Hospital NHS Trust who suggest, "You only die once", and who focus on ensuring that each person's death is in accordance with their wishes. End of life care is genuinely everyone's business and touches virtually all registered services. In acute hospitals it is inspected as a separate core service and for hospices supporting people to a good death it is their core purpose (whilst recognising early input from specialist palliative care teams can extend both the quality and quantity of life).

Levi

I still remember being taught about good end of life care on the respiratory unit at Great Ormond Street. On reflection, I can see it set the standard by which I measure all other provision.

If I could remember the full details of Levi's care and treatment, I suspect it might show it was 'of its time' and there would be room for improvement, if viewed through lenses that offered a current perspective.

I know at the time that we made every effort to afford the children and families that we worked with every possible respect and comfort. My education about respectful end of life care was taught by a night-sister called Dorcas. She was a truly kind and knowledgeable nurse. I was a senior student in charge of the ward, and we had a very unwell, but beautifully smiley, six-month-old baby called Levi, who had a rare condition that affected his breathing. We knew, and the parents knew, he wasn't expected to live very long. Dorcas came to do rounds and I explained that Levi seemed 'off colour', he'd been with us a few weeks, so I knew his usual patterns of behaviour. He was off his feeds, sleepier than usual, a little clammy and 'just wasn't himself'.

She went into the cubicle to see him, tickled his tummy and spoke gently to him. She then said I needed to phone for his parents to come over from the flat they were renting near the hospital, as Levi really was very unwell. She stayed with me and we tidied the room and Dorcas brought a lamp from somewhere, so there was a gentle warm light. She told me to get Levi's drugs a little earlier, so that he stayed comfortable, and then to ring someone from an adjacent ward to complete the 10pm drug round. She meanwhile made a phone call to ask the Rabbi to attend, as soon as possible. By the time his parents arrived Levi was unrousable and floppy; barely breathing. He had oxygen but his skin still had a grey tinge and his lips were darkening.

His parent's arrival was followed shortly afterwards by the Rabbi with two nurses that I didn't know and a doctor from another ward. Levi was lifted gently into his parent's arms. The parents asked for a lock of hair and an instant photograph to be taken, using the ward camera.

Very few words were spoken that were not Hebrew prayers. Dorcas had found some Jewish staff to come and support the family, as their own community was too far away to provide immediate support. We slipped outside and I was sent to fetch a white flower from the front desk (there were always white flowers at the front desk for these times), to check the two juniors were coping and to ensure we had the necessary items to care for Levi after he had died. Then we slipped into the cubicle as Levi slipped from life. The Jewish doctor confirmed death and the Rabbi led the post death care. We simply stood by, unhurried but present.

After some time, we walked with Levi, his parents, the Rabbi and the Jewish staff to the mortuary where we were taken to a quiet room and Levi was lifted gently, by the Rabbi, from his parent's arms. We had no words that would comfort the parents. Platitudes seemed irrelevant in light of their unimaginable anguish. We left them to the care of the Rabbi and the grandparents, who had arrived by then.

It was both the saddest and, in an odd way, the best night of my nursing career. I remember feeling fairly useless and too inexperienced and young to offer much. I am also certain that, because of Dorcas, however sad the situation was, no child or parents could have had better or more personalised care. A few weeks later, I received a thank you note that I have still. It said that simply being there, providing a quiet and reverent presence was more appreciated than I could know.

Dorcas taught me that good care is about delivering what is right for the patient and their family, that sometimes doing little is as important as rushing around doing lots of things. It is all about attitude.

In adult social care services, end of life care is contained within the judgement about responsiveness, which is why it sits here. Inevitably, it cannot be delivered or assessed in isolation from other aspects of care and must be considered as part of other domains, too. Appropriate use and governance of opioids is a safety issue; nutrition and hydration sit within the effective domain.

We've become unaccustomed to death and somewhat fearful of it, despite it being the only certainty throughout life. We expect modern medicine to treat, to heal, to cure and usually hide death away in unspoken words. At some point, we have to recognise our own mortality or that of people we love and those providing health or social care services need to be prepared to step in, to open up the conversation, to give permission to discuss fears and to acknowledge truthfully that life is finite. In my experience, the unknown always creates more anxiety and more unhappiness than dealing with reality.

Euphemisms may help if you meet someone with a dying relative in a supermarket, but they have no place in health and social care services when discussing someone's approaching death. A lack of clarity leads to misunderstanding and mistrust.

From the Adult Social Care Key Lines of Enquiry

How are people supported at the end of their life to have a comfortable, dignified and pain-free death?

The Daffodil Mark

The point where many people first acknowledge or hear that they may have a condition that may be (or may be perceived as being) life limiting is with their GP. People who have been healthy all their life may find themselves in the GP surgery in older age; people with progressive disease may find themselves needing an increased level of support and treatment, pregnant women faced with the unimaginable pain of a difficult decision around an unborn child diagnosed with an anomaly that is incompatible with life may turn to the GP they trust to help them find the answer.

Some GP practices will now display a yellow daffodil mark because they have committed to improving end of life care. This is a new partnership between the Royal College of GPs and the terminal illness charity Marie Curie. The practices involved agree to improve their care in three of the eight standards each year. Over a three-year period, all of the eight standards should have been reviewed and the practice should be able to demonstrate improvement.

The eight Daffodil Standards are:

1. Professional and competent staff
2. Early identification of patients and carers
3. Carer support – before and after death
4. Seamless, planned, coordinated care
5. Assessment of unique needs of the patient
6. Quality care during the last days of life
7. Care after death
8. General practices being hubs within compassionate communities

These are specific to GP practices, but it wouldn't be difficult for other service types to take the same standards and consider how they could improve against them, would it? Not all would apply to all services, but some would apply to most providers. A care home for people with learning disabilities might want to ensure staff had training in end of life care; a domiciliary care agency might want to set up a formal support system for carers who had been involved with an elderly person for several years before their death; a mental health inpatient unit might want to ensure that there is proper guidance, resources and training to enable staff to provide care in the last few days of someone's life. An independent healthcare hospital might want to introduce ReSPECT forms and assessments for people admitted for end of life care, or for whom it becomes clear they need end of life care during their admission.

Namaste Care International

Namaste Care International is a not-for-profit membership organisation for the global promotion of Namaste Care. In 2016 they launched an initiative to bring Namaste Care into the global mainstream of care provision. Namaste Care International is a member organisation open to individuals and companies in all areas of healthcare. They have Namaste Care Champions in England, Greece, Australia, Iceland, Canada, the Czech Republic, Scotland, the Netherlands, Singapore and the USA.

The word 'Namaste' means 'to honour the spirit within' and Namaste Care honours the individual receiving its services. Developed and pioneered in the USA by Professor Joyce Simard, it was originally developed to help improve care for people with advanced dementia. The two basic principles of Namaste Care are creating a calm environment and providing all activities and interactions with an unhurried, loving touch approach. Namaste Care helps people with advanced illness to live, not simply exist, for as long as possible. It improves the end of life experience for the person with a terminal disease, their families and carers.

In common with many of the very best examples of care, the resources required are minimal and the financial cost is low.

Care homes and end of life care

End of life care is clearly an essential consideration for every care home. A good home has clear strategies and policies to guide staff and ensure the best possible care is provided as people's lives draw to a close. Many care homes provide particularly good end of life care in a calmer setting and with a very gentle approach by staff.

One of the first things that should perhaps happen, is supporting the local GP practice to meet and improve against Standard 8 of the Daffodil mark – general practices being hubs within compassionate communities. A care home team and the local GP practice should be working together to improve the end of life care for people using the service. There is little point in a care home having an anticipatory medication policy if the GP won't prescribe anticipatory medicines. Similarly, there is little point the GP spending time talking to service users and their family about delivering the right care, at the right time, in the right place and their ceiling of care if the care home staff insist on calling an ambulance to someone in their last days of life who starts having a Cheyne Stoke breathing pattern. Care home staff and GPs need to work together.

Every care home provider needs to have a clear strategy that is known to staff and service users (or their families), and which is created in collaboration with other providers of services to people resident in the home. It should detail how the home will provide personalised care to those who are dying, drawing on the national guidance and encouraging the dying person to make as many of their own decisions as possible.

A trained member of staff should have a conversation with the person or their families well ahead of the last few days of life. Can you imagine if you'd attended services at a Cathedral every week since you were 16, but nobody thought to ask you whether you'd like a vicar to come and give a final Holy Communion? What if your children had chosen a non-faith-based path through life and couldn't remember your favourite hymns but wanted them played at the funeral – wouldn't it be better if someone had thought to ask? Imagine you had been married for 40 years and nobody thought to suggest a photo of your spouse was with you when you died.

I remember caring for a woman in late middle age in the last few days of her life; her daughter had brought a disposable razor and some shaving gel and wanted me to shave her dying mother's top lip. To me, it seemed a bit of an odd request and I think I said as much, probably reassuring them that it wasn't something to worry about and that nobody cared about a few dark hairs. Her daughter just looked at me as if I were a numpty who knew nothing about caring for her mother – which in fairness and on reflection, held some truth. She explained in carefully enunciated words that her mother was quite image conscious, she liked to be fashionable and well-groomed at all times. Her mother had hated the dark shadow that appeared on her upper lip and had always had it waxed regularly; it was very important to her. Her daughter asked me (in a nice way) who I thought I was, to dismiss it as not worth worrying about. Her mother, she said, would want to be well-groomed as her life closed as much as when she was full of life.

She was right. It was not for me to determine what was important to the patient or her family. The last photograph the family had taken together should show their mother as being beautiful and moustache free. It is so important for health and social care staff to understand what is important to the person rather than assume they know what the patient needs.

"If you want to be happy, practice compassion. If you want to be happy, practice compassion."

Dalai Lama

Dorset Integrated Care System in collaboration with Easier Inc NHSE Personalised Care Group

The BMJ Opinion published an article, 'Personalised care: what matters to you?' in March 2020 about an end of life care collaborative that focused on improving end of life care in Dorset. The article written by Saskie Dorman, a consultant in palliative medicine and Andy Brogan, a founding partner of Easier Inc, shared the story of a patient who was failed, but which led to a review of how personalised care was delivered.

"A 90-year-old woman near the end of her life is hoisted from a hospital bed, semi-conscious, for staff to take a photo of the pressure sore on her bottom. Two hours later, her husband arrives on the ward to find that she has died.

"How did we end up here? When looking through healthcare records, why is it more normal to see photos of pressure ulcers on backsides than photos of faces?

"This patient had been taken to the hospital that morning because staff felt it was unsustainable for her to stay at home. She'd become weaker over the past few weeks and developed incontinence. Her husband, also 90, found this hard to manage. She knew that she was dying, and we knew that she preferred to stay at home. But somehow the system didn't seem able to support that. Her needs weren't particularly specialist or complex, but somehow admission to hospital seemed like the least bad option from the perspective of the nurse visiting her.

In their 90 years, this couple hadn't used the health service very much. When they did need it, we fell short. Despite everyone involved caring deeply — from the nurse who arranged to take her to hospital, the paramedics who wanted to set up a drip en route, the ward nurse who took the photo, the regulator who wants care to be above all safe and to protect people from avoidable harm—and despite everyone doing their best to do their job — we let this couple down."

A terribly sad story of someone not being afforded a good death.

I am delighted to say that the regulator's framework has been updated and has a far more holistic approach to end of life care in hospitals – there is still a need to ensure that the underpinning basics are being delivered safely, with good medicines management and a culture that learns from mistakes but the balance has changed to include assessment of how well providers are listening to people and their families and enabling personalised care.

The collaboration has changed the focus to one of 'Results through Relationships'.

The authors go on to describe the benefits of good end of life care to individuals and to the system. I cannot improve on their writing:

"Of all our lifetime healthcare costs, a third is spent in the last year of our lives. Healthcare costs—particularly hospital costs—rise dramatically in the last weeks of life. With stories like this, it's easy to see why this may happen. Care which focuses on tasks—rather than what matters—costs more overall and tends towards outcomes that no-one wants.

"We can do better than this.

"We can create a world in which it's normal to ask each other and talk to each other about what really matters to us. We can give each other the time, knowledge, confidence, freedom and support to respond in highly bespoke ways to the people and circumstances we find. And we can make it normal to find out and do what matters most to a patient rather than just what's expected.

"Creating that world may not always be easy and will take some courage. It will mean stopping doing some of the things we do now, some of the things which we have become accustomed to doing and that may make us feel safe.

"For the patient we described above, this would mean the chance to stay at home on the last day of her life, and for her husband to be with her when she died—even though the circumstances were not as we had anticipated. It would mean being able to rest in comfort rather than being hoisted to have a photo of her pressure sore—recognising that her dignity and comfort were more important than following the 'standard protocol'.

"It will therefore mean not only challenging the ways we care for the people, families and communities we support but also the way that we care for each other within our institutions. Only then may we feel like doing what really matters is doing what really matters here."

They have worked with stakeholders across the local health economy to consider what people were saying was important; they have really listened to the people they serve and developed a new way of looking and a new way of working. They have moved from a narrow focus on the last days of life with a task orientated approach to a broader understanding of end of life as the last year of life. The focus has changed from intervention to relationships and living rather than dying.

They talk about moving from OVER testing, treating, diagnosing, referring, prescribing to UNDER standing.

Their key message is that learning to do ALWAYS, ONLY and EXACTLY what matters is both better and cheaper...

Ethel and Percy

Some 45 years after I cared for her, I can still see Ethel's face clearly. She was a sweet and gentle woman who had been admitted to hospital after falling at home. Her husband, Percy, was already an inpatient on a different ward. Ethel was fairly confused and being cared for in a side room, as she was quite noisy and this disturbed the other patients. She was physically quite well, but hadn't been eating properly for some time, so needed 'building up'. We used to indulge her sweet tooth with milky hot chocolate drinks and jam sandwiches.

Sadly, Percy died and there followed a lengthy discussion about the funeral arrangements and whether there was any benefit to Ethel attending. The consultant had told Ethel about Percy dying but, while upset at the time, she didn't seem to retain the information and was rapidly back to enjoying the extra puddings we sneaked to her.

I and a couple of others felt quite strongly that she should attend her husband's funeral. They had already celebrated their diamond wedding and it felt wrong to deny her the chance to say 'au revoir'. There was a significant voice from others who felt there was little purpose and too much risk, that she might be unsettled or might fall, and we'd be held responsible.

Luckily, the ward sister was aligned with the 'she should go' side and only wanted to understand how those who supported attendance might ensure that Ethel was accompanied, and that the ward was still adequately staffed. The consultant sat on the fence and agreed that it wasn't really a medical decision as she was well enough, but that it would do no harm.

In the end, I took Ethel and the consultant offered to drive us. It was a somewhat bizarre event, both sad and moving but with a slightly surreal edge. Ethel insisted we sat at the back of the empty chapel at the cemetery. There was a congregation of seven, which included Ethel, her niece and her niece's husband, the consultant, two of the funeral director's staff who agreed to make up numbers and me. Ethel thought the flowers we had persuaded the hospital flower shop to donate were beautiful and that it was a lovely service. She kept asking who was 'in the box' and became momentarily upset on hearing it was her beloved Percy, but quickly rallied and said she'd need to, "Tell Percy when she got back, as he'd have wanted to come, if he could".

Why was it important and was it the right decision? To this day I have no regrets about taking Ethel. She had an absolute right to say her final goodbye, in whatever way she could. Percy was the most important person in her life and dying well is about consideration of what is important to people. Percy would have wanted her there. Her niece knew that and was pleased we had made the effort; she left the funeral tea in the ward day room knowing that Ethel was being cared for with genuine compassion and that Percy was laid to rest surrounded by the most important people in his life.

Do we deny people living with dementia the right to say goodbye, I wonder? I hope not.

Two Rivers Medical Partnership

The GP service is a training practice with four partners based in two medical centres in north Hampshire. They are currently rated as 'Good' by the Care Quality Commission.

One of their GP registrars was asked to visit a nursing home where someone was very unwell. The doctor realised the person was dying and wanted to phone the family to ensure the person had someone with them and that the family were involved in their final hours, if possible. Unfortunately, the number held by the home was not answered, despite numerous attempts throughout the day. The home did not have any other contact information for relatives.

The doctor felt uncomfortable not making contact and looked for other options; they noticed a water bottle shaped as 'Our Lady of Lourdes' – a white plastic Madonna wearing a blue crown lid, adorned with roses and carrying a golden rosary: something only a committed Catholic was likely to keep in a prominent place beside their bed. The person had lived all her life in the local area, so the doctor felt it was worth a call to the local Catholic priest to see whether he might know the person and possibly have contact details for her family. The doctor balanced the risks of sharing confidential information against leaving someone to die alone and decided the sharing of limited information was better than having nobody familiar with you when you are dying.

The priest did know the woman very well; she had been a parishioner for many years. He didn't have contact details as she had not had children. He was aware there was a nephew, but the home already had his number and there was no response. The home care staff were very busy with a number of quite unwell residents, the doctor did not want to leave the person to die alone and it was arranged that they would stay whilst the priest drove over to the nursing home. The woman received the Sacrament of Anointing of the sick, which is often especially important to practicing Catholics as they approach death, and clearly recognised the priest. The doctor ensured the woman had appropriate drugs and that the home staff understood fully what the plan for symptom control was overnight, before leaving. The priest was given a comfortable chair and stayed beside the woman throughout the night, holding her hand and talking gently to her about things that were familiar. She died early the next day, slipping gently from a peaceful sleep into the arms of her God, knowing she was with someone who cared deeply for her and whom she trusted completely.

She had what most aspire to, a good death.

What made it good?

- Having professionals in the GP practice and nursing home staff who cared enough to make a difference.
- Staff with an attitude of finding solutions and thinking outside the box.
- An understanding of the importance that good care is holistic, never more so than at the end of life.
- Effective multi-disciplinary working

End of Life care during the Coronavirus pandemic presented enormous challenges for patients, for staff and for relatives across the globe. There are plenty of truly tragic stories of people dying too young who were without those that were most important to them close by. We lost an inspirational colleague to metastatic cancer but because she died at the height of the pandemic in London, none of her work family could attend the funeral and offer personal support to her actual family.

The sadness crosses the world despite a commitment from health and social care staff to remain compassionate and to offer the best care they are able.

Jordana Horn writing for Kveller

Kveller.com is a Jewish parenting website. The account needs no narrative from me for people to understand the pain when people can't follow their chosen path when someone they love dies.

On Sunday morning, my husband and I drove down empty highways to the cemetery, some 30 miles away. It was my longest trip out of the house in weeks. The funeral director approached our car, standing at a distance of six feet from our window. She told us that, due to restrictions on the numbers of people at the cemetery, the hearse and casket would have to go to the gravesite before we did. Once the casket had been lowered into the grave and the gravediggers left, only then could we proceed to the grave.

We waited in the cold rain, a triangle of six feet of distance on each side – my husband and I at one point, our rabbi at the second, and my husband's brother and his wife at the third. The two brothers couldn't even embrace. We stood in the cold, hands only warmed by rubber gloves, waiting for the gravediggers to finish their work.

The gravedigger foreman, mask over half his face, came over and told us brusquely that only three people in total would be allowed at the grave due to the prohibition against gatherings. Apparently, all my husband's prior discussions were for nothing. And those three people, the gravedigger said, would be the funeral director, the Rabbi, and one mourner.

The not-so-pleasant 'discussion' with the foreman over this point took 20 minutes, at the end of which he stated that he would take only three people to the grave – and then he would take his leave, "and what you do then is up to you".

"That guy needs to work on his bedside manner," I muttered to my husband in spite of myself as we headed to the grave, once we saw the foreman beating his retreat.

"I think you mean 'dead side manner,'" my husband offered.

Any comfort provided by humour, however, was gone by the time we got to the grave, keenly feeling the absence of all those who would otherwise have been there – the grandchildren, my siblings and parents, my father-in-law's long-term caregivers, my husband's friends and those of his brother. The wooden coffin lay at the bottom, separated from us. It was not lost on me that we were also separated by six feet.

In Jewish tradition, the mourners shovel the first dirt into the grave, covering the coffin. Not only could we not share embraces with each other in these strange times, we were also told before arriving that we could not even share a shovel: we were instructed to either bring our own shovels or simply throw handfuls of earth into the grave.

The thumps made by the sound of earth hitting the coffin were excruciating. I have always felt shaken by that sound at funerals past: each 'thump' sounds like an emphatic period at the end of a life. But the sound brought tears to my eyes this time as I realised that, in a 'socially distanced' funeral, this was the only small bit of contact permitted us: only the casket and the earth were allowed to touch.

There was no traditional meal of consolation awaiting us when we got back to our house, and no mourners pulling up to the curb to spend time with us as my husband sat shiva. During the seven days of shiva, mourners are supposed to have every physical and emotional need met by their community. Friends and family sit with you, feed you, and share your stories or your silence. Mourners are never supposed to be in isolation – they are always supposed to be surrounded by community.

Instead, we sat in front of a computer screen as 'visitors' dialled into a Zoom shiva room. Like some sad version of The Brady Bunch on a monitor, people from all points in my husband's life dropped in and out to pay their respects.

Shona, Zoe, Lorna and Corinna

I don't know where these four members of staff work, I don't know their surnames or paygrades. I think maybe they work in Berkshire, so am guessing it's the Royal Berkshire County Hospital intensive care unit, but I could be wrong. I know throughout the difficulties they faced caring for dying patients in the pandemic they remained compassionate and considered the needs of patient's families. They recognised the fears and anxieties of relatives who wanted to be close but couldn't. They used a simple brown box with a simple message signed by the four staff. The message said:

"The nurses wanted you to know that your relative was not alone when they died. We sat with them and held their hands. The box contains a wooden heart with their fingerprint and a lock of their hair tied with a ribbon. We are so sorry for your loss."

It was then signed by hand by the four nurses.

Darent Valley Hospital

A similar brown box was given to someone in the Gravesend area. I don't know the nurses named but their little brown box contained a heart, a handprint with the person's name, date of birth and date of death, and a card with seeds that will grow as plants for years to come. This message was handwritten and said:

"Firstly, can I say I express our greatest sympathy to you and your family at this time. As I mentioned on the phone, here are mum's keepsakes. My email address is .... should you wish to get in touch about meeting some of the staff when the hospital re-opens to the general public.

Warm regards from all the staff on ITU."

Apparently, the consultant called the daughter a few days after her mother's death to see how she and the rest of the family were coping, they then called a month later to see how they were getting on.

As with most aspects of excellence, it is about attitude and a culture of kindness.

Spiritual care

Spiritual and cultural care is often an overlooked, or uncomfortable consideration when thinking about the holistic needs of people. It's an issue that many staff won't see as important or even relevant in everyday life, and not much to do with healthcare. The best providers might help staff understand that because it is not important to them, it doesn't mean it is not important to the people they serve. It can be incredibly hard for some staff to understand. They may eat pancakes on Shrove Tuesday but have no idea where the tradition comes from. They probably call it pancake day not Shrove Tuesday. The 2011 Census showed that almost 60% of people living in the UK considered themselves to be Christians, 4.4% followed Islam. There were 1.3% who were Hindu and 0.75% who were Sikh. Another 0.45% were Jewish. Just over 25% of people said that they did not have a religion. In 2003 an Ipsos MORI poll reported that 18% were "a practising member of an organised religion", which means that an awful lot of people who identify as having a religion don't practise but might well want consideration of their beliefs when facing their own serious illness or the end of their life or that of someone they love.

All too often the question asked (often with a glazed expression) is simply, "Religion?"

That rather devalues what may be an intrinsic and important aspect of people's care. It depersonalises a very personal subject – few people can say they are observing all aspects of their own religion or cultural norms.

There are Catholics who use contraception, divorced Catholics and gay Catholics. I know Muslims who drink alcohol, who wear bikinis and eat bacon sandwiches. The degree of observance amongst the Jewish communities will vary enormously from those who tend to orthodoxy to others who celebrate the major festivals of Judaism but who do not routinely observe the Sabbath. Not all Jews obey the dietary laws, or 'keep kosher'; sometimes their observance depends on what denomination of Judaism they belong to. Most Reform Jews consider the laws of Kashrut to be an outdated ritual and ignore them completely. Others keep kosher at home, but not while dining out or at someone else's home. There are atheists who find time for quiet contemplation within a Christian church and atheists who attend Catholic Mass because they enjoy the music or to support their spouse.

A person's spiritual beliefs may be complex and unexpected. A response to the question, "Religion?" may give a completely erroneous understanding of the person. They may have been born a Jew, raised in a convent and become a Quaker in later life but still want to celebrate Hanukah and enjoy listening to the Ave Maria.

At key moments, and particularly as life's end approaches, people's perspective can change, and they may want to start asking questions about what happens at and after their death. The families of someone who is dying or who has died may find comfort in religious rituals having not been near a place of worship in many years. It is really quite important that staff are sufficiently comfortable discussing spirituality and religion and sufficiently interested to allow the people they care for or treat to feel comfortable to ask those questions. It can't all be left to a chaplain or a visiting cleric. I'm not suggesting all staff need a theology degree, but they do need to be respectful of people's beliefs and practices and skilful enough communicators to listen. It is such an integral part of so many people's lives.

I am sure we can all think of people who have been able to find comfort from believing they will be reunited with their adored spouse in the afterlife. I imagine most people will know parents who have told children that granny is twinkling as a new star in the night sky. I can't count the number of times I have been to the beautiful chapel at Great Ormond Street to find parents who have found solace in lighting a candle and quiet contemplation while their child was having major surgery.

Do we tell patients and relatives where the chapel is? Do we tell Muslim patients what facilities there are for prayer and offer a Qibla compass? Do we even keep a Qibla compass on wards where there are likely to be Muslim patients?

What about in care homes? How do you provide for the needs of someone who held a strong religious belief throughout their adult life? Does dementia mean their religion is no longer important?

Healthwatch Suffolk

Healthwatch Suffolk produced a report in 2017 called *What does spiritual care look like within three care homes in Suffolk?*. It aimed to share good practice.

Within the report is a foreword by the Chaplain of St Elizabeth's Hospice, the Reverend Jo Perry, which explains:

"St. Elizabeth's Hospice has moved from the language of 'chaplaincy' to one of 'spiritual care'. As the Chaplain, the ribbon I wear holding my badge bears the words 'spiritual care'.

Within the Hospice we have changed how we view spirituality. People have a wide range of beliefs, some are Religious, others are Spiritual but not Religious (SBNR being the academic term). We're adapting rather than holding on to a conservative view of spiritual care.

We seek to recognise where people are at and what their needs might be, because people in our care, whether relative or patient, are facing the biggest challenge of their lives, which brings spirituality into focus.

A challenge for the spiritual care team and the Hospice is that a patient or relative may not be spiritually articulate. Before the illness they may not have recognised themself to be a spiritual person.

When having to face mortality questions can arise. Such as, what is important in life? And what isn't important in life? This can happen to anyone having a big life change or illness, whether terminal or not. None of us are as prepared for that as we may think we are, we can all have an awakening of spirituality at that time

Good spiritual care encompasses all beliefs, religious, non-religious, and none. Those with no beliefs still go on a journey and exhibit a spiritual need – they may be coming to terms with the life that has been, which may not always be the life they wished for."

Lois Hickley, a mental health lecturer at the University of Suffolk, says in the Healthwatch report that spirituality has broadened in its meaning beyond religion. This new perspective being drawn from themes in literature include a sense of purpose, a sense of 'connectedness' to self and others, with nature, 'God' or a quest for wholeness. It can be seen from this that a patient need not have a belief in God or a religion to experience spirituality. Much of the research on spirituality is in the field of palliative care, for at this time spirituality can come into sharp focus.

Seckford Alms houses and Jubilee Hall

The Healthwatch report asks the question, "How are people given the care and support they need, in terms of their age, disability, gender identity, race, religion, belief or sexual orientation?" They give the answer in a description of what they found:

"A prominent feature in the Seckford Alms house's is the Chapel, which is part of the local Parish of St. Marys.

Prayers are held in the Chapel on Wednesdays and there is a monthly Anglican service on Sundays. There is an adjacent Chapel Lounge. On the day we visited there was a funeral service taking place in the Chapel for a resident who wished to have their service there.

There is a fortnightly Quaker meeting held at the home. The Head of Care explained how all staff are very attentive to people's needs, especially at the end of life stage, adapting their support and care for both the resident and their relative's needs.

For example, for a resident who was a very devout Christian, a member of staff offered to say prayers with her and ensured she had the music and flowers and a wooden cross in her hand, as she had wished for. These wishes had been discussed with the resident beforehand and were in the resident's care plan. The staff, as a team, collectively helped ensure the resident's wishes were respected.

When a resident has died an electric candle and a card are placed in the hall, to let everyone know.

Some residents attend church services and faith-related groups elsewhere in the locality.

The manager gave several examples of sensitivity to individual needs. There is a tradition of Christmas gifts being given by the Home to each resident. Planning starts in October with staff pooling ideas to match the gift to the individual.

The manager shared an example of a gentleman who was a resident who had a Jewish faith, and how they listened to and respected his preferences, offering an appropriate choice of menu, for example, and supporting him in choosing his time for prayer, and discussing with him how he wished to take part at Christmas.

At Lent, especially for residents who were used to fasting and giving alms, there is the opportunity to have a Lent Lunch, for example soup and a roll, and to choose to donate. The residents choose the charity to benefit.

The Head of Care explained that they endeavour to see each person as the individual they have become through the story of their life so far, to thereby be best able to support them on their continuing journey."

Nightingale House, Wandsworth Common

Nightingale House is a care home that can accommodate up to 215 older people across six self-contained units, each with separate adapted facilities. Three of the units specialise in providing nursing care to people, while the three other units were residential and provided people with personal care. The majority of people living at Nightingale House were living with dementia. In August 2018, the home was rated as 'Outstanding'. The report is a truly inspiring read; I could copy the whole thing as an example of personalised and thoughtful care. I recommend using an internet search engine and reading about the work they do and the attitude of providing the best care. It's humbling.

The home serves the Jewish community and the spiritual and religious aspects of the home centred around the Jewish faith. The report recognises the importance of this for many people who were living at the home:

"People told us staff understood the Jewish faith and culture. One person said, 'They celebrate all the main Jewish holidays and festivals here, just like my family and I would do at home'. A relative also told us, 'The bonus for us is that this is a Jewish home, so our faith which is really important to us as a family, is very much supported and celebrated here'. Information about people's spiritual needs was included in their care plan.

The provider had their own religious coordinator and on-site synagogue. People and their relatives told us the synagogue was always open and they could visit whenever they liked. Staff told us if people were too frail to attend the synagogue the religious coordinator would visit them in their room or unit.

Staff received equality and diversity training as part of their induction which had included a module about understanding what it means to be Jewish, and Jewish Faith and culture in general. The registered manager told us several specially trained volunteers regularly presented seminars to people living in the home, their relatives and staff on Jewish history, and specifically the Holocaust.

The catering staff demonstrated a good understanding of how to prepare kosher food to conform with Jewish dietary law. For example, the chef was aware the main kitchen and pantries on the units all had specially designated areas for preparing and cooking meat and milk separately, so these two food groups were never mixed in accordance with the Jewish Faith.

Staff received end of life care training, which included a specific module on understanding death and dying from the perspective of the Jewish faith. They demonstrated good awareness of the special candlelight ceremonies (known as 'Yahrzeits') that were often held in the home to commemorate the lives of people who had died at Nightingale House".

St Catherine's Nursing Home

It's shut now, but I visited a nursing home in West Sussex many years ago that was run by a religious order. The employed nursing staff were supplemented by young nuns who travelled from India to work in the home as part of their training. Many went on to register as trained nurses and some were already registered but completing adaptation programmes, having recently immigrated.

These additional nursing staff allowed an exceptional level of personalised care and meant there was no rush to get everyone up and dressed each morning. Baths, showers and personal grooming were at the pace that residents wanted; there was time for hair styling, make-up and nail varnishing, if people wanted it.

Most but not all residents were from a Catholic background and felt extremely comfortable being cared for by nuns. There was a corridor through into the parish church and daily Mass, which people were supported to attend regardless of their disabilities or level of dementia. People from the local community attended and brought the community into the home; they shared coffee and cake after the service and chatted with residents, some they had known for many years.

It was interesting to see the effect of the familiarity of the Mass on people who were living with quite advanced dementia. Sons and daughters could join their elderly parent at the Mass and see them connect, remembering the words to prayers perfectly and knowing when to sit, when to stand and when to kneel. When I tried to connect with the same elderly people over lunch, they were disengaged and unable to respond much at all.

As people approached the end of their lives, they were supported by the staff they knew well. They were never left alone and one of the nuns sat up through the night in case they woke or were distressed. The sisters gently sang the words of familiar hymns and shared their vigil with family members, whenever possible. Everything about the environment was familiar to a practicing Catholic – the sounds, the smells of incense, the rhythm of prayers.

When death finally took over, the person remained in the home (assuming the family wished it) and the person made their final journey from the home, through the link corridor for their funeral in the adjacent parish church. The funeral was the usual daily Mass and the family, the nuns, any residents who wished, and local parishioners attended. I remember people telling me that it was reassuring to know they would be looked after by people they trusted and who would walk beside them as they reached their earthly journey's end.

Are they well-led?

Key messages

- Good leadership sets the standard for an organisation and is worth investing in.
- A compassionate culture is the foundation stone of high performing organisations.
- Leadership is not something that can occur in isolation from the rest of the team; leaders are part of the team.
- A shared and explicit vision of what excellence looks like in your service, or area of a service, is key to moving in the right direction.
- A leader's role is to support the staff to deliver high-quality services by setting the standards and helping them achieve their goals.
- Vision alone is not enough; there must be efficient systems to identify gaps, to monitor quality and safety and to drive continuous improvements.

"A leader is a dealer in hope."

Napoleon Bonaparte

"Leadership is the art of getting someone else to do something you want done because he wants to do it."

General Dwight Eisenhower

"Great leaders are almost always great simplifiers, who can cut through argument, debate, and doubt to offer a solution everybody can understand."

General Colin Powell

"It is better to lead from behind and to put others in front, especially when you celebrate victory when nice things occur. You take the front line when there is danger. Then people will appreciate your leadership."

Nelson Mandela

"I didn't get there by wishing for it or hoping for it, but by working for it."

Estee Lauder

"You can design and create and build the most wonderful place in the world. But it takes people to make the dream a reality."

Walt Disney

> ## Well-led
>
> By well-led, we mean that the leadership, management and governance of the organisation assures the delivery of high-quality and person-centered care, supports learning and innovation, and promotes an open and fair culture.
>
> The leadership, governance and culture are used to drive and improve the delivery of high-quality person-centered care.

Are leaders born or made? Can we all be inspiring and effective leaders? Indeed, are we leaders or managers? How do we get to be good leaders? What influences us?

This is an area staff at all levels would do well to reflect on. Leaders are not just those in senior management positions. Managers may even find they have staff working for them who have a greater influence on service delivery and their teams than they do themselves. There are great leaders at all levels within most organisations, regardless of their experience and sphere of influence. How do you best harness this 'natural leadership' to ensure it is used positively?

The well-led question is so important to how well services meet the needs of the people who use it, that it is inspected as a stand-alone domain. Within the hospital directorate, there is a separate part of the inspection process focused exclusively on leadership at all levels within an NHS trust. For Primary Medical Services there is recognition that leadership is key to other areas of care. There is guidance, for example, about using the questions in leadership interviews to provide assurance on the safe domain. The importance of building a positive culture is recognised by the Chief Inspector of Hospitals, Professor Ted Baker who said in an interview in March 2019, ahead of the GS1 UK Healthcare Conference, "Culture is the core that needs to change if we are going to be able to keep moving forwards on safety".

Some people talk about leadership and management as separate things. Both are essential for a successful health or social care service. As Peter Drucker suggested in 2007, management is doing things right; leadership is doing the right thing. In health or social care settings the dividing line is very blurred.

There are non-negotiable reporting procedures that are imposed by providers and external agencies (including the Statutory Notifications required by regulation, for example). Oversight of these sits clearly with management, doesn't it? It may be, however, that persuading staff to complete the required reporting processes is probably more about leadership than management.

A memo posted on a noticeboard or a policy on the intranet is not going to persuade most staff to check that fluid balance charts are totalled or that the results are acted upon. Monitoring a patient's fluid balance to prevent dehydration or overhydration is a relatively simple task, but fluid balance recording is notorious for being inadequately or inaccurately completed (Bennett, 2010). Simply telling people to do this everyday task is rarely going to be enough. The true leader will work with the team to find a way of ensuring more regular and accurate completion. They will understand that solutions and improvements devised and owned by the team are far more likely to be sustained. The leader might ensure that staff understood the importance of monitoring fluid balance as a means of identifying acute kidney injury but will not necessarily impose a solution that is simply to remember to fill in the charts.

Similarly, in a GP practice, an all-staff email from the practice manager is not going to persuade busy, salaried GPs to check liver function after starting a patient on statins. A leader allowing discussion at a practice meeting might hear how the GP registrar had seen a good reminder system in place at their previous practice. One of the partners might then take responsibility for setting up a pilot and carrying out a before and after audit with the GP registrar.

The obvious outcome is improved outcomes for patients on statins. The add on outcomes are a staff group that felt listened to and shared accountability for improved patient care.

Primary Medical Services

"Where the decision resulting from an Annual Regulatory Review (ARR) is that: there should be an inspection, and the focus of that inspection does not include the safe key question

You can still gain assurance about Safe through asking a set of trigger questions when inspecting well-led.

These questions are designed to test whether a provider's governance arrangements continue to ensure that safe is at least Good (as previously inspected and rated).

This approach is only applicable to practices that at the last inspection were rated 'Good' or 'Outstanding' overall and 'Good' or 'Outstanding' for both safe and well-led."

Self-awareness and reflection are probably more critical to leadership than to any other aspect of running a successful service. Unless you understand yourself, unless you understand how you formulated the views you hold and how you react to individuals and groups, you are going to struggle to lead a service to excellence.

You need to understand what your personal view of excellence is and whether this is a commonly held or shared view (and if not, whether your view is reasonable and achievable or a bit 'left field' for your staff team). If your view and vision is quite extreme and differs hugely from the norm for the sector or corporate perspective, you might need to consider whether it is the right vision for a service; perhaps you need to listen hard to the people who will be delivering on the vision.

That is not to say left-field visions and ideas are to be discouraged – some of the seemingly wildest ideas have led to the greatest innovation. Nobody wants to stifle innovation in health and social care, but it will never reach fruition if you cannot persuade others to share your view.

If Jean-Henri Dunant (a Swiss businessman) had not been in Solferino in 1859 and had not had the idea to convince the population to service the wounded without regard to their side in the conflict, and also to secure the release of Austrian doctors captured by the French to assist the wounded. There would be no International Red Cross Movement and there would be no Geneva Conventions regarding the humanitarian treatment of people in war.

Today, the International Federation of Red Cross and Red Crescent Societies (IFRC) co-ordinates activities between the 190 National Red Cross and Red Crescent Societies. On the international stage, the IFRC organises and leads relief assistance missions after emergencies such as natural disasters, manmade disasters, epidemics, mass refugee flights, and other emergencies. As per the 1997 Seville Agreement, the IFRC is the Lead Agency of the Movement in any emergency which does not take place as part of an armed conflict. No small achievement for someone who just had an idea.

Understanding your organisation, the people and the context is also key to driving improvements and creating a positive culture. There is no single effective leadership style. Leaders need to adapt to the people around them and the task to be most effective and avoid having a detrimental impact. We all tend to have a preferred management or leadership style: what is important is to recognise that and understand how we need to modify our approach depending on what needs to be achieved and by whom.

I've been fortunate to work with some excellent leaders and teachers; to see the very best in action and benefit from their guidance and support. Some who had a significant impact on me were very humble and unassuming and probably wouldn't recognise their talents. I am a little sad that I cannot remember all of their names – I can picture them still, but as part of a generation who called teachers, 'Sir' or 'Miss' and who trained when ward managers were simply called 'Sister' and referred to by the ward 'Sister Observation', they must remain unnamed.

Not all the managers I've worked for have been the kindest or the most effective – one or two I would actively avoid still. A few years later and I can see they helped teach me what sort of leader I wanted to be by showing me, very clearly, the behaviours I knew were unacceptable.

Bryn

Bryn is the reason I know that kindness and consistency, clear expectations and compassionate support really do work better than criticism and condemnation. Our involvement with him taught me so much. He remains the ultimate example of how changing a culture that people are exposed to really can change individuals. I learned from him that kindness and compassion are not synonymous with weakness – exactly the opposite, in fact. He is also a clear example of how education and learning are the most effective tools for change.

I'm not sure we ever set out to foster teenagers (indeed, I know we didn't), but it happened because it's impossible to turn away a child that is frightened, wearing saturated clothing, hungry and very angry at 2 o'clock in the morning. At the time, my (then) fiancé, Toby, and I were both working with children living in incredibly challenging circumstances. Toby was teaching in special education and Bryn had been in his class a few years previously. We knew Bryn had been through a tough time growing up and had been excluded from several mainstream and special schools, but we also knew he was 'salvageable' because we'd seen the relationship he had with his elderly step-grandfather and the loyalty he showed friends and teachers he respected.

That night Bryn couldn't return home as he'd just destroyed his stepfather's brand-new car; he'd been wandering the streets until he thought of somewhere he could safely turn up to at 2am. We were living in a multi-agency residential children's resource and assessment centre, so he knew where we were and that we might have a spare bed and some food. We sorted him out and let him sleep until we called his parents the next day. His parents refused to have him home or to speak to him. His mother was simply too frightened to talk to her husband about their parental responsibility. The local authority wouldn't take him because he wasn't currently in danger; they knew we were unlikely to throw him out onto the streets and he did have a family to return to. They had no alternative suitable placements for a young man of 15 with challenging behaviours. He stayed with us for about six years, until he was 22 years of age.

The precipitating factor for him breaking up his stepfather's car with a crowbar was being involved in a road traffic accident that had horrific consequences. He had a bit of a habit of 'taking and driving away', stealing motorcycles and riding them through town onto an area of rough ground for 'a bit of a laugh'. He couldn't read but could strip any engine down and rebuild it; starting cars and motorbikes came easily to him. Tragically, Jack, the friend he was with, rode the motorcycle, without a helmet, across the bonnet of a car travelling at speed and was seriously brain injured. Jack spent a good while in intensive care whilst his father, who also had learning difficulties, took up residence at the hospital. It was probably the first time in his life that the father or Jack had felt cared for.

Bryn was really distressed at having witnessed his best friend changing beyond recognition. He showed his distress in the only ways he knew, through violence and extreme anger at a world that had allowed him to watch his mother be beaten with the slats from his bed and which tolerated him being hurled from a moving lorry when much younger. His cultural norm was violence. Toby sat as the appropriate adult, with a good solicitor doing pro-bono work, through numerous police interviews. We became used to our doorbell ringing at 5am and finding the local police sergeant on the step; we knew him well from our professional roles. He was a kind man and could always be persuaded to have a cup of tea whilst one of us woke Bryn, rather than forcing his way in to arrest him.

Unfortunately, Bryn was charged with a string of offences and we were fairly certain he was facing a custodial sentence. We also knew that would destroy him. Inside he was a vulnerable and muddled child that felt the whole world hated him; a youth custody centre wouldn't change that view.

We were fortunate to have a good friend in the local police sergeant, the one who regularly arrested Bryn. He was completing a PhD in restorative justice at the time and was keen to use Bryn as a case study, if he could persuade the court. The outcome of the trial was that Bryn escaped a custodial sentence, but that there was a programme of restorative justice he had to complete. As a condition, he was required to live with us; we were given responsibility for his care and welfare until he reached 18 years of age. We were in our 20s, just setting up home together and didn't seek that, but could hardly refuse.

The recordings of the calls he made to a young policewoman were quite harrowing to listen to. I can only imagine how frightened she must have been. I do know that locking him up with other offenders would probably have increased his involvement in criminal activity rather than reduce it and would not help him understand the impact of his behaviour on others.

Bryn refused to attend a special needs college course; he was very rude about those he had been at school with and the opportunities such a course might offer him. He did agree to attend a 'normal' (his word) car mechanics course.

We worked hard with him. We negotiated with the local college and succeeded in securing a place on the course but with the proviso we arranged his work placement. Toby taught him to read using his obsession with VW campervans and car magazines (basic literacy and numeracy was a prerequisite of course admission set by the college).

We bought a battered VW campervan and spent many weekends camping and visiting rallys and other likely venues to see VW vans with Bryn and his only other friend, plus the brain-injured Jack's 12-year-old sister (who also moved in with us, having fallen through a gap in service provision before we fostered her, too). I know far too much about air cooled engines, safari windows and splitties from those days. We found a garage owner prepared to give Bryn a chance as, "He'd been a bit wild once too". He took Bryn under his wing and taught him his trade but had exceptionally high expectations. He worked long hours and Bryn used to cycle the eight miles every morning, come rain or shine. No excuses were allowed, and Bryn arrived home very cold, covered in oil and paint, with cracked and sore hands and hardly able to keep his eyes open. We ran him a bath, laundered his clothes, cooked warm, filling suppers, and then he had an hour doing reading practise. We would have let him have half an hour watching television, but he usually just wanted to go to bed. He certainly didn't have any time for him to get into trouble or go off and 'hang around' town.

We set a no smoking inside the house rule and no alcohol except maybe a beer when camping. We filled weekends with structured activities, so there was still no time for him to creep back into crime. He became accepted as part of our family and joined us for all family and friend celebrations and events. He learned a different set of social norms and behaviours. Rather amusingly, when we went away at New Year with a large group of friends, it included the police sergeant (now retired chief inspector) who used to arrest Bryn and a superintendent from the Metropolitan Police who we knew through running children's camps. As our norms became Bryn's norms, he chose to distance himself further from his origins. He gave up smoking, changed his style of clothing, passed his driving test, became a role model for some of the children we were working with and was comfortable joining us at formal supper parties. He continued to work for the same garage owner and passed his exams. He was, finally, a motor mechanic and had body work repair qualifications too. He joined Gerry on breakdown recoveries to earn a bit more money and saved hard. We could not have been prouder of him.

He was an usher at our wedding and looked quite dashing in a morning suit. He knew we trusted him completely when he was tasked with looking after our two-year-old daughter, when our son was born. It was a lovely moment when he arrived at the hospital, to say hello to our latest addition, with a tiny girl on his shoulders.

She had most of her clothes on back to front and inside out and her legs were bare in November. She was plastered from head to toe in melted chocolate, but they were both beaming from ear to ear. Woolly tights were apparently an ask too far!

Bryn is now in his 40s. He has never committed another crime, except possibly speeding (but he's never been caught). He is gentle and kind, with a very well-developed sense of humour and a strong work ethic. He set up his business renovating VW cars and vans and reselling them and is reasonably successful. When we moved from the area, he decided, with some difficulty, to stay behind as he had a good job and wanted to care for his now frail and elderly step-grandfather, who had been the one kind influence in his life.

I have no doubt whatsoever that it was learning to read fluently and being supported to achieve through kindness from numerous people that allowed him to escape being another sad prison statistic. I also have no doubt that this early exposure to the impact of kind leadership and role modelling taught us more than it taught Bryn.

Role modelling

Role modelling is so important for leaders. Absolutely no use setting up an organisational vision underpinned by explicit Values and a Behaviour Framework if leaders don't live by them. There is absolutely no point telling your care staff or junior doctors to be kind if you, as a leader, enter a ward, department, GP practice, clinic or other service and see dirty mugs on a tray in the reception area and start an inquisition to determine who was at fault. It is damaging to the organisation to shout at the culprit in public because they answered a call bell or the telephone rather than clear away immediately. How much better to pick the tray up yourself and load the mugs in the dishwasher? Role modelling, setting an example, shows how much nicer an organisation becomes if leaders live the values (assuming the values are appropriate) rather than just impose them on others.

One of the other people that has had a significant influence on how I developed my understanding of leadership was a ward sister, Anne, who guided me in my first experiences of leadership. She was firm but fair and would never have expected of us a standard that she would not have upheld herself. She was unfailingly kind to those around her; patients, parents, students, her staff nurses, housekeepers, the doctors, everyone. It is that kindness that made her an exceptional ward leader. She set reasonable expectations but also allowed staff to have fun; she understood that happy babies and supported parents were more important than tidy linen cupboards – at a time when tidy linen cupboards were considered essential.

I still have incredibly happy memories of being told to sit and rock a crying little one rather than tidy linen cupboards. If she sent a student on 'errands' such as a trip to the milk kitchen or to another ward to find a tin of tomato soup, we suggested they took one of the bored long-stay patients with them for a change of scene.

We were encouraged to make a shared pot of tea on Sunday afternoons, around the nurses' station desk with the resident and visiting parents. It helped build relationships, trust and understanding, and it taught us to see the young patients and their families as individuals with a life outside the confines of the unit. This in turn meant we could provide more personalised care.

East Surrey Hospital

One of the best examples of a senior member of staff role modelling, providing a positive example and 'living the values' took me by surprise. It was the Chief Operating Officer of a busy NHS Trust. I had seen the COO in action and thought she had clear control over the operational performance of the hospital. It was the role modelling that caught me unawares and which made me see that this organisation didn't just say they had a good culture.

The COO ran the site meetings twice a day. She chaired in a way that I would describe as 'efficient'. The first time I tried to attend the site meeting I was five minutes late and it had already finished. Absolutely no wasted time and an expectation that everyone attending came with the necessary information to support decision-making, and that they concentrated in the meeting. I knew she managed flow through the hospital incredibly well and that she had a good grip on the hospital activity. I knew she was a rapid thinker and able to juggle conflicting demands. I could see she had the respect of the staff and authority over the meetings. I would have described her as efficient, effective, delivery focused: I wouldn't necessarily have used fluffy words to describe her until I followed her along a corridor, later in the inspection.

My view of her changed as I walked. She was well ahead of me and deep in conversation with a matron. They were just approaching the door to the medical assessment unit where a porter was struggling to get a trolley through the doors, whilst also keeping hold of numerous bags belonging to an elderly patient. The patient had dropped one of her bags and, in so doing, the blanket covering her had moved and her leg was exposed above her knee. Without a second glance and without breaking her stride, the COO moved over to the trolley, introduced herself with a warm smile, shook the patient's hand then picked up the belongings and sorted them out whilst also 'tucking in' the blanket. She then held the door wide for the porter. The COO didn't know we were following behind and had seen her; it was clearly second nature and something she just did because it needed doing. That one incident made me reconsider my view of the COO and while I was truly impressed with her strategic and operational oversight of the hospital, I was left smiling at how she could be such a strong chair one minute and then chatting sweetly and gently to patients the next, without so much as blinking. A fantastic example of leadership.

Culture and speaking out

Why is it so vital that organisations listen? What happens if things are such that concerns raised by staff are ignored or worse?

The Public Interest Disclosure Act

The Act protects workers from detrimental treatment or victimisation from their employer if, in the public interest, they blow the whistle on wrongdoing. The Act protects most workers in the public, private and voluntary sectors. The Act does not apply to genuinely self-employed professionals (other than in the NHS).

The Act protects workers in several ways, for example: if an employee is dismissed because he has made a protected disclosure, it will be treated as unfair dismissal. Workers are given a right not to be subjected to any 'detriment' by their employers on the grounds that they have made a protected disclosure, and to present a complaint to an employment tribunal if they suffer detriment as a result of making a protected disclosure.

For a disclosure to be protected by the Act's provisions it must relate to matters that 'qualify' for protection under the Act. Qualifying disclosures are disclosures which the worker reasonably believes tends to show that one or more of the following matters is either happening now, took place in the past, or is likely to happen in the future:

- a criminal offence
- the breach of a legal obligation
- a miscarriage of justice
- a danger to the health and safety of any individual
- damage to the environment
- deliberate concealment of information tending to show any of the above five matters

Dr Raj Mattu

In April 2001, Dr Mattu and several colleagues raised concerns about what they said was the dangerous 'five in four' practice at a hospital in Coventry. The hospital was putting a fifth bed in a bay of a cardiac ward only designed to take four. Their concern was that the practice would leave vital services such as oxygen, suction and mains electricity harder to reach in the event of an emergency. Tragically, a patient suffered a heart attack and died after staff could not reach that equipment in time. But that produced no changes in practice. It did, however, lead to a chain of events which ended with Dr Mattu's sacking in 2010.

An employment tribunal subsequently ruled that Dr Mattu had been unfairly dismissed. His former NHS trust had spent £6m pursuing about 200 allegations against him – which later proved to be false – including using private detectives to investigate him. He had been vilified, bullied and harassed out of a job he loved.

Sharmila Chowdhury

Having enjoyed an unblemished 27-year career with the NHS, Sharmila Chowdhury was sacked after blowing the whistle on senior doctors who were moonlighting at a private hospital while being paid to treat NHS patients. The radiology service manager had repeatedly warned the hospital's senior managers that doctors were dishonestly claiming thousands of pounds every month and that the trust had lost £250,000 of public money through such arrangements.

The hospital failed for two years to take any action against the two doctors, who were later accused of fraud at a tribunal hearing. Instead, Ms Chowdhury was suspended after a counter-allegation of fraud made against her by a junior whom she had reported for breaching patient safety.

The allegation was never proven and in July 2010 the employment tribunal judge took the unusual step of ordering the trust to reinstate Ms. Chowdhury's full salary. However, the trust made her post redundant and offered an out of court settlement.

Kim Holt

Kim Holt, a consultant paediatrician, told managers about serious failings at the clinic where Baby P was later treated just days before his death at the hands of his mother and her boyfriend. Along with three colleagues she wrote to managers in 2006, warning that understaffing and poor record keeping posed a serious risk to patients' safety at the clinic in north London, and that a child would die if action was not taken. But bosses ignored her warnings and removed her from the clinic.

Baby Peter Connelly was seen by an inexperienced locum doctor at the clinic in the summer of 2007, three days before he was killed and after Ms. Holt and her fellow whistle-blowers had left. The inexperienced doctor failed to spot signs that the 17-month-old boy, who was already on the child protection register, had been physically abused. Ms. Holt was reported as saying: "If our concerns had been taken seriously at the time, we raised them, then we could have prevented the death of Baby Peter. Several of the failings found by the inquiries into his death were 100 per cent the same as the failings we complained about the year before he died."

She also said the hospital had offered her £120,000 to withdraw her complaints in the wake of Peter's death – a claim the hospital denied. In 2011, the providers that co-managed the clinic formally apologised to Ms. Holt. That was five years after she raised concerns.

In all three examples given above the costs of not listening were far, far too high. There were no winners.

- Patients died.
- The whistle-blowers were subject to appalling treatment and lost their livelihoods. Some were lost to the NHS.
- There were huge financial costs to the NHS.
- Their treatment undoubtedly stopped others speaking up about poor practice.

An organisation that is unwilling to look at mistakes openly, that hides errors or shortfalls, that doesn't listen to staff when they come up with ideas or raise concerns is not going to be amongst those rated the highest. Sometimes (particularly in small organisations, with low staff turnover) there is an accepted way of doing things. Sometimes national guidance or societal expectations change but organisations don't, and the way of working becomes outdated. Sometimes risks are ignored and not acted upon early enough. Sadly, sometimes staff raise concerns, but the leaders have not built a culture where staff are listened to and the staff stop raising concerns because they don't believe anything will be done. Historically, there are examples where staff concerns have been dismissed but time has shown the staff were right and that people suffered harm, even death, because nobody listened.

Good leaders and good organisations listen. There is a culture of learning and mitigating risk. No organisation gets it right all the time. Those human factors mean mistakes happen, even in the best services. The real problem is when a mistake is ignored, dismissed as 'just a one off' or worse, hidden.

Sally

Unfortunately, as I am no longer in contact and cannot ask her permission, I have had to rename the whistle-blower as 'Sally'. I say unfortunate because her courage deserves to be named. She spoke out against a culture despite ongoing intimidation and ridicule. She must have felt very alone and vulnerable. She remains one of the bravest people I have ever had the privilege of speaking with.

Sally made a phone call that was put through to me, a good few years ago (before the current legislation came into being). She was a senior member of staff at an independent hospital; it was obvious from her language and knowledge of the service that she knew what she was talking about. Sally was upset that she had tried to raise concerns and had been dismissed as a troublemaker who was being unreasonable. She had, sadly, tried to contact the Commission several times and not had much response. Nobody was listening. She was quite distressed on the call and said to me, "I just know someone is going to die if things don't change". She had been through every avenue imaginable and received brush offs and ridicule. I spoke to her for about two hours. She was credible, was willing to be named, could give times and dates of incidents and still nobody had listened.

We carried out an unannounced inspection just before Christmas. The report made the national press. I'm not easily shocked but I was shocked by what we found and heard at that hospital. We had nursing and theatre staff coming to us in tears, confirming the truth of the issues Sally had raised, but frightened for their jobs. We found some significant safety issues and saw quite well-hidden records of seriously ill patients who were mismanaged. It included a child with a pulse of 40 who had not been transferred out for six hours for fear it would look bad. We were told by the then matron, that oxygen and suction was not connected in the rooms of patients returning from surgery because they "didn't want it looking like an NHS hospital". One woman had to undergo an emergency hysterectomy because the hospital managers had not listened to their staff. Another woman, with breast cancer, had an invasive procedure carried out in the outpatient department because theatre staff had told the consultant that the patient's blood tests showed that her white cell count was too low to allow the operation to continue safely.

We suspended their children's service, we took enforcement action and made referrals to both the General Medical Council and Nursing and Midwifery Council. Sadly, Sally was forced out of the organisation rather than used to help bring about changes.

The Francis Report

Sir Robert Francis was invited to conduct a second inquiry into the care provided at Mid Staffordshire NHS Foundation Trust to highlight the contributory factors and make recommendations to try and prevent similar occurrences at any NHS hospital going forward. The preceding inquiry had reported that between 2005 and March 2009, conditions were such that appalling care was allowed to flourish in the main hospital serving the people of Stafford and the surrounding areas. A mortality rate higher than that of other similar trusts had been an initiating factor but the team also found a lack of basic care. Drinks were placed out of reach, patients were left in excrement for many hours, they were not assisted to eat or drink when necessary and they were denied privacy and dignity (even in death).

The report of Mid Staffordshire NHS Foundation Trust Public Enquiry report says:

"It is a story first and foremost about the appalling suffering of many patients. This was primarily caused by serious failings on the part of the provider Trust board. It did not listen sufficiently to patients and staff to correct a series of deficiencies brought to the Trust's attention.

"It is clear that a staff nurse's report in 2007 made a serious and substantial allegation about the leadership of accident and emergency. This was not resolved by the Trust management. These issues were not made known by the Trust to any external agency."

It also highlights a culture of fear about repercussions which meant many shortfalls in care went unreported. The organisational drivers were said to be hard targets and financial savings over the quality of care.

What is sad – beyond sad – is that had they focused on the quality of care and supported quality improvements, the costs would undoubtedly have been lowered and patients and staff would not have suffered from the organisational neglect.

In 2015, the Trust received the largest ever group fine of £500,000 plus £35,000 costs following four avoidable deaths. These were deaths that were not only avoidable but were easily avoidable. Lapses in the real basics of care and treatment; falls, missed insulin doses, a person given penicillin despite the relatives telling the medical team they were allergic to it. These deaths were in an acute NHS trust, but it is easy to see that this could happen in most types of services (albeit not on the same scale).

Sadly, not everyone who is brave enough to raise concerns is valued and listened to. There are numerous cases where individuals have suffered harm from speaking out, although the legislation and requirement to have a Speak Up Guardian has brought about significant improvements.

Gosport War Memorial Hospital

It is over 27 years since nurses at Gosport War Memorial hospital first voiced their concerns. It is at least 20 years since the families sought answers through proper investigation. The persistence of those families means that they have discovered that experts who had found reason for concern had been ignored or disparaged. The investigation panel found that in 465 patients, there was evidence of opioid use without appropriate clinical indication. The Panel's analysis demonstrates that the lives of over 450 people were shortened as a direct result of the pattern of prescribing and administering opioids that had become the norm at the hospital, and that probably at least another 200 patients were similarly affected.

Concerns were first raised by a staff nurse working at the hospital. A fellow staff nurse also wrote to their manager in February 1991 expressing concern over the prescribing and use of drugs with syringe drivers. The documents the panel reviewed showed that, between the first concern being raised and January 1992, several nurses raised concerns about the prescribing specifically of diamorphine. In doing so, the nurses involved, supported by the Royal College of Nursing, put the hospital in a position from which it could have rectified the practice. In choosing not to do so, the opportunity was lost, and premature deaths resulted. Gosport is a story of individual poor practice and an institutionalised regime of prescribing and administering 'dangerous doses' of a combination of drugs not clinically indicated or justified that led to lives being shortened.

Winterbourne View

Winterbourne View was a facility providing healthcare and support for people with learning disabilities. The BBC sent a letter to the provider on 12 May 2011 which gave details of concerns raised by a whistle-blower. The charge nurse had written by email to the acting manager earlier on 11 October 2010 giving details of their concerns. The letter alerted the unregistered manager to the disrespectful, confrontational and aggressive stance of named staff; delays in securing emergency treatment for a patient with arm lacerations; the harmful consequences of corralling patients in a sitting room; and bad staff attitudes. No action was taken, and the concerns were shared with the BBC.

The abuse revealed at Winterbourne View hospital was criminal. Staff whose job was to care for and help some of our most vulnerable people instead routinely mistreated and abused them. Its management allowed a culture of abuse to flourish. Warning signs were not picked up or acted on by health or local authorities, and concerns raised by a whistle-blower went unheeded.

The two examples are not, sadly, isolated. The Report of the Morecambe Bay investigation into maternity services published in 2015 showed heard evidence from two whistle-blowers. Both interviewees were deeply disappointed and disaffected by how they considered they had been treated by managers and colleagues at the trust following what they regarded as a brave step to whistle-blow. Both expressed their distress that fellow clinicians did not share their concerns, even when they suggested that there was evidence to support their claims.

Every example has in common evidence of missed opportunities and warnings unheeded. They are more than that though. They provide salutary warning of what happens when organisations fail to listen and where the culture does not support speaking out. While perhaps on a different scale, there are examples in all provider services, from care homes to GP practices, from independent healthcare to community services. Ensuring patients, staff and relatives can raise concerns and that they are listened to (rather than dismissed) goes far beyond keeping people happy and being 'nice'. It has the potential to save lives, stops mutilating surgery and sexual assault, and prevents the torture of our most vulnerable.

Freedom to Speak Up Guardians

The National Guardians Office is an independent, non-statutory body with a remit to lead cultural change within the NHS so that speaking up becomes 'business as usual'. The National Office provided leadership, training and advice for the Freedom to Speak Up Guardians in all NHS and Foundation Trusts. The office was established in response to recommendations made by Sir Robert Francis following the Mid Staffordshire Enquiry.

The National Guardian's office also supports trusts by reviewing their speaking up culture and handling concerns where they have not followed good practice.

All NHS services are required to appoint a Freedom to Speak Up Guardian by the 2017/2019 NHS Standard Contract. This is mandated by NHS England for use by commissioners of all healthcare service contracts.

There is additional guidance for NHS primary care providers issued by NHS England in 2016. It recognises the challenges of appointing a Freedom to Speak up Guardian who is a named individual who is independent of the management chain, and is not a direct employer of the Freedom to Speak Up Guardian. There are suggestions made that primary care providers could consider making arrangements with the local NHS trust, the CCG, the NHS England responsible officer and or arrange with another local provider, such as a neighbouring GP service.

Between April 2017 and March 2018 there were 7,087 cases reported to Freedom to Speak Up Guardians in NHS Trusts which related to:

- Bullying and Harassment (45%).
- Elements of patient safety and the quality of care (32%).
- Raised anonymously (18%).
- Staff suffering detriment because of raising concerns (5%).

The Freedom to Speak Up Guardians are not a legislative requirement for care homes, for independent hospitals or other non-NHS regulated service. There is, however, nothing to stop providers developing this provision in their services. If you are committed to listening to your staff, to using feedback to drive improvements and to addressing concerns raised by staff, why would you not appoint a Freedom to Speak Up Guardian, to help provide assurance that staff felt listened to and that concerns were addressed in timely way? Creating a culture where staff feel able to voice concerns and to address poor practice is vital when driving patient safety and preventing abuse.

Freedom to Speak up is growing within the independent healthcare sector. It seems a small step to develop the role within adult social care settings, dental clinics, call centres and independent ambulance providers. It certainly helps support the message that you are a provider or leader that welcomes staff speaking up about poor practice or other concerns.

BMI Healthcare

During 2018, BMI relaunched their Raising Concerns at Work Policy and established the role of Freedom to Speak Up Guardian. Freedom to Speak Up leads were appointed in each hospital. There is also a BMI corporate Guardian and the involvement of the Medical Director, who has executive responsibility as the Freedom to speak up lead. They recognise there is more to do but are committed to ensuring staff feel safe to raise concerns.

Spire Hospitals and Spire Cardiff

Spire Healthcare launched its Freedom to Speak Up initiative during 2018 and was the first independent acute provider to work with the National Guardian's Office to deliver training to their guardians. It is included as part of the mandatory training programme.

Spire Cardiff has a team of seven speak up ambassadors, but it is the Freedom to Speak Up Guardian who takes concerns to senior managers and ensures that the issues are explored. In the Cardiff hospital all concerns are submitted electronically and the Guardian is the only person in the hospital who can see the submissions. The Spire Corporate Guardian also has sight of all concerns raised within Spire and uses the information to troubleshoot where there are recurring issues and to escalate patient safety concerns.

Benenden Hospital

The Quality Accounts for Benenden Hospital 2018-2019 show that, while they demonstrate a commitment to supporting staff to speak out safely, they are intending to rebrand their Speak Out Safely policy as the Freedom to Speak Up initiative and are introducing Freedom to Speak Up Guardians and to offer engagement sessions.

Castle House Nursing Home, Somerton

This service, a care home for elderly people, was inspected in September 2019. The inspection team found that the provider was exceptional at helping people to express their views, so that staff and managers at all levels understood their preferences, wishes and choices. Speaking up isn't only about serious concerns. It can also simply be about listening to people.

The report says:

"For example, people had 'Freedom to speak sessions' where staff met with people individually every month. This gave people the opportunity to express their views and staff to take steps to make specific arrangements just for them. The provider shared the positive outcomes for people who attended these sessions. This included an improvement in one person's mental health by helping her work through her 'bucket list'. Another example was arranging for a local knit and natter group to come to the home so one person continues their interest and shares this with others."

Denise and Solomon

Denise and Solomon are Freedom to Speak Up guardians. They are both passionate about ensuring that concerns raised by staff are carefully considered. Denise spoke about a project that she and other staff were involved in at the trust to help interpret the values into more tangible form that made explicit behaviours that were unacceptable. This new initiative was called 'Above and below the line'. It had come about in response to a member of staff who wanted to share a concern about 'casual racism' by a doctor when referring to an Asian patient's possible food preferences. The member of staff had felt uncomfortable but as it was a meeting with several other staff, they didn't feel they knew what to say or how to address it without making it a huge issue.

Part of the initiative was for a group of staff to come up with several possible responses for when something was said that made someone feel uncomfortable or where it was felt to be inappropriate. These phrases were quite simple, and were not accusatory so unlikely to escalate the issue. They allowed a response that made it clear it was unacceptable without creating conflict. These were simple things staff could say such as, "That's not an OK thing to say".

The initiative was rolled out to staff via their health and safety training face-to-face update sessions. It was incorporated into inductions as well. While not technically health and safety, the reasoning was that putting it in the health and safety programme gave wider staff coverage and supported broad dissemination. It was a bit of thinking outside the box to get something across. The phrases might not be health and safety in themselves but encouraging a culture where all staff felt able to speak out was a very important health and safety improvement tool. If staff hold back from addressing racism, are they going to also hold back when the wrong implant is about to be inserted in someone's eye? Will staff hold back if they see a team leader behaving inappropriately towards a young person with learning disabilities

How do you encourage staff, relatives and patients to speak out? It's not that difficult where the senior managers and providers want it to happen.
In some larger organisations with deeply entrenched and mistrustful cultures (or even just pockets of resistance) it can take a good while to change attitudes and educate people to new ways of being, but the investment really does pay off in all sorts of ways. The basic means of changing remain the same with both large and small organisations, but the scale may differ.

It makes it sound simple, no? It is quite simple. I've seen it happen in quite large organisations, quite quickly. If we expect it to take years and years, there is a risk we'll give up and return to the old ways. There must be executive level commitment and determination. There must be senior role modelling. Shabby behaviours must be addressed. There must be accessible ways to voice concerns and there must be sharing of changes made where concerns have been shared. Openness and transparency are key. Listening is key. Respect is key.

Registered manager

Care Quality Commission (Registration) Regulations 2009

Registered manager condition:

1. Subject to paragraph (2), for the purposes of section 13(1) of the Act, the registration of a service provider in respect of a regulated activity must be subject to a registered manager condition where the service provider is—

   a. a body of persons corporate or unincorporate; or

   b. an individual who—

      i. is not a fit person to manage the carrying on of the regulated activity, or

      ii. is not, or does not intend to be, in full time day to day charge of the carrying on of the regulated activity.

Another issue from Winterbourne View was that there was an absence of a registered manager. Under the Health and Social Care Act 2008, the Commission registers managers to manage the regulated activities. The requirement for providers to employ a registered manager is imposed as a condition of registration.

In smaller services, the registered managers are key to the provision of services that go above and beyond expectations. They are the people that set the cultural norms among the staff group, who recruit and build their team and who have day-to-day oversight of the service.

In larger, corporate providers, the regional or area managers will have impact and oversight, but it is one step removed. Often their impression of the service quality comes from secondhand information such as a manager's report or statistical data such as the number of incidents. The number of incidents is only going to be an accurate reflection if the manager supports and encourages staff to report them. It's entirely possible for a manager with less understanding to discourage reports for fear they make the manager and the service look bad – when in fact a high reporting of low harm is a good thing.

NHS trusts don't usually need a registered manager, although if an NHS trust provides a care home or similar service then they will need one. Failing to employ a registered manager is a criminal offence. The offence is an offence of failing to comply with the conditions of your registration (Section 33 of the Health and Social Care Act 2008). This offence can be dealt with by way of a fixed penalty notice (£4,000 fine) or a prosecution (unlimited fine).

That's quite a big sanction and one that needs to be taken very seriously. It's not imposed lightly or as a money-making venture for the Commission. It is because a registered manager is legally accountable for the safety and quality of the services being provided. It is someone who should be qualified and suitably experienced to run the service well and should afford protection from poor practice. Registered managers can be prosecuted for care failings; unregistered and interim managers cannot (although they might be held to account through their professional bodies).

Health and Social Care Act 2008 (Regulated Activities) Regulations 2014: Regulation 7

7.— A person (M) shall not manage the carrying on of a regulated activity as a registered manager unless M is fit to do so.

M is not fit to be a registered manager in respect of a regulated activity unless M is—

■ of good character, has the necessary qualifications, competence, skills and experience to manage the carrying on of the regulated activity,

■ able by reason of M's health, after reasonable adjustments are made, of doing so, and

■ able to supply to the Commission, or arrange for the availability of, the information relating to themselves specified in Schedule 3.

In assessing an individual's character for the purposes of paragraph (2)(a), the matters considered must include those listed in Part 2 of Schedule 4.

In 2013, 3,900 locations were identified as not having a registered manager, a quarter of which had been vacant for over two years. Enforcement action in the form of fixed penalty notices focused on providers without a registered manager in post for over two years.

The ratings characteristic guidance for inspectors of adult social care services states that there are several limiting factors – the limit being to a rating of 'Requires improvement'. This includes where the location has a condition of registration that it must have a registered manager, but it does not have one, and satisfactory steps have not been taken to recruit one within a reasonable timescale. The reasonable time is generally taken to be six months.

Who should you appoint as the registered manager? The regulation is quite clear that it must be someone that is qualified and fit to meet the requirements of the role. A person who is very competent to be the registered manager of a day hospital providing elective surgery, who has a strong background in theatre practice, may not be ideally suited to managing a substance misuse service. It is about someone having the skills and experience of the specific regulated activity they are looking to be registered to manage.

I would suggest that if you want a service to be among the absolute best, then the manager should be among the best rather than someone just slotted in because there is a gap. An outstanding manager is worth paying for.

Research published by Saleh *et al* in 2018 to explore the nature of leadership styles used by the nursing management team, as perceived by nurses working at the bedside, showed that the leadership style employed by nurse managers has a major impact on nurses' satisfaction, turnover, and the quality of patient care they deliver.

Similarly, research carried out by Firth-Cozens and Mowbray, published in the *British Medical Journal* showed that leadership skills can have real benefits to patient care. To the authors, it seemed clear that certain traits such as arrogance, authoritarianism, and strong competitiveness may be prejudicial to good leadership, and that sociable, confident people who work well under stress have a head start in making good leaders. Just as important is their suggestion that any assessment of good leadership needs to go beyond performance monitoring and to look at the effects on staff well-being, the ways in which staff are used and developed to enhance their strengths, and the ways that leaders can show they are able to recognise and learn from the errors and inadequacies which will always be a part of healthcare.

Becoming a registered manager or appointing a registered manager is not something to be taken lightly.

A Suffolk care home owner and manager were fined at Ipswich Magistrates' Court in January 2018, after admitting they failed to provide safe care and treatment. The home was fined £16,500, plus a £170 victim surcharge, and its manager was fined £1,000, plus a £170 victim surcharge, in a prosecution brought by the Commission. The prosecution was brought against the company and registered manager after an investigation into the death of a resident who was found dead outside the home in 2016 after falling from his second-floor bedroom window which, at the time, did not have window restrictors. The home had undergone previous health and safety audits when the need for window restrictors in residents' rooms was highlighted.

The prosecution's case was that the accident resulting in the service user sustaining fatal injuries was entirely avoidable and that the overall responsibility for health and safety lies with the registered provider and registered manager, who both had a clear role in ensuring that safe care and treatment was provided.

Birchwood Grange Nursing Home, Harrow

Birchwood Grange is a nursing home that provides care and accommodation for elderly people, many of whom are living with dementia. The report comments on the registered manager and shows the impact they have on the culture and quality of services:

"The registered manager constantly strived to empower staff through effective delegation and provision of opportunities to develop skills. Staff were assigned to be 'champions' for specific roles they were interested in, which clearly had a positive impact on their confidence. They spoke positively about the nature of support. A member of staff said, "I want to thank management for this opportunity. They have taught me and trained me and have been so supportive. This isn't just my job; it's my life and I love it here."

Home Instead Senior Care, Tavistock

Home Instead Senior Care is a homecare agency providing care for people in their own homes.

"Staff were incredibly positive and motivated by the management and leadership of the service. Telling us, 'They are both very dedicated, they live the values and ethos of the organisation', and 'She (the registered manager) is incredibly motivated and has heaps of energy. She is approachable, kind, and very effective and very understanding'. A recent staff survey showed that 100% of staff were proud to work for the provider, with 94% of staff expressing a very strong motivation to carry out their role".

Courage and resilience

"You will never do anything in this world without courage. It is the greatest quality of the mind next to honour."

Aristotle

"Courage is not the absence of fear, but rather the assessment that something else is more important than fear."

Franklin Roosevelt

Great leaders throughout history share the personal characteristics of courage and resilience. Their belief in doing what is right persists and continues to be their driving force. They take risks along the way and never lose sight of where they want to end up.

For Martin Luther King Junior, it started with a dream, like it always does. A dream for change and a dream for a better tomorrow. Martin Luther King Jr. was an activist and a leader in the civil rights movement of the USA. He was also a member of the clergy. He is known for the non-violent ways in which he advanced and led the civil rights movement. He fought for racial equality and showed the people a picture of a better future where all people are equal. Courage, perseverance and the will to fight for what's right till the very end made him a great leader. His first major protest was the Montgomery, Alabama, bus boycott of 1955-1956, when he, along with Rosa Parks, protested conditions that African Americans faced on buses in that city. At that time, African Americans were forced to move to the back of the bus in Montgomery and other southern cities when whites boarded. From the outset, Dr. King faced hostility from segregationists and his life was threatened repeatedly. For example, during the bus boycott his house was bombed. And he was arrested during a campaign to desegregate the city of Birmingham, Alabama. He was jailed several times during his lifetime.

Emmeline Pankhurst was a leader of the UK's suffragette movement and a political activist. She has been one of the most influential people of the 20th century. In 1886 Pankhurst was involved with the strike of girls working in the Bryant and May match factory. The girls worked 14 hours a day and were fined for dropping matches on the floor. She was also concerned with the conditions in workhouses in Manchester. She began organising meetings in a local park, which were soon declared to be illegal. Emmeline was arrested on many occasions although often released because of poor health. She sometimes refused to eat and was force-fed. She started wearing a disguise to avoid arrest. Her courage and resilience paid off and universal suffrage was introduced for all over 21 years of age in the year of Pankhurst's death in 1928.

Nye Bevan is a name that must be known to all who work in healthcare in the United Kingdom. He was a social reformer deeply committed to socialism and the presiding spirit behind the founding of the National Health Service. Two thirds of the adult males in the town where Nye Bevan grew up worked underground for the Tredegar Iron and Coal Company, and in November 1911, the month he turned 14-years-old, Bevan followed his father and elder brother down the pit. Aged 31, Bevan entered Parliament at the general election on 30 May 1929 as Independent Labour Party member for Ebbw Vale. He proved a memorable parliamentary performer as he relentlessly championed the cause of the poor and unemployed, but he had major brushes both with the parliamentary authorities and with his own party. In April 1937 he was suspended from the house 'for disregarding the authority of the chair' during a crucial debate on the so-called 'Special Areas' of social deprivation; and in March 1939 he was expelled from the Labour Party for his constant opposition to the policy of non-intervention in the Spanish Civil War.

He oversaw the building of over a million new houses before 1950, and in 1946 the government steered through the National Insurance Act, which created the infrastructure of what was to be the Welfare State. There would be mandatory contributions from employers and employees towards financing welfare provisions for old age pensions, unemployment, sickness, maternity and widows' benefits. Then, in 1948, the National Health Service Act, which Bevan had seen through Parliament, became law. This allowed for people to receive, free at the point of use, medical diagnosis and treatment at home or in hospital, as well as dental and ophthalmic treatment. He died in 1960, having transformed the healthcare and life chances of the nation.

Great leadership isn't necessarily easy. I am not sure it's meant to be. A leadership team or leader that goes unchallenged isn't allowing their team or the people using services to help share the future. If you are a leader and never receive any criticism, no suggestions or challenges and everything just coasts along comfortably, then chances are you are not leading very effectively.

Without ideas from the team or feedback from people using services, you may well miss opportunities to introduce brilliant ideas that will revolutionise how you do things. Something complicated could well be simplified if you hear what the staff are saying. More importantly, if a healthcare assistant, support worker or housekeeper shares concerns about a consultant or senior manager and nobody listens, then poor or even abusive and dangerous practice can continue. A good few years ago I inspected an independent hospital where the matron refused to have oxygen and suction put out ready for post-operative patients returning from theatre as "It made it look like an NHS hospital". None of the staff felt able to tell her not to be so silly and the practice continued until exposed on inspection after which she lost her job. She lacked courage as well; she allowed maverick consultants to continue to perform outside good practice guidance because to challenge the status quo (even as a senior leader) would have been unthinkable for her.

Willow Lodge

One of the first things I did when I moved from clinical practice to work for a local authority children's service was to assume responsibility for Willow Lodge. This was a children's home that admitted children with the intention of providing a short period of intense assessment and worked to address the issues that had resulted in the child coming into care. The idea was to turn around the situation and prevent the need for the children to be looked after long-term.

I had moved from working with children in a fairly structured hospital environment, which always focused on the needs of the children and their families. From the day we stepped over the threshold of the Charles West School of Nursing we had the mantra, "The child first and always" drilled into us.

My belief to this day (after many years living and working with some very troubled youngsters) is that all children need kind and attentive adults who are good role models, a clear set of expectations and boundaries, and a structure and routine to help them regulate their lives. I believe education is the greatest tool for social change at both individual and organisational levels. Education sometimes means challenging the old ways and bringing fresh ideas.

I had plenty of fresh ideas but am not sure whether I was courageous or naive in the way I implemented them. I suspect naive. I certainly learnt a lot and, in the process, gained a distinction for my dissertation.

On my first visit, I rang the doorbell at about eleven in the morning and was let into an entrance hall where the paper was peeling off the wall and there was graffiti and letters scratched into the paintwork. A thick fug of cigarette smoke hit me. It was a sorry building that lacked any sense of welcome. A member of staff opened the door to the sitting room and shouted, "She's here", and then I was abandoned and ignored by the three adults sitting on dingy velour sofas, between four children who appeared to be in their early teens. They were all smoking and there were tins of cider on the table.

I wandered around the building and found a filthy kitchen full of empty ready meal packets and an overflowing bin. Upstairs there were three more children who were still in bed.

My first staff meeting for the home was brought forward to the following day, I knew I needed to be decisive and to stand by what I knew to be right. I asked all the staff to attend and most came out of curiosity more than anything else, I think. After a few introductions, I laid out my expectations very clearly and was greeted with looks of horror and contempt. There was much eye rolling and sideways glances at each other. My rules, I felt, were entirely reasonable:

- No smoking on the premises.
- No alcohol on the premises.
- Children should be taken to school each day.
- Food should be cooked from scratch, with the children helping.
- Staff should be appropriately dressed for work.
- Unless a child was unwell, the television should not be on during the day (this was pre-internet).
- The staff rota needed changing to have the highest number of staff on duty when the children were out of school.

Next day I had 14 of the 16 staff members arrive in my office to tell me they were all putting their notice in unless I rescinded the new rules. It was the smug look on the face of the team leader, who had applied but was not appointed to my role, that did it; I smiled, thanked them for coming to see me and asked them to put their resignation letters on my PA's desk on their way out. Then I breathed out and started shaking. It would have been wrong to reduce my expectations simply because the staff had grown a culture that accepted poor childcare. Could I have introduced a no smoking or alcohol rule more slowly? Probably not.

From that day forward the rules changed. The two remaining staff said it was the best thing that had ever happened, despite having to work goodness knows how many extra hours. I virtually moved out of my own home to work nearly full time at the home. The children sulked initially and then accepted there was a new way of doing things. They ate better food, had more positive attention, had merit badges from their schools and some went back to their families. It took about three months to recruit high-quality new staff and it was hard during the intervening weeks, but I never once regretted doing the right thing.

There was an improvement in behaviour, there was more laughter and we all benefitted. My PA offered piano lessons, we arranged riding lessons, the staff used their own time to offer children age-appropriate holidays and activities. Instead of smoking they went ice skating, instead of cider they made cupcakes. We bid for funding to redesign and redevelop the garden and to refurbish the inside so that it looked more loved. Nicer decoration and furniture inevitably meant the children respected it more.

Some children still had their 'moments' and there were still sad situations, but the staff worked together as a team to find solutions and held fast to their expectations. It became a pleasure to drop in for a coffee or to have a small group turn up at my office to plead for money for an ice cream.

Was it courageous leadership? It might have been had I realised the tempest I was stirring up, but I went in without great foresight or planning and survived because of a strong conviction and unwavering message about what was in the best interests of the children.

Would I do it again now? Almost definitely.

The executive team at East Sussex Healthcare NHS Trust

This could sit under culture; it could sit under speaking up – in truth, the two overlap so much it is impossible to separate them. I think it sits best under courage and resilience though, and goes a long way to show that kind leadership is not synonymous with weak leadership.

This isn't from the latest report but from an inspection when the CEO had been in post just a few months. The trust was not in a good place and there were some courageous decisions made and some true resilience and determination from some of the longer serving members of the team – notably the Director of Nursing, Alice Webster, and the Company Secretary, Lynette Wells.

The trust recognised engagement and communication with staff had historically been a serious concern, which had impacted significantly on the culture of the organisation. The Chair and Chief Executive acknowledged that when they took up post, East Sussex Healthcare NHS Trust was an organisation with which they had had to build bridges and regain the trust of the staff. Some staff had been treated very poorly under a previous regime.

The trust's strategy, vision and values led to a change in culture to one which was patient centred. Staff felt much more positive and were prouder about working for the trust and with their team. Staff felt able to raise concerns amongst their peers and with leaders. Leaders understood the importance of staff being able to raise concerns – not all was perfect but culturally the organisation had come an exceptionally long way in a short space of time. Staff now spoke positively about the organisational leaders and felt them to be both recognisable and approachable. The trust had held a series of roadshows with staff to reach as many employees as possible.

The board recognised that there had been a divided consultant body. There was also a culture of bullying behaviour, and many consultants appeared to role model a 1960s way of working: directive, remote and quick to apportion blame). The CEO met with the many members of the consultant body within his first two days in post. About 150 out of the total 230 attended a meeting where the new expectations were set out explicitly. These included:

- The trust was dependent on the consultants for clinical leadership.
- A divided trust was not an option and there was to be no relationship divide across the two sites.
- Any inappropriate behaviour would be dealt with.
- It was necessary to involve consultants in the wider leadership issues facing the trust and that the board was keen that they work together with the consultants.

A clear example of taking swift and strong action to deal with poor behaviour towards other staff was given by several people we spoke with at the time. The message was clear: that consultants shouting abuse at other staff would not be tolerated. This message had spread and reached all levels of the organisation quickly.

The CEO talked to us about pockets of issues that had been 'festering for years' without being properly addressed. It was clear that action needed to be taken to ensure that the cultural norm of bullying and nepotism that these managers and staff created was no longer tolerated. Swift, formal action was taken in several departments where there were longstanding concerns.

The medical director had dismissed two consultants, which demonstrated that the trust acted where behaviour or clinical competence was an issue. We were also told about an issue in which a doctor was not adhering to best practice and trust policy around being bare below the elbows. The medical director had intervened and made it clear that the anaesthetist was required to follow the trust policy and idiosyncratic behaviour would not be tolerated.

The minutes of the Trust Board meetings showed that there had been six disciplinary hearings in a six-month period. Two cases resulted in dismissal, three in a final written warning and one had no sanction applied. This demonstrated that, although the trust wanted to build a positive culture, they were prepared to act to address poor practice and inappropriate behaviour when necessary. It sent a very strong message that staff would be protected from bullying.

The CEO and other trust staff used social media to spread positive messages about the work that staff were doing. One campaign, #our marvellous teams, celebrated the work of staff and volunteers across the trust. The Freedom to Speak Up Guardian was the most prolific user, but other staff did post celebratory messages. The posts were as diverse as sharing the 'Sock it to Sepsis' campaign, the pharmacy team having a baking day for Macmillan, critical care unit and ward staff celebrating International Nurses day and spinning classes for staff.

The trust had appointed a Freedom to Speak up Guardian in line with the principles and role profile produced by the National Guardian. The CEO met monthly with the Speak Up Guardian and was said to have responded to any concerns that required support. This gave another clear message to staff that speaking up was a good thing and that staff would be heard.

It took a lot of courage for the chair and CEO to take on a trust that had such an oppressive culture. It took courage and resilience for the longer-standing board members to jump aboard after they had been through such a hard time under the previous regime. But they did, and they worked with the new team to bring about improvements, while providing some stability and a sense of security in a rapidly changing environment.

Dr Nicola Brink and the Guernsey response to Coronavirus

The channel island of Guernsey has led the way in managing to become Coronavirus free. Without wishing to become too political, this has to be about leaders on the island recognising and utilising the advantages that being an island state with a small population affords. It is about the political leaders on the island recognising the knowledge of others, sharing the leadership and using the skill of experts to ensure that they reduced the impact of the virus.

On May 31, *The Times* reported that, "The island had no active cases of the virus last week because of the efficiency of its 'test, track and isolate' approach launched nearly three months ago. Any travellers arriving in Guernsey after March 19 were ordered to self-isolate for 14 days with a full lockdown introduced on March 24." Their Covid-19 strategy was led by an expert, a virologist, Dr Nicola Brink, who according to Guernsey's chief minister, was "the only one of us here who has trained all her life for this".

This was courageous and decisive leadership. Imposing unpopular restrictions but ensuring the population understood why it was necessary. Dr Brink had spent a lot of time preparing for a pandemic as part of her work as the director of public health and so, by the time Guernsey's first positive Covid-19 case was confirmed on March 9, there was already a strategy in place with a proactive test and track programme.

By late March, everyone who tested positive was called within 24-hours by someone from a team of contact tracers who worked seven-days a week, 24-hours a day with clear instructions on what they must do. People who tested positive were also asked for a list of contacts. Those people were contacted, asked about their condition and instructed on self-isolation.

Apparently, Dr Brink also read an online children's story to provide reassurance to the island's children.

Leadership styles

Geese

I like simple things – I believe that if you can't explain something using simple language then it is probable that you don't understand it fully. Theories about the development of organisational culture abound. Some are common sense for reasonable people wrapped up in jargon. Some are very complex, and research based, but not readily accessible for the average leader in health or social care settings.

Read this from Wikipedia:

"Different concepts of culture, stemming from two distinct disciplines (anthropology and sociology), have been applied to organisational studies since the early 1980s. These two underlying disciplines represent different paradigms in Burrell and Morgan's (1979) framework and have contributed to the emergence of the different theories and frameworks of organisational culture in the academic literature. Anthropology takes the interpretivist view and sees culture as a metaphor for organisations, defining organisations as being cultures. On the other hand, sociology takes on the functionalist view and defines culture, as something an organisation possesses. Despite the separate definitions of organisational culture, there seems to be a movement towards a consensus.

"The most widely used organisational culture framework is that of Edgar Schein (1988), who adopts the functionalist view and described culture as a pattern of basic assumptions, invented, discovered, or developed by a given group, as it learns to cope with its problems of external adaptation and internal integration, that has worked well enough to be considered valid and, therefore is to be taught to new members as the correct way to perceive, think, and feel in relation to those problems."

It may not have you mesmerised and buying in to the idea; it probably won't grip many of the staff you work with. It doesn't engage me or tell me much that I can apply in practice. It isn't tangible.

Most people can relate to geese though.

This isn't an original thought; it's very well-known and I can't find who the original author was. I first heard about it from Andy Buck, a teacher and National Leader of Education who worked with my husband at the National College for School Leadership. He went on to write and created two organisations: Leadership Matters and #honk. I think many of his messages that are aimed at education leaders translate very well into health and social care settings.

The lesson we can learn from geese derives from their habit (usually of the Canadian variety) of flying in a V formation and the sound of honking. I say familiar because our home in West Sussex allows us to walk our dog on the incredibly beautiful East Head beach all year round. It's Franky's favourite place, so we visit often. The adjacent fields are full of flocks of geese. We frequently see the perfect V formation and think about the theory and how it applies to organisations we know. Every now and again Toby takes a photo and sends it to Andy with the simple message #honk.

Those important lessons are about how to get the best out of a team of people. The underlying ideas aren't difficult to understand but it can be difficult to persuade your middle managers (or indeed senior leaders) to use them as their default setting. It's much easier in many ways to set the KPI around some numerical value and then use that measure to reward or beat staff with. KPIs are just that – an indicator. They measure things. They tell us how well we are doing and where our performance is pretty good and where there are potential shortfalls.

Just stating the achievement percentage as measured against a KPI is never, not in a thousand years, going to get your team to deliver to their absolute best. People go the extra mile because they care about relationships, they have an altruistic streak, they want to do the right thing. Very few people say, "I am so proud that we reached 92% on the hourly lavatory cleaning checks this week that I went home and baked a cake for the team". They might, however, say, "I am so proud that the team supported each other, and several people offered to stay on and support the evening shift staff to ensure that people weren't waiting too long after that minibus crash". Success in most things is down to relationships and mutual support.

People work hard for others not for numbers. Anyway, those geese and what we can learn from them.

Sharing a common goal

As each goose flaps its wings it creates 'uplift', an aerodynamics orientation that reduces air friction for the birds that follow. By flying in a V formation, the whole flock achieves a 70% greater flying range than if each bird flew alone. The lesson we can learn here is that people who share a common direction and goal can get where they are going quicker and with less effort because they benefit from the momentum of the group moving around them.

Leaders need to set a direction and end point and make sure that all staff know where they are meant to be heading. Clarity helps ensure staff buy in to the idea; they need to know where they are going before they buy the travel ticket.

In practice, a staff group who know and understand the simple shared goal will work towards that if shown the right steps to take and the direction they need to move in. In a residential setting, clearly the vision and goals should be set by the residents or their families working with staff. All services should involve service users, but that is even more important where the service is the person's home for a long period of time.

Benenden Hospital, Kent

Benenden has a clear and simple message about its strategic goals.

Staff are aware of the three strategic goals, which are printed on staff lanyards. The strategy for core services feeds into the hospital's strategic goals.

The explicit goals are underpinned by shared values that were developed collaboratively and are known to all staff. The hospital shares the vision and strategic goals with staff in open sessions. The hospital also provides written information on the vision and values to new staff.

The provider's Quality Account 2018/2019 shares the values publicly:

"Our Values

Our values were defined by our people based on the principles of how we like to work here, and that's why we are so proud of them. Our values and behaviours give us a common language and a framework to help us in our everyday business interactions. Our values are the very essence of Benenden, and they define what makes us unique. We ask every colleague to Be Caring, Be Connected, Be Brave and Be Smart everyday so that Benenden can continue to thrive over the years to come.

Be Caring

- We know what we do matters
- We're proud and enjoy what we do

- We promote a culture of care, respect, compassion and well-being
- We protect the mutual ethos

Be Connected

- We collaborate and share across teams, departments and the business
- We listen to understand each other and our members' needs
- We support one another by having open and honest conversations
- We recognise that we're strong together

Be Brave

- We embrace change
- We challenge and ask 'Why' as well a 'Why Not'
- We always want to learn
- We are not afraid of trying new concepts and ideas

Be Smart

- We approach problems with a solution mindset
- We actively seek to improve and be better and we learn from our mistakes
- We spend members money wisely
- We're invested in the future of our business"

Nothing too complex, nothing that most healthcare professionals would not accept as a sound basis from which to provide service and reasonable expectations of staff. The provider makes it easy for staff to share a common goal because they have helped create it and the 'ask' is entirely reasonable. The visibility of the message reinforces the expected and agreed values; it's a strong and positive message that encourages the notion that the staff can and do achieve.

Leaders can't do it alone

At first it appears that geese have it all figured out; the strongest goose will lead the gaggle. Perhaps this head goose was born to be the leader through his strength and size; undoubtedly they received no training in such a leadership position. From this, one might think that the leader goose is born and not made. If this is true, then the geese have answered our question about the origin of leadership skill.

However, there is more to this leadership story. It turns out that the head goose is not always the same. When the head goose tires, it falls to the back of the V formation, where it can expend less energy. Another goose then flies up and takes its place, having more energy saved from being elsewhere in the V formation. So it turns out that the leadership role in this flying gaggle is shared among several, if not all, of the geese.

In good organisations and strong teams, there are always examples of this happening. If you are an NHS trust following a formal QI process across the whole organisation, it isn't the CEO who leads on the individual work streams or presents the updates to the executive. Different staff lead on different areas of improvement work. Staff of all grades and disciplines are involved in leading areas where they have the expertise or brilliant ideas.

Charlotte

We have an inspector, Charlotte, who has significant leadership skills but who, having re-entered the workforce after having children, wanted to spend some time consolidating her knowledge while retaining a reasonable work-life balance. Technically, she isn't a 'leader' in the sense that she isn't employed in a leadership role. That has not stopped her using her undoubted skills to help build and develop the team. Her leadership skills have been critical to the development of our team culture.

If you use a search engine to determine what the essential leadership skills are you might come up with something like:

- Patience
- Empathy
- Active listening
- Reliability
- Dependability
- Creativity
- Positivity
- Effective feedback
- Timely communication
- Team-building
- Flexibility
- Risk-taking
- Ability to teach and mentor.

Charlotte is probably a bit too self-deprecating to see herself as one of the leaders of our regional team. She doesn't do the scheduling or lead on mortality and safeguarding. She is, however, the person people are likely to trust with their worries, the person people talk to, to share concerns with and to ask for help from.

She also 'goes the extra mile' when considering the needs of the team. She once opened her rather nice beachfront home for a team-building barbecue – doing all the shopping and planning (including press-ganging her children and husband into helping too). The entire team were there, and all had a lovely day which was underpinned with team-building activities that made people work with those they didn't perhaps know very well and to share experiences in a fun way. It was such good team-building… but I still think the other team may have cheated when it came to the scavenger hunt on the beach; I am not a sore loser at all.

Every now and again Charlotte creates high tech quizzes which are far better presented than our local rugby club quiz nights. All flashing, musical, animated creations that are used at our regional days as light relief between the serious stuff. She wouldn't see it as leading on team-building, she certainly might not see it as organisational development. It absolutely is though. It is the near perfect example of a team goose moving to the front to lead and to reduce the workload and relieve the pressure on others.

Increasing visibility
Flying in a V formation increases the visibility as every goose can see what's happening in front of them.

The lesson here is to make our organisations visible in both directions. Having top-down visibility enables leaders to stay connected with the edges of the organisation and allows them to make better informed decisions. Bottom-up visibility enables employees to see the bigger picture, engages them, and empowers them to better align themselves with the organisational objectives.

I think lots of leaders are quite good at the top-down visibility and a few are now looking at ways of ensuring bottom-up visibility (the workforce becoming visible to the leaders).

Guy's and St Thomas' NHS Foundation Trust
In 2019, 130 members of staff celebrated the trust reverse mentoring programme, which sees people in junior positions mentor someone more senior. The programme offers mentees – usually a senior leader or manager – the opportunity to see things from a different perspective and discover new ways of thinking. It also allows mentors to share their ideas while gaining valuable skills and knowledge along the way. It works towards avoiding a 'disconnect' between leaders and frontline staff.

There are a few trusts that I have visited which have similar schemes – often linked to work around Workforce Race Equality Standards (or equality and diversity more widely). Where the schemes are in use, it allows the organisational leaders to understand how their decisions might impact or be received by their staff. It would not be difficult to develop a similar programme in services as diverse as independent hospitals, corporate care home providers, large GP practices or hospices.

Having humility to seek help

When a goose falls out of formation, it suddenly feels the friction of flying alone. It then quickly adjusts its mistake and moves back into formation to take advantage of the lifting power of the bird immediately in front of it.

The lesson we can learn here is to be humble enough to admit the challenges we face and to seek help as soon as we get stuck. Leaders don't know everything. Asking for help is a strength. This humility will enable you, your team, and your company to move faster and achieve more. My experience is that people like being asked to help. They like supporting others and showing how something is best achieved.

Not long ago I had a phone call on a Thursday afternoon from another Head of Inspection. They had a team who were struggling on an inspection visit because surgical treatment was being done so badly that it put people at significant risk of harm. Indeed, the reason the team were at the service was because we had been told about a woman who had died in a London hospital a week after having surgery at this centre, which was not in London. I think the team knew and I knew as soon as I entered the premises that it was not a suitable place for surgery to be carried out. The team had done some really good work but wanted to be certain that all the necessary safeguards were in place before they left and that they had collected sufficient evidence, in the correct way to be admissible. They phoned their 'Head of' who wasn't able to get to the site that day, the Head of Inspection phoned me to ask whether I could get there. I dug out my ID badge and drove to meet the team. I didn't have to do much except to be a reassuring presence, for them to talk through what they had done and what their plan was.

Their own Head of Inspection wasn't able to be there. It wasn't about their skills or knowledge; they would have done exactly what I did. It was logistics, but regardless of the reason, they needed help and were prepared to ask directly. I could step in, the team felt supported by us both and people who may have used the service were protected because the team felt confident to act. The service closed that day.

Empowering others to lead

When the lead goose in the front gets tired, it rotates back into the formation and allows another goose to take the leadership position.

The lesson here is to empower others to also lead. Micro-managing and keeping tight control will cause 'burn out'. It will also disengage and demotivate others around you. People have unique skills, capabilities and gifts to offer. Give them autonomy, trust and a chance to shine, and you will be surprised with the outcomes.

I know the very worst leaders are those who lack the confidence to trust their teams. Constantly checking up on staff, looking at their diaries or delegating a task without giving control has a truly detrimental effect on performance. Nobody likes to feel that their manager doesn't trust them. Nobody wants to think someone is seeking out failings. That is not to say that where there is cause for concern that you don't act but that you don't need to dig and dig until you find a minor transgression.

How do you empower others to lead?

Across most areas of work, command and control is making way for a more collaborative way of leading. Most work places are demanding innovation at such a rapid rate that endless ideas are needed in order to thrive. These endless ideas cannot only come from a leader but must come from everyone else involved. The first step is to recognise that and show you value everyone's ideas. Throughout history there are examples where people with little formal education have gone on to become world leaders in their fields.

Henry Ford is best remembered for almost single-handedly creating the American car industry. Ford had only a basic education. He was born near Detroit, where he worked on a farm with a father who believed his son would someday take over from him. Instead, Ford became an apprentice with a machinist in Detroit at the age of 17. He went on to establish a career path that led to him becoming a very rich and successful industrialist who created the first mechanised assembly line. Imagine if someone had said to the young Henry Ford, "No, we'll do it my way or no way".

You need to Live the behaviours that you want staff to embrace. It's no use having organisational values such as 'Compassion to all' or 'Honesty' pinned as a laminated poster on a practice wall if a senior GP partner then asks a receptionist to tell a patient enquiring about why the pharmacy hasn't got their prescription that they are, "Sorry, there has been a problem with the computers but it should be done by the next day", when the truth is the GP simply missed the message about it.

Role modelling follows on quite nicely from living the values. Don't have an objective about managers prioritising regular one-to-ones with their direct reports if you cancel or change their one-to-ones every other month. Don't allow it to be culturally acceptable for some senior staff or leaders to exhibit shabby behaviour without censure. Whether that is surgeons with practising privileges in an independent hospital not adhering to the Bare Below the Elbows Policy, a shift leader in a care home sitting drinking coffee while the care staff are run off their feet with calls bells ringing for extended periods or a Chief Operating Officer being ten minutes late for every site meeting.

Give your team the autonomy to make decisions, share ideas and have more freedom than you are entirely comfortable with. They will usually repay you many times over.

Beechcroft Green Nursing Home

This is the home my mother lives in and which I visited recently. It was sleeting and very windy; when we went for lunch at a nearby beachside café after the visit, the waves were crashing right across the road. Not a day most people would choose to venture out, but one resident was quite distressed, saying they needed to get out and banging on the door repeatedly. Their cries became louder and louder. The shift leader tried to calm the resident, but to no avail. In the end the care assistant explained to the resident that it was wet and cold, that it was not very nice at all but, if she was adamant that they go out, then the care assistant would take her. I could overhear what was happening from my mother's room. The resident said yes, they definitely wanted to go out despite the weather. The shift leader was uncertain but said if the care assistant really thought it might help calm the person then give it a try.

I then watched them out of the window. The care assistant and the resident were wrapped up well, with the resident being tucked up under blankets and plastic sheets in a wheelchair. It really was horrible weather, but the care assistant took the person for a short spin in the chair, getting soaked through and working physically very hard to push the chair against the wind. I wouldn't have enjoyed the experience, but the resident was smiling very happily and was much calmer after their brief outing.

What was good was the care assistant felt able to raise the idea, the shift leader listened and weighed up the risks and discussed the idea without dismissing it out of hand. The care assistant had understood that a short period of discomfort might be effective in showing the resident that the idea of a walk along the seafront was not the best idea given the weather. They both understood that to truly personalise care there has to be consideration of the risk threshold that staff, leaders and providers are willing to hold and how that balances with empowering staff and people using services to make decisions.

As an aside, I don't know whether they'd just had training in the Mental Capacity Act 2005, but it certainly felt like they innately understood the fifth principle. This states that where a decision is made (or an act done) on behalf of a person who does not have mental capacity, it should be the least restrictive option of the person's rights and freedoms.

Always recognising great work

The geese honk to recognise each other and encourage those ahead to keep up their speed.

The lesson here is to make sure we praise people and give them the recognition they deserve. Lack of recognition is one of the main reasons people are unsatisfied at work and leave. It's quite common for people's efforts to go unnoticed by their peers in a busy and fast-moving work environment. However, remembering to constantly provide recognition and encouragement is vital and keeps teams motivated to achieve their goals.

I don't think there is a trust in the country that doesn't have some sort of formal recognition awards. This is often a monthly 'star award' which culminates in an awards evening or similar. That's a positive thing but it's not enough. It affects very few people and only really recognises a couple of dozen from a workforce of potentially thousands.

There are as many possible ideas as there are people working in healthcare. I can't believe there are any leaders who are incapable of thinking of how to recognise their staff's achievements and efforts on a daily basis. It doesn't have to be about ballrooms and black ties. It can sometimes be as simple as a, "I can see you are working really hard and haven't had a break, FY2 doctor, so I made you a cup of coffee and brought you a biscuit. You do have it black, don't you?" Hopefully, you'd use their name rather than FY2 doctor though.

What do we do in my team at the Commission? Do I walk the walk or just talk the talk?

- At an organisational level, we have letters sent out by the CEO thanking staff who are nominated by their managers for a specific achievement or effort.
- We have online or printable thank you cards on our intranet for staff to use.
- The Recognising Outstanding Contribution (ROC) award enables anyone in CQC to nominate a colleague or team for special recognition.
- In the Head of Inspection weekly message there are Values Nominations for people to suggest colleagues who have 'lived the values' in some way in the preceding week or two.

- We do Paper Cup Awards at our Christmas lunch; some are silly or teasing but some are recognition of genuine achievement. One inspector, Catherine, received a Kate Grainger award for driving the introduction of the 'Hello my name is' campaign in the Commission and another received an award for the most effective enforcement when they had driven the closure of an unsafe cosmetic surgery service.

- Jacquie Lawson e-cards are used by several managers to send thank you, well done notes and birthday, Eid or Happy Hanukkah cards to their teams. The subscription isn't particularly expensive and the cards are always well received.

- I always send a handwritten thank you postcard to each member of the inspection team, regardless of how big the team is. I always give personal feedback in it so that people can use it in their professional portfolios, for revalidation or just to support reflective learning. Other managers send a personal email the following day. It doesn't matter. What matters is that people do receive a thank you and that it is personal.

- We sometimes have e-pinboards where people can write a note to pin onto the noticeboard and share when someone deserves recognition.

- Obviously we make cakes, give presents and sign cards for leavers, for babies, for bereavements, for serious illness or engagements and weddings.

- We also make sure that we tell people when they've done something well.

For recognition to be effective it can very rarely be 'You are all fabulous' type comments; these are platitudes not recognition. It's fine as the ending statement on a training day; it is not fine as a way of acknowledging a job well done. Recognition is about individuals and teams and is always specific. It needs to be to the person or people involved and detail what is being recognised.

Many organisations would be better places to work, and to receive care or treatment, if a few more people honked regularly!

Offering support in challenging times

When a goose gets sick or wounded, two geese drop out of formation and follow it down to help and protect it. They stay with it until it dies or can fly again. Then, they launch out with another formation or catch up with the flock.

The lesson here is to support each other in difficult times. It's easy to always be part of winning teams, but when things get difficult and people are facing challenges, that's when your support is most needed. On the whole, those given support and time to recover pay back in terms of organisational loyalty and commitment. Those who have experienced support will usually offer support to others at a different time. This is around life events such as bereavement or relationship breakdowns, it's around illness and disability, but is also about the everyday life challenges that many people face from time to time.

Imagine if you had a call to tell you that a very close relative was critically ill in a distant country. You'd want to go and be with them, to make sure you had some time together. What happens if you have no annual leave left? Does your manager say, "Bad luck, you have no more days to take"? I hope not. What's the risk?

The risk of that lack of empathy is that the draw of a very sick family member may be such that they go off anyway. Maybe on sick leave or maybe they just go knowing they can probably find another job in health or social care relatively easily. The organisation ends up unable to plan, possibly having another vacancy, or at best a disengaged and resentful member of staff. Potentially a team who thinks that the decision to say 'bad luck' was unkind and unreasonable. Not good for morale, and recruitment is expensive.

Now consider you say, "Don't worry, go anyway. We'll sort how we manage the time off once you know the situation and how long you'll need. Can I do anything to help? Do you have outstanding work that needs sorting? I'll do the rota you just go and call me to let me know you've arrived safely and what the situation is."

That member of staff feels supported and can go to deal with the situation. Other staff see a kindly manager who puts staff interests high on their list of priorities. It might be a bit hard to persuade others to work overtime or to cover the additional work, but they will be more willing knowing there will likely come a time when they need to ask for help. The staff member phones you and is grateful. They say their relative is on the mend and they will be back, having had eight days off. They turn up for work when they say they will. You don't need to recruit anyone else. You save the recruitment costs. The member of staff volunteers to work over Christmas, as they know the other staff did extra when they needed the time off. They make up the days by doing an additional shift every fortnight for a few months. This saves the cost of using agency staff and the people using the service benefit from greater continuity of care. It feels like everyone wins; not least the manager who gets lovely feedback in the staff survey.

South Central Ambulance Service

This ambulance trust is one of ten ambulance trusts within England. They provide emergency services and patient transport services, using their own call centres to plan and dispatch crews and vehicles. They have good training and try to reduce risks to their staff. One of the ways they do this is by offering staff who are unable to work on frontline operations the opportunity to work in the call centres, either as call handlers, planners or clinical advisors. They value their staff's experience and want to ensure staff returning from a period of sick leave, who have developed a long-term condition that prevents them lifting or driving or who are pregnant, are protected until they are fully fit to work on the frontline again.

Staff appreciate this and know they are likely to be offered alternative employment that protects them when they need it.

The Commission

The Commission has generally been very supportive of staff during the pandemic. Akin to many services, the Commission's staff has faced significant personal and logistical challenges during these testing times. The response was to ensure staff safety as a priority by stepping back from the inspection schedule and only making site visits where there was a significant risk to people. Time has been spent looking at alternative ways of monitoring services and gaining assurance from providers.

Staff are not classified as key workers, so some are having to juggle children and work. The attitude is one of flexibility and support to do as much as possible, to allow staff to cope without applying too much pressure.

It is recognised that these are hugely stressful times and the very clear message is that staff well-being is a priority. There are regular check-in calls from managers, optional team contact calls, reading groups and training that all allow an escape from the effects of the Coronavirus pandemic. Staff are encouraged to make time to get outside and walk, run, cycle or swim.

Many staff felt they wanted to support frontline staff by returning to clinical practice at the Nightingale, in local GP practices, and in local trusts. Some chose to accept secondments to the pandemic response teams and work more closely with NHS England or Public Health England. Some are not able to take on those roles, for whatever reason, and have been encouraged to support through sewing scrubs or collecting food and prescriptions for vulnerable neighbours. It all helps staff feel valued and involved rather than irrelevant.

There have been mindfulness sessions, quizzes, virtual birthday drinks; lots to maintain team cohesiveness and to encourage staff to stay well so that they are able to step back into their full range of duties as soon as possible.

Staying committed to core values and purpose

The geese migration routes never vary. They use the same route year after year. Even when the flock members change, the young learn the route from their parents. In the spring they will go back to the spot where they were born.

The lesson to learn here is to stay true to your core values and purpose. Strategies, tactics and products may change for an organisation to remain agile, but great teams always stick to their core purpose and values.

I'll use an example organisation that has been used previously, partly because I know it well and partly because the simplicity of the message chimes so well with their staff.

Patient First – Western Sussex Hospitals NHS Foundation Trust

Their headline is so simple that it's almost impossible not to understand the message being delivered from the very outset. No other words are necessary. Patient First

Patient First is their long-term approach to transforming hospital services. Whether it's small steps or complex changes, it's a continuous process of improvement within existing processes and pathways that leads to measurable improvements for their patients and staff. It's about empowering front-line staff to make improvements themselves – by providing the training, the tools and the freedom to work out where the opportunities are, and the skills and support to make change happen and to make it sustainable.

There are several underpinning principles but the most obvious one is that the patient is at the heart of every element of change. There is an explicit commitment that everything that any member of staff does, that any changes anyone makes, should always contribute to improving outcomes and experiences for the people using the hospitals. This is the 'True North' of the trust – the one constant towards which all staff set their direction of travel in order to achieve their vision.

There are big changes around pathway redesign, there are small changes around providing earplugs or nurses wearing soft-soled shoes, but what they have in common is that True North focus. The staff understand what their role is in improving patient experience and outcomes. They know changes are made for the good of patients. It unites the entire staff team across the trust.

A survey was developed and published by Kouzes and Posner in their book, *The Leadership Challenge* (2002). It asked people what characteristics of a leader they admire and would cause them to follow. From this came the Leadership Participation Inventory; a list of the characteristics that were identified and which many people could demonstrate without much thought. The list of things people want in a leader is remarkably similar to all the management consultancy traits listed when you type 'qualities of a leader' into a search engine. It seems staff really do know what good leadership looks like.

Role model: A leader needs to be an exemplar, presenting themselves to show what is expected of staff and how actions should be performed. The leaders should be setting standards by adhering to organisational uniform policies, handwashing and ensuring people's privacy and dignity is respected. They should be courteous and supportive of other staff at all times.

If a site manager is wearing a long-sleeved cardigan and going from clinical area to clinical area, then the staff will follow the lead. If a surgeon is shouting at people in theatre, other staff will see that as acceptable behaviour. If a care home manager is smoking on the doorstep, others will join them.

It seems so obvious.

Inspiration: People need to be inspired but with a goal. They need to see that there is a specific point to aim for. Leaders need to be able to stand firm in the face of adversity and know that the goal, the end point, remains the same, but that the route may need to make a slight deviation to avoid potholes.

If a service goal is to reduce the number of falls but for one month there has been an unexpected increase in the number of falls with harm, you will still want to reduce the number of falls by 60% and so the goal isn't moved. You may want to look at whether there are any connections between the falls – a loose carpet, lower staffing levels or someone 'tidying away' walking aids – but you don't want to simply accept more falls.

Facing adversity: Leaders cannot be deterred by difficulties or challenges. They need to be resilient and calm whatever the team might be facing. Courage is a gold hallmark of good leadership.

I'm not going to be so crass as to give examples of courageous leadership in adversity when health and social care service leaders across the country are showing such resilience amid the Coronavirus pandemic. Daily examples are shared on social media about staff and leaders who have been incredibly courageous and put the needs of others first.

Empowerment: Leaders get others to act by supporting and encouraging others to step up. They listen to, learn from and validate the idea and opinions of others.

Generates enthusiasm: A vital component of leadership is not only getting others to act, but the need to act with passion. Sometimes that can be about generating a bit of fun. Sometimes it can be about encouraging reflection and empathy.

It feels like quite an achievable thing to be a good leader based on what other people want from a leader, doesn't it?

Situational leadership

This is the one theory that I remember (without looking it up) from my formal management training at Portsmouth University many years ago. It's another one that resonates as a very simple and obvious theory that leaders would do well to include on that shelf in their brain where they keep leadership tools.

Leaders are essentially people who know what they want or need to achieve and who can influence the thoughts and actions of others to garner their support and co-operation to achieve goals. In the case of longer-term goals, the leader may not achieve the realisation of their vision in their tenure but may be the guiding hand that keeps the organisation on track and working towards the end point.

Ever since time began and people lived in small, close groups that hunted and foraged, they had leaders who led their expeditions and took greater risks than the rest of the group members. In turn, they received a larger share of the kill gaining respect and a higher status. With changing times, how leadership is perceived has also changed. Command and control as a leadership style is rarely acceptable in a modern, forward-thinking organisation that wants to excel – with the proviso that sometimes a Control and Command style is essential to ensure a good outcome to a specific task. It's why it is called situational leadership. If anyone tells you they never use Command and Control, they are either in a very dull job or they don't understand good leadership.

This theory says that the same leadership style cannot be practiced in all situations: depending upon the circumstance, the skills and motivation of the people involved and the context, the leadership style needs to adapt to be successful. The pioneers of this theory were Ken Blanchard and Paul Hersey.

If you are ever asked in an interview what your leadership style is, you probably need to explain that you don't have a single style and it entirely depends who you are leading and for what purpose.

As an example, if you are an anaesthetist in charge of a resuscitation attempt, or a Naval Officer bringing a £3 billion-pound aircraft carrier through the narrow entrance to her Portsmouth Harbour home, you might not use your best consultative style to discuss the full range of options to progress the task. It might, in this situation, mean the best outcome can be achieved by using the less popular Command and Control, with the designated leader giving clear commands and making decisions rapidly, without consultation but with their ears attuned to hear any concerns raised.

The model encourages the leaders to consider a situation and then lead in the most appropriate manner, suitable for that situation. Experienced, good leaders do this automatically without a long pre-amble or dissection of the best leadership style to use. It becomes a deeply rooted part of themselves. The three aspects that need to be considered in a situation are:

- Staff competences.
- Motivational levels of the employees.
- Complexity of the task.
- Leadership style.

Not too many variables and not too complex to use regularly. Most people are fully capable of adapting how they lead or manage, if they know something as simple as this can change the performance of individuals and a team.

In this model, the leadership style is divided into four types:

- **Telling:** Telling style is associated with leaders who closely supervise their staff, constantly instructing them about why, how and when the tasks need to be performed. It isn't necessarily a bad style of leadership, but it only works where there is a certain set of variables including staff who may not have the specific skill required but who display a high level of commitment towards the task they have to perform. It might be a new foundation programme trainee doctor learning how to suture; they want to do it but need a clear direction about how to do it well. It might be a nurse who has moved from an acute hospital to a hospice and needs to set up a syringe driver to deliver pain relief. They will gain confidence more by being told clearly how something is done well than by being left to work it out for themselves.

- **Selling:** Selling style is when a leader provides controlled direction and is a little more open and allows two-way communication between him/herself and the staff, thus ensuring buy-in to the process and work towards the desired goals. It is best used where staff have a certain level of competence which might be sufficient to do the job, but they are for some reason low on commitment towards the tasks. Despite having relevant skills to perform the task they seek external help when faced with new situations. The leader needs to sell them the benefits of the task to boost their buy in and consequently their performance. An example of when this might be applicable is, perhaps, a large care home needing an interim shift leader but having no applicants from among the nursing establishment. The leader might talk about the opportunity in a team meeting and suggest someone appointed would be in a strong position when applying for a substantive post. They might talk to individuals about the greater autonomy and control they would have as well as the better rewards package. They might offer a mentor and opportunity to shadow a shift leader in another of the provider's homes.

- **Participating:** This style is characterised when the leaders seeks the opinion and participation of the followers to establish how a task should be performed. The leader in this case tries creating relationships with the staff, who have the competence to do the job, but their commitment level is inconsistent. They also tend to lack the confidence to go out and perform tasks alone. It's about shared working as a means of providing that confidence and growing the individuals and the team.

  If you have a fairly complex task, such as completing a staffing rota for the next three months or introducing an induction framework, you might ask someone who is very able but often chooses to stay in the shadows to help you. You might have someone else who is also quite capable on a day-to-day basis but never really seems to 'go the extra mile' or put their hand up when volunteers are needed. You could ask the same willing person who will be able to do it with their eyes closed and standing on their head – but nobody will learn much and those able but under involved staff might feel further disengaged. If you involve a small team (so, not giving any one person full responsibility) with a clear task that isn't something they would normally take on, then they learn and become more engaged in the work of the wider team. Performance improves.

- **Delegating:** Possibly the scariest thing to do is to trust some of the staff and let go of the reins. That is not to say you give up all responsibility – we are talking delegation not abdication. In this style, the leader plays a role in decisions that are taken but passes on or delegates the responsibilities of carrying out tasks to one or more staff. The leader, however, monitors and reviews the process. For delegation to work it has to be done with a sense of justice and desire for the person(s) to succeed. Delegation is not about giving all the unpleasant tasks that you don't want to do to someone in a junior role to you. It is not about feeling overloaded, so you simply overload someone else. That is very shabby leadership and in nobody's best interests. Delegation is a carefully thought through process used to develop and enthuse your most able and most motivated staff. I would caution against delegation to those who feel press ganged into accepting the responsibility. It should be a task or process that will allow development opportunities, that give a degree of 'stretch' and personal challenge. There must be a clear remit and explicit success measures. Any 'rules' or inflexibility in the task must be made known at the outset. There's no point asking someone to knit something, waiting until they put in a huge amount of time and effort and just have the buttons to sew on the sweet little yellow cardigan before mentioning it has to be a green jumper. Tasks you might delegate are as varied as the plants at Kew Gardens. It might be that one of the practice nurses wants to have a wider role and that you feel he could lead on the travel clinic service. It might be that you have a care support worker who loves singing and has mentioned setting up a community choir in the care home for residents, staff and visitors to attend.

Clearly in both these situations, you don't just say, "Oh, go on then". There need to be ground rules; there needs to be a discussion about parameters and limitations. There will need to be ongoing monitoring and agreement about how this will be done. There needs to be consideration of any training and resources needed to allow them to succeed.

If you do it properly, then every Saturday afternoon you might have a volunteer pianist and 15 members of the local community coming along to join eight of your residents and three of their family members in a medley of songs from West End musicals. How lovely would that be for those who sing and those that listen? How lovely for the staff member to feel this was the outcome of them suggesting something and agreeing to see it through to fruition.

Servant leadership

"Whosoever will be chief among you, let him be your servant."
Matthew 20:27

This is another quite simple leadership model that feels almost intuitive to me. The term 'Servant Leadership' became popular in a book called *Servant Leadership* by Robert Greenleaf (1977). The idea of 'a leader who serves' has been expressed in many different ways for very much longer. Perhaps the earliest notable reference to servant leadership is recorded in the Bible – hence the quote above. This broad leadership concept of prioritising the interests of those being led, is of course seen in other religious texts and teachings.

For me it seems very obvious that the only role of a leader or manager is to support those being led to deliver their job which should be focused on the core purpose of the service. A Director of Nursing is not much use without a team of nursing staff to lead towards high-quality delivery of nursing within a service. A CEO sitting alone in a boardroom isn't of any real value without a team who actually delivers the core purpose of the organisation.

The caveat is that the term 'support' is broad. I am not suggesting that the role of Medical Director is to personally do a ward round on every ward every day or to make junior doctors' lunch, that they then deliver. It might be nice if they did go to wards and make junior doctors a mug of tea and biscuit while they had a brief chat about how they were finding things but that isn't their key role.

Support may be ensuring that the service is properly resourced, setting safe staffing levels or liaising with a community trust and CCG to ensure that a nursing home receives proper support from a tissue viability nurse specialist or palliative care physician.

There are many and various examples of 'servant leaders'. These are leaders whose service towards others is the leader's driving force. I suspect most clinical leaders in health and social care services can identify with this idea.

The examples below are examples of this leadership philosophy:

- Florence Nightingale
- Mary Seacole
- Jean Henri Dunant (founder of the International Red Cross Movement)
- Nelson Mandela
- Dalai Lama
- Dr Thomas John Barnardo
- Martin Luther King
- Leo Tolstoy
- Barack Obama
- Aneurin Bevan

The basic idea of servant leadership is simple: that the leader serves their followers (or a cause, which benefits the followers in some way).

A servant leader is not leading for reasons of status, wealth, popularity or power. They just want to make a difference. I have lost count of the times that I have been told by exceptional leaders in health and social care that their motivation is the desire to 'make a difference'.

I'm slightly reluctant to name particularly good leaders and managers that I have come across in regulated services – there are so many who do such a good job and the variation in how they work is enormous. It's probably that variation that makes them stand out, as these are people who are incredibly well suited to lead the specific services that they work in.

I've seen and experienced a few shockingly behaved leaders in my time, but they are in the minority. If you stay the course with a poor leader (and most choose not to) then you can learn from them through reflecting on what they are doing wrong and why. It can teach us how not to lead but it can also be so destructive that people give up their jobs and their careers. It isn't the best way to support learning in an organisation.

The people below are mainly from healthcare, as that is where I work. I have come across incredible leaders working in adult social care but a good while ago, and I cannot, sadly, recall their names. Working with hospitals we tend to spend more time engaging and get to know individuals better, perhaps. There is no suggestion that leaders in hospitals are necessarily better than leaders in other settings. Some are and some aren't.

Catherine

To say Catherine was responsive to the inspection team was an understatement. When I first met her, she was a Director of Nursing and Patient Safety in an acute trust which is now rated 'Outstanding' but wasn't at the time.

On one inspection, one of the team mentioned that they thought the elderly care ward was very boring for the patients and pointed out that many couldn't see, hear or even turn on the above-bed television and telephone consoles. Within an hour or so, Catherine had found several, very large televisions, had them plugged in and set to an appropriate programme. She'd also redirected a few volunteers to talk and play dominos or cards with patients and started a more formal programme of regular volunteer befrienders and activity supporters on several wards.

She was always completely upfront and honest when things went wrong. She never tried to put a spin on bad news, never tried to minimise care shortfalls and had always taken decisive action even before we could ask the questions.

With Catherine, if something needed doing, it got done and she gave off the feeling that no task was ever beneath her while having a strong grip on the wider needs of the service. Staff knew her and respected her, she was very visible and visited most areas of the hospitals frequently. She knew the service exceptionally well and was incredibly proud of the work the staff were doing.

Durab

Durab is a Divisional Head of Nursing working as part of the triumvirate that leads the Medical Division within an acute hospital. He was waiting by the lift doors when we exited onto the medical floor of the trust, ready to show and tell us everything about his service. His pride and excitement at showing off his team was palpable; he formed a barrier between us and his wards until we'd heard exactly how fantastic his team were. Nobody else could get a word in, in a good way. His colleagues looked sideways at each other, wondering whether his volubility would hinder rather than help their ratings.

Later, after a site meeting, he found us again and talked even more about things he had forgotten to mention until someone called him away. There was no escaping; he was going to give us the evidence we needed.

Far from being a negative force, he was an absolute star performer; telling us what was good about his service and giving concrete examples to support his opinion. Everywhere we went we were introduced to his staff and told very specifically what was brilliant about each person. He did much the same with patients and introduced us to people with warmth and a positive comment about everyone.

No suit from Saville Row, no self-publication or smugness, but a humble recognition of the good work of others that resonated with his team and earned him their respect. It's those geese honking again.

Alison

Alison was, and is, a Director of Nursing. When I first met her she was working in a very challenged trust that was put into special measures. The trust has evolved into a much better place and Alison has moved on to a new opportunity, in another trust with its own challenges. At the time, what she offered was the ultimate servant leadership to the staff at the trust, who had been through exceedingly difficult times.

Staff knew Alison and respected her; stakeholders also knew and respected her. She was described as a safe and steady pair of hands – exactly what the staff knew they needed to steer them through a hugely tumultuous period. Her biography from her new trust describes her as, "being committed to ensuring that staff in all of our settings are supported in delivering the best support to our population that they can." Throughout all the changes that she helped lead the trust through, Alison was always the person staff spoke about as being on their side, as being calm and measured and of being trustworthy and supportive.

Excellence in leadership isn't always about pointy elbows and driving fast-paced change. Sometimes it is recognising that the staff and the service need stability and the reassuring presence of someone they trust, who brings people with them gently. A strong and steadying hand at the tiller in stormy waters.

Dan

Dan is a consultant in acute medicine and a geriatrician. He is chief of medicine at an acute trust, responsible for leading the services within the medicine division, ranging from the emergency department and cardiology to therapies and pharmacy.

He comes across as passionate about the delivery of efficient, safe, high-quality care. He is a powerful advocate for listening to the staff who work in his division.

Part of his role is around transformation and quality improvement across the trust. One could be forgiven for thinking he might talk to us about the Standardised Hospital Mortality Indicator or the National Lung Cancer Audit, but he didn't: he talked to us about diarrhoea. He talked passionately and with real conviction about the work his team had done after a suggestion was made by a health care assistant. The idea was about as simple as it comes, so quite easy to dismiss, but it wasn't. It was piloted as part of the quality improvement methodology and shown through the collection of data to save staff time, reduce costs and improve the patient experience. It probably reduced the risk of pressure damage and falls too, although that wasn't evidenced at the time.

The idea was simply to create a diarrhoea management pack that had everything necessary to help someone who had experienced an episode of diarrhoea, in one place. No running around trying to get wipes, gloves and disposal bags from different places – just pick up a pack and attend to the patient. It meant the patient was sorted out much more quickly, there was less time in horrid mess, it was more dignified and reduced the risk of a patient falling when trying to sort themselves out. For the staff, it was less stressful than knowing someone needed help but having to rush around trying to find equipment. Everybody wins.

Dan was able to describe in detail to us how this lowly but important task had been transformed, and explained the impact on costs, staff time and the patient experience; he attributed the idea to the correct person and identified the team effort. He didn't take any credit, but as a leader what he had done was listen to his staff, consider the ideas of someone much junior to himself and supported them to deliver on the idea. Improved outcomes were delivered by the team who would be using the packs daily. Strong leadership is sometimes about allowing and empowering others to lead – it's in the lessons from geese.

Elizabeth

Elizabeth is the Volunteer & Community Liaison Manager of a local Healthwatch branch. She has developed a diverse team of committed volunteers, who undertake activities like 'enter and view' to support services by helping them recognise what they are doing well and where there is potential for improvement. Healthwatch work closely with local people and organisations to make sure that the voices of local people are heard and used to inform how services are provided.

As a leader, Elizabeth is a skilled communicator and ensures the voice of Healthwatch is heard by providers in her patch and beyond. She is sufficiently courageous to stand up for what is right and insist that local people are listened to. She works tirelessly and passionately, and her passion is infectious; her team of volunteers are drawn to her commitment and positivity.

She allows others to take the lead sometimes, and even manages to persuade her volunteers and a CQC inspector to venture out at night to engage with people from some of the very hard to reach groups.

She sets the direction and stays true to the organisation's sense of purpose – another lesson from the geese.

Fiona

Fiona was the registered manager of a small independent hospital when I first met her. She is now the Director of Clinical Services and Caldicott guardian sitting on the board of a corporate provider. What singles her leadership style out is her willingness to step in, to support her team and take responsibility when there are problems, and her willingness to step back and trust her staff at other times.

The day before an announced inspection, I asked whether we'd see her the next day. Without any hesitation at all she said, "No, the registered manager is perfectly capable and can call me if you want to know anything she can't answer". A much better message to give the staff who form your team than any suggestion that they are not trusted, or able to present the service well.

Sometimes an inspection team turns up to a service, the manager or shift leader calls the provider, regional director, or other senior person and before the visitor's book is signed, several corporate representatives arrive to try and take control of the inspection process. It's a poor message to send to the inspection team and the staff.

It's often a mistake because it signals a lack of trust in the staff providing the care or treatment. The corporate representatives then try to follow the team around, sit in on every conversation and hover in a way that invariably makes one wonder what it is they are worried about. What do they think staff will tell the team that shouldn't be said? It reeks of central control rather than local accountability and innovation; it suggests oppression rather than support.

It has the potential to hide some really good work that is going on by only permitting staff to use words that appear on the corporate song sheets. Staff become wary and fail to show the enthusiasm and commitment that they usually have for the work they are doing.

Shalini

Although Shalini was her given name, she was known universally as Joy; she felt it was easier for 'her ladies' to say and she wanted to do anything she could to serve them. That was her mantra, 'Here to serve always'. She said it often and whenever anyone was hesitant about asking for something, whether that be her staff or one of 'her ladies'. She used to run a small residential home for 14 ladies and was insistent that only the best would do. She didn't talk of a vision or values but was clear what they were – everyone gets everything they need and want; nothing is too much trouble. Underpinning that quite profound vision were expected behaviours – compassion, kindness, fun, respect and attention to detail.

On my first visit as a very green regulator, I was invited in like an A-list celebrity. I was shown into one of two sitting rooms and introduced with some excitement and hand clapping, then I was offered a seat at a table with two of the ladies and a member of staff and told they would look after me. We were brought tea, cake, biscuits, fruit, homemade lemonade. I chatted for a short while and asked about what it was like living at the home, what involvement people had in planning and what activities were provided.

Apparently, the ladies ran the home and decided most things. If someone wanted to go to the shops, a member of staff took them. If someone wanted to go to the library, a member of staff took them. Joy spent her time checking people had everything they wanted, offering staff help, and making sure that the 'hidden jobs' of the home were completed. When I was eventually shown records, they were immaculately presented, with detailed diaries of the care everyone had received.

What the home offered more than any other home I have ever visited was fun and laughter. I found myself being persuaded to dance with the ladies when a musician and dance teacher arrived to show us all how to do the Macarena. It showed me far more about the quality of care being provided than any paper record could ever have done. A rather large but very gentle dog spent his day wandering between the ladies, being petted and given too many treats.

Lunch was another enlightening experience. I, along with all the care staff, was expected to sit and eat with the ladies – "No, I'll look at the fire safety log now" simply wasn't an option. It was a tiny home, but the choice was phenomenal. The chef was expected to lead and kitchen staff came out to take orders from the diners. A menu gave several hot dishes, salad, sandwiches, soup, omelette and several puddings. I was told if nothing appealed then the chef would always make something else. When a visitor arrived to see a relative, they were also announced with much excitement and persuaded to join the meal.

The staff were all long serving and thought Joy was wonderful. They had training to achieve NVQs and other care qualifications, but Joy had also paid for a couple to have driving lessons, so they could take people out more easily in the home's adapted car. The laundry person had been offered sewing lessons so that they could repair the ladies' clothes, If necessary. The chef had been sent on a professional cake decorating course, so they could make a truly incredible cake for the Queen's Golden Jubilee.

There were no ratings back then, but Joy offered truly outstanding leadership to those she served – and there was no doubt in her mind that her role as leader was to serve and encourage others to achieve their potential. She was perhaps the ultimate head goose; encouraging and supporting others, a clear sense of purpose and direction which promoted a commitment to shared values and recognising and building on good work.

I drove away with a picture of what residential care should look like. Joy and a couple of 'the ladies' stood waving farewell to me from the door.

Kiara and Daniel

Kiara and Daniel are two trust ambassadors from an acute trust – they are two of many in a similar role. During inspections they seem to become omnipresent and ever willing. They have 'day jobs', but what makes them stand out as excellent examples of devolved leadership, where not all leaders are senior managers, is their commitment to promoting a positive culture. They genuinely shine, physically; they wear beaming smiles the whole time. They usually help the inspection team find their way around and willingly sort out any job that needs doing or information that the team wants. Nothing is too much trouble, whether that means popping to the shop to get a diet cola or having something photocopied. The cynical on the team question whether it is just to improve the ratings that they are around so much, but walking around the hospital with them it becomes clear this is not the case.

They have pride in their service exuding from every pore. They greet every person, it seems, like a long-lost friend. They seem to know all things about everyone. "Hi Maria, how is your daughter, has she had the baby?", "Hi Simon, is it busy downstairs? I've some chocolates to drop off for the team from an ex-patient." Almost everyone including patients and relatives is greeted in a personal way. "Mrs. Burrell, hello! How are you doing now? Are you OK finding your way? Did the surgery help your knee?" Their warmth and interest are reciprocated and every person they engage with goes on their way with a smile on their face. We make slow progress because they seem to hug everyone. Slow but important progress because walking beside them shows us so much more about the trust culture than any bar graph could.

As they walk alongside us, they tell us about the people they come across and usually have some story to give a favourable impression. It's a hard sell wrapped up in loveliness but has also pointed us towards evidence that we wouldn't otherwise know about. One example included telling us about the work of the Chaplain in finding where the stillborn child of an elderly woman had been buried. We followed up on the lead and discovered an incredible story of a tenacious chaplain researching and using strong persuasive powers to track down a baby that had died 65 years, or so, previously and arranging for the mother to visit the place they were buried.

Leading isn't always about being designated as 'being in charge'. Through their role modelling, supporting others in challenging times and providing recognition when things might otherwise go unnoticed, they built a culture of kindness that spread throughout the trust.

Governance

"Good governance depends on ability to take responsibility by both administration as well as people. While transparency reduces corruption, good governance goes beyond transparency in achieving openness. Openness means involving the stakeholders in decision-making process. Transparency is the right to information while openness is the right to participation."

Narendra Modi (Indian Prime Minister).

What even is governance and why does it matter?

The need for governance exists anytime people come together to accomplish something. There are three key things that matter in good governance: authority, decision-making and accountability.

Governance determines who has overall authority, who makes decisions and the level of decision each person involved can make, how others can make their voice heard and how the information and outcomes are delivered.

Flixton Field Camp

I think I first became aware of the need for an organisation to have systems in place to ensure that boards remain accountable for the quality of care and that they consider the risks through my work with the children's charity. We'd started off as team leaders responsible for the entertainment and welfare of about six children. Over a couple of years, we'd become a bit concerned about variation in the quality of care, idiosyncratic local control and a lack of oversight from the board, which we felt had potential to leave children at risk. I was commissioned to write a set of basic policies (which didn't meet with universal approval), we introduced staff training and then we negotiated a programme of camp visits. Some called them inspections and were very hostile to the idea, some were more accepting and could see merit in peer review. Seasoned leaders were cross and felt the programme had been imposed by 'whippersnappers' who lacked their experience. We felt uncomfortable fronting an organisation where children became invisible for a fortnight. This was ten years after the inquiry into the death of Maria Cowell at the hands of her stepfather had highlighted a serious lack of co-ordination among services responsible for child welfare. I'd heard Arnon Bentovim talking about child abuse at Great Ormond Street, but child protection and the wider acceptance of child abuse was not on most people's radar. The child protection register, first known as an 'At Risk Register', wasn't established until 1975, as a national requirement for local authorities to improve contact in such situations. It remained very much a local authority issue until quite a bit later.

Our visits programme started off as a nice tour of the country visiting holiday camps, big and small. It took us to Suffolk, Devon, Gloucestershire, Northampton, Hampshire, Essex and Yorkshire. We saw some beautiful parts of the country and on the whole, enjoyed a couple of days at each camp understanding how it was run, checking the basics were sound and playing with children. Most were having a fabulous time, running under sprinklers, building campfires, playing cricket and making daisy chains. The facilities varied from site to site, the food had significant variability but, generally, the children were having huge fun in the English countryside. We had a few debates about managing homesickness and the best way to settle children at night, but nothing too awful jumped out at us.

Then we visited a beautiful site just outside a small Cotswolds village at the head of a green valley through which a gentle brook flowed, on its way to join the River Stour. Truly idyllic, with the most noise coming from cricket of both varieties and the repetitive popping of a tennis ball on a grass court. We found the camp with two lines of army tents on either side of a large field, a sports pavilion and a marquee strewn with bunting. The children were queuing for lunch when we arrived; a veritable feast of colour and smells, served by smiling women in flowery aprons. We had onion tart and salads, the children we sat with had whatever they wanted. We all had huge slices of chocolate cake and homemade ice cream. It seemed like a perfect holiday with the children telling us about riding lessons, milking goats and swimming at the 'big house'.

Then the vicar's wife came around the tables to talk to the children. She gave each group leader a piece of paper which we thought was for an after-lunch treasure hunt. It seemed not, as she was giving directions around the village as she spoke with each group. We were curious and asked what was happening. It seemed that the list was the 'bath and shower list'. Twice a week the children were allocated (a bit like evacuees) to villagers. This was to allow them to have a bath or shower at the host villager's house. One or two children, aged between 7 years and 13 years, were dropped off at each house and spent the evening there, having a bath or shower, getting laundry done and being pampered. Some chose to spend the night at the host's house.

Criminal Records Bureau checks for people working with children were still at least a decade in the future. We spoke with the camp organiser and said the practice had to stop; it was far too high-risk. They genuinely could not see any problem at all with the practice. We were told that it had been going on for years without problem and all the hostesses were good people, who were known personally to the vicar and his wife. It took a bit of explaining but the charity agreed that the practice was outdated and must stop. Sadly, the villagers decided it was too much interference and decided to stop offering holidays rather than compromise.

I don't know if any children were harmed when staying with the villagers; to the best of my knowledge none raised any concerns, but this was a time when children tended not to be believed. I'm sure most had a fabulous evening of total indulgence, but that could not be allowed to outweigh the risks that such a practice posed. I think all of us that were involved in the camp visits programme quickly realised that organisational oversight (or governance) needed to be more than just writing a report about the quality of food. It should be used to identify risks, to consider the threshold of risk the organisation is prepared to carry and to bring about improvements. Ensuring that staff understand that good governance should be far more than checking boxes and filling out forms, goes a long way to encouraging them to support and use the governance framework.

The United Nations Development Programme offers five key principles of good governance which relate to governments, but which are readily transferable to health or social care settings:

- Legitimacy and Voice: The United Nations Development Programme suggests that people should have a voice in decision-making, either directly or through legitimate intermediate bodies which represent them. Such broad participation is built on the idea of freedom of association and speech, as well as capacities to participate constructively.

- Direction.

- Performance: Including both responsiveness in meeting the needs of Accountability: Health and social care providers are accountable to the public, to external stakeholders and to several regulators. This accountability will differ depending on the organisation and the decision or action necessary. Transparency is built on the free flow of information about the service. Processes and information should be directly accessible to those who use or who are considering using the service as well as key stakeholders. Information should be provided to allow people to understand and monitor the service; people includes staff, service users, families, the public, external stakeholders and regulators.

■ Fairness: Good governance considers and promotes equality. It allows for anomalies related to people with protected characteristics to be identified and addressed, for example.

Governance is very variable and dependent on the type of organisation provided. A private ambulance service with two vehicles offering patient transport only, will have a vastly different governance framework to a small home for people with learning disabilities or a large NHS community mental health trust. They all need appropriate governance systems, but some will be far more complex and will collect, analyse, share and respond to far more information.

This is not the place to go into the full detail of the NHS governance processes; there are clear requirements set out in various documents that all trusts will be aware of. There should be a Board Assurance Framework that provides detailed information about the way that a trust board assures itself that they are meeting the legislative and contractual requirements. It's a whole other book. Where trust staff can use this information is probably to build on their information and involvement at team and department level, seeking the views of patients and families about the care and treatment provided by specific teams or specialties.

Governance, including clinical governance, is a way of benchmarking services, with the intention of improving the service by responding to specific measures and changes in outcomes. Those outcomes might be clinical or may be the wider service provision. The best services identify areas of their services which fall short of expectations in some way, through effective governance and they then respond to the shortfall and implement plans to ensure that aspect of a service improves rapidly. Governance is not simply a way of measuring and recording data; it should be a cycle that responds to variation in the data recorded by putting in support to improve the situation.

There is sometimes an awful lot of waffle around governance and seemingly endless spreadsheets feeding different stakeholders, yet it should be a very simple cycle in which the provider or board sets strategic goals from which operational objectives are agreed. How those objectives will be met and measured is agreed and implemented. The staff delivering the agreed actions record the data, which is collated and shared upwards (possibly through several tiers), becoming less detailed as it joins with information from other areas of the service, until it reaches the provider or board who see a wider picture of performance overall.

I think I may have just made that sound quite complex, so will give a specific example.

The corporate provider decided, using information they received from a service users survey, that people were not getting enough opportunities for physical activity to maintain mobility and core strength.

They set a strategic objective: 'We will improve access to physical activities for all service users'.

The executive team meets with the managers of their six care homes for older people and agrees operational goals.

- Each care home will have a planned programme of optional activities that will include four physical activities each week.
- Each care home will assess each resident's potential walking ability and support them to increase the distance they walk three times a week, wherever possible.
- Each care home will offer all residents an hour's supervised and supported, individual activity weekly.

Care home managers take the operational goals back to their individual services and discuss with staff what the intention is; they involve a member of the local frailty team, to help staff understand the importance of maintaining core stability and core strength.

They agree to discuss this with residents and their families at each service's Home Meeting.

Feedback from the meeting is positive. People are clear they would like a tea dance and opportunity to swim regularly. Some would like to walk to the corner shop but are frightened to do so on their own.

The member of staff feeds back from the Home Meeting to the staff meeting and possible solutions are identified, and an agreement reached about piloting a few activities. Staff are asked to record in individual records the distance people have walked and any increase over time. A rota is set up to offer each person an hours individual, supervised, physical activity overseen by a physiotherapist.

An annotated copy of the weekly activities programme is saved as evidence of which activities are offered and provided.

After two months the home managers meet again and bring the information about the increased activity goals. One home manager says it wasn't popular and nobody really wanted it, but they do not provide any evidence this is the case. Two home managers say the physiotherapist has worked with individuals, but staff haven't had time to help people walk more. Their activity programmes are incomplete but show the usual bingo, singalong and vintage afternoon tea. One home manager is absent.

The remaining two home managers can show new programmes that include weekly dancing added into the singalong session, a fortnightly minibus trip to a private hydrotherapy pool with relatives joining the residents to provide additional support in the water, and a new series of yoga and outdoor tai chi classes.

One has changed the accommodation around to move the dining room further away and encourages residents to walk there rather than automatically be pushed in a chair.

They say that it's too early to say, but they feel that people are sleeping better and are more mentally active during the day.

Additional help is provided to the homes struggling to make the changes and they too develop a series of more physical activities including helping put up decorations and introducing action songs to the singalong. One has started offering a trip for afternoon tea at a country park with a petting farm where residents must walk from the car park to the café and can also walk to a bench near the pond to feed the ducks.

Over time the services can demonstrate that they have more engagement with physical activity and can show improved night-time sleeping, fewer falls and less daytime sleeping through a process of daytime observations.

A specific resident, staff and relative survey provides evidence that the changes are universally popular with staff saying how nice it is to get out to the farm park and how much more involved they feel.

The data is collated into a report to feed up through the executive to the corporate provider. The corporate provider is able to share in their annual report that this has been a positive initiative and that falls within the participating homes have reduced by 28%.

The provider writes to staff in each home congratulating them for their work and sharing that the individual physiotherapy input will be funded as a permanent arrangement.

Good governance, strong evidence and few spreadsheets!

Governance is simply a system of using data to identify and mitigate risks, of understanding how well your service is performing and using that understanding to bring about improvements.

It is data from complaints, from incidents, from observations, from resident or patient group meetings, from staff or service user surveys or other feedback mechanisms, from audits and from improvement projects. It is about where your hazardous substances are stored and how well you manage records and medicines. It is about how clean your service is and about infection prevention and control. It can be huge and seem overwhelming, until you reduce it to bite sized chunks and share the responsibilities.

Nobody can possibly manage all the data, even in small services, without support and sharing the load. Governance, like safeguarding and end of life care, is everyone's business. People need to know who is responsible for what and what they are personally accountable for. That might be knowing who is responsible for checking and recording that the fridges are clean and the food is in date. The key aim is, of course, to avoid an old, half-eaten tub of prawn cocktail contaminating the ham sandwich it is next to, but it is also so that a pattern of potentially contaminated food being left open alongside fresh food can be addressed and the long-term risk reduced.

Virgin Care Services Limited

Virgin Care Services Limited are one of the Virgin brand providers of health and social care in England, with over 400 services under their umbrella. Virgin Care has a clear line of accountability flowing from the Board and Chief Executive through the management structure to individual practitioners and staff. They have one of the most comprehensive governance systems that I have seen with local teams taking responsibility for the governance in their areas.

Strong systems and processes are in place to provide assurance on the delivery of high-quality and safe care, to identify and manage risk and share good practice and learning. When Virgin Care takes on a new service it pledges to make that service better than it was before so that everyone can 'feel the difference'.

In 2017, I wrote their provider report which said, "Virgin Care have demonstrated through documented evidence that following acquisition of services it has managed to bring about sustained, significant improvements to patient care and that the leadership, management and governance were outstanding".

How do they do this?

One of the tools they had developed as part of their assurance framework was Internal Service Reviews, a comprehensive account of the way services were provided, completed by each team every six months.

The web-based tool used the CQC five key questions and Key Lines of Enquiry as a basis for assessing each area of care provided by Virgin Care Services Limited. Staff were required to complete the very comprehensive assessments, with supporting evidence to the governance team for analysis and benchmarking against other similar services or regions. Kit was detailed but as it was ongoing, it wasn't overly burdensome and gave a clear picture of improvement over time. It also meant any potential deterioration in services was picked up quickly and acted upon.

Where services rated themselves as anything other than 'Good' based on the responses to the questions and using a scoring matrix, then a review of why the score was less than 'Good' was held and the team were supported to make improvements. It wasn't punitive, there was no 'battering with KPIs' but an exploration of what the information was saying and how the team could best be supported to address any shortfalls.

The Board saw the review tool as both a monitoring tool and a development tool. Front line staff had worked with subject matter experts to create the review tool. Where services were new in scope, additional support and resources were made available to enable them to reach the benchmark of at least 'Good'.

If you are lucky, the person inspecting your service and drafting your report will be satisfied with a description of your governance policies and processes. Most experienced inspectors, however, will want to see the impact and effectiveness of those policies and systems.

There is absolutely no point having medicines management audits that identify the same problem with, say, illegible drug charts month on month, if nothing is done to change the situation. Little purpose in having an action plan that isn't completed and which doesn't bring about sustained improvements.

What governance would you expect in a smaller service?

Chiswick House, Norwich

The report says:

"Staff told us they could easily speak with managers who were open to and interested by new suggestions and ideas. Staff were actively encouraged to contribute ideas to shape the service through staff meetings, staff surveys and daily open communication with the management team. Staff were empowered to care in a way that they would care for their own family. They were encouraged to hold group meetings without members of the management team and to think creatively. An example of a member of staff following this direction from management was given. We were told the cook spoke with everyone to discuss and develop the menu. They took the creative approach of cooking example dishes as part of the discussions. This developed into people helping to cook their favourite dishes and producing recipe cards for the cook. The benefit of this was that people using the service contributed to the creation of dishes they enjoyed."

While on first consideration the paragraph above might not even be considered governance, it is a good example of sound governance. It is an idea that has evolved from giving people using the service and staff a voice. The ideas were piloted, and everyone had an opportunity to participate. Performance improved because people were having food they wanted and had chosen. It was a fair system that anyone could contribute to. I have no doubt that the cook also monitored food serving and storage temperatures; it's rare that someone goes above and beyond while ignoring the basics.

The report goes on:

"The service worked creatively to empower people living in the home to influence the care they received. For example, there were various mechanisms for people to express their views on the people who looked after them. The service's recruitment process included a 'resident recruitment panel'. This panel interviewed appointable candidates for the registered and deputy manager positions and their views determined the candidates selected. This ensured that the people living in the service had confidence that their care would be managed by someone they had previously met and liked.

The service also actively sought feedback from people about staff performance. The feedback was used to inform any areas of good practice or to highlight if any areas of performance needed to be addressed. The involvement of people in this way showed them that their views mattered and that they had some control over the way they were looked after."

Again, this might not on first read be considered governance but of course it is. It's quite brave governance to offer people using the service the opportunity to feedback on the support they receive from individual staff members. The governance is around measuring that which is hard to measure numerically. It offers a voice to people using the service and is quite empowering. It gives the leaders an accurate picture of staff performance which no tick box in the world could provide. The cycle can then be joined up with a report to the corporate provider as a percentage of positive comments, and any concerns can be escalated, then a discussion with the team about any trend or patterns can be identified. Direct feedback to individual staff is a real benefit, if managed well and used to coach improved performance. Of course, concerns raised should be addressed but such an open and inclusive culture is less likely to have hidden pockets of poor care.

The section below is the part of the report that most people would recognise as being about governance – the numerical data collection. It is important to make sure that the basics are in place, and that will involve checklists, but good governance goes beyond that to the next level. Assurance is about having the evidence, about collecting the numbers; governance is about service improvement.

"We saw excellent governance in practice. Internal audits demonstrated that the service benefitted from a robust and effective quality assurance mechanism, which ensured continual service improvement. Listening, learning and improving was central to the way the service functioned. Information was readily available, easy to follow and actions required to address any issues arising were promptly addressed. The service was compliant with regulatory and legislative requirements."

Your monitoring systems do need to be effective. You do need to comply with various bits of legislation. You are not going to get an 'Outstanding' rating if your governance systems do not identify and address shortfalls in basics such as:

- Fire Safety
- Electrical and equipment safety
- COSHH
- Food safety
- Cleanliness
- Consent and the requirements of the Mental Capacity Act 2005
- Equality and Diversity
- Safe staffing levels
- Staff training, including mandatory training completion
- Environmental risk
- Infection prevention and control and hand hygiene
- Record keeping
- Medicines management
- Incident reporting, management and learning
- Waste management

- Basic care needs assessment and management – pain, skin integrity, falls, nutrition and hydration, continence,
- Outcomes
- Engagement
- Statutory Notifications

All the above should be firmly embedded; they are about the minimum expectations of a good service. They are around the fundamentals of care. My hope is that providers will have all these and then can take the next steps, to challenge themselves and improve further what they offer. The difference between a sandwich made with a supermarket's value range loaf of bread with jam – nothing wrong, perfectly edible, fills bellies – but it's not the same as a hand-crafted sourdough bagel filled with local crab, avocado and tomato with a little chilli.

The sandwich analogy means you get to pick the sandwich at your next staff meeting – what quality of care do you and your staff want to deliver? It is almost entirely a choice about attitudes and commitment.

Quality Improvement

Most services and most staff want to deliver excellent care, I hope. In order to reach and sustain a point of excellence, it is necessary to adopt an attitude of continuous learning. Being good at something rarely happens by accident or without effort.

Gary Lineker, who I am told is one of England's most successful strikers of all time (I think this translates as pretty good at football), says, "I wasn't obviously outstanding as a young player. There were so many kids that were much better than me... I wasn't even the best in my own Sunday league team." He was dedicated and he worked hard. Like learning Spanish when he moved to Barcelona, he says, "You've got to commit the whole way".

It's the same with improving your service or your own practice; you have to work at it in an ordered and planned way. Wild card ideas can make a difference but sustained, planned effort is likely to see greater improvements that are sustainable.

There are all sorts of commercial Quality Improvement methodologies out there. Some are fairly incomprehensible and speak a different language. Some are quite simple. For smaller organisations, I would go with simple. Small steps, planned steps, steps everyone knows to complete the marathon. I'm not going into the detail of every QI process but think that whatever you use it should follow a consistent pattern and be directed towards improving a specific aspect of quality. That leads to the question about what quality is, I guess.

Please don't think that because you can't afford to send staff to Japan to learn from Toyota that you can't introduce a Quality Improvement culture to your service.

I would think 'Quality' in health and social care was the extent to which a provider met the five key questions about the care and treatment being delivered, as set out by the Care Quality Commission:

- Is it safe?
- Is it effective?
- Is it caring?
- Is it responsive?
- Is it well-led?

Most other considerations that might form part of the definition are contained within these five key questions. Consideration such as whether the service is person-centred or whether it is an equitable fit within the Commission frameworks. Where do you begin?

1. **Understand your service**

   I would suggest you begin by understanding your service and yourselves very well. Individual and group reflections on aspects of your service are an excellent starting point. Of course, I am going to suggest using the Reflective Journal that forms part of the Towards Outstanding book series. Spend time knowing what you do well and why and then use that as a foundation to build better practice on.

2. **Identify areas for improvement (problems)**

   Specific, easy-to-understand improvements. Not something as vague as 'improve mealtimes', for example. An issue such as 'Reduce the number of complaints about sandwich suppers' is a specific goal that everyone can understand and work towards, and would be easier to show improvement. Avoid overload.
   A small team of 15 staff can't drive improvements in all aspects of the service at the same time. Overloading staff will see disengagement and incomplete improvement projects. At the outset, I might be tempted to find a few 'quick wins' where improvement activity is simple, where staff and people using the service can see or feel a difference. A positive result at the start is going to motivate people to further improvements.

3. **Collect data**

   Collecting data will help you understand the nature of the things you identify as a problem. It should help you know how many steps you need to travel and at what speed, how to scope the improvement work, to reach the intended goal. Clearly, if you have identified that 62% of the Do Not Attempt Cardiopulmonary Resuscitation forms are incomplete, you might want to increase the resourcing of the project to bring about swift improvements. If, however, your staff thought that patients finding it difficult to get through to make an appointment was a problem they could improve on but the data showed that 87% of patients were happy with how easy it was to make an appointment, you might want to consider whether this was the most important area to focus on.

4. **Understand the pathway**

   You cannot bake a decent cake if you don't understand the recipe. You can't make the cake better unless you can reflect on the recipe and see where you perhaps didn't follow or where you could change it to make it even more delicious. This doesn't necessarily mean a referral or treatment pathway. It might be that you have seen a high level of medication errors, confirmed by data, showing that there have been three errors each week for the past month. Tracking the pathway for medicine administration, looking at when they happened, where they happened and where perhaps the correct process wasn't followed, might lead to potential solutions and improvement. Imagine that all the drug errors happened at lunchtime in the residents dining room; there would be little point introducing double checking of drugs administered overnight as a solution.

5. **Discuss the steps to reach the goal and identify the tools needed to get there**

   Again, you can talk at this in a complicated language, using highly technical QI systems, or you can follow a simple plan. The team or a small group from a wider team discuss the problem and the pathway. They consider as widely as possible what sustainable steps could be taken to bring about improvements. They agree an end point – a measure of success – and interim measures, if it's a big project affecting a large number of staff. They agree how to measure improvement, what data to collect. The steps for the raised incidence of medicines errors might feature staff training, improved oversight with weekly audits or medicines charts. They might feature a 'Do not disturb' message on the medicine trolley or on a tabard for the person responsible for dispensing the medicines. They might be increasing the number of staff in the dining room so people have someone to ask for help who isn't involved in handing out medicines. It might be changing the timings of medicines so that the staff aren't trying to manage them at the same time that pudding is being served. It's not for me to tell you the best way to sort the issue – the staff who know and understand the service, or the people who use the service, will have the answers.

6. **Monitor and evaluate**

The idea of a quality improvement model is that you can embed and evidence improvements. In the medicines example above, just telling staff to make sure they check that everyone has their midday tablets isn't going to bring about sustained improvements, and even if it did, you couldn't prove that.

At the planning stage, the measures of success should be agreed. Data should be collated over the duration of the project and then reviewed. If the changes have resulted in improvement, then consideration of how to keep the changes as 'usual practice' need to be considered. If the changes haven't seen improvements, then they probably weren't the right changes to practice: the process needs revisiting and new ideas tried.

In larger organisations, you may want to trial or pilot a new way of working or new practice before rolling it out across the whole organisation. Having a QI lead is an excellent opportunity for a member of staff to 'step up' and build their own leadership skill base. In very large organisations there may well be a whole QI team, and people with formal qualifications - that being the case, you don't need me to tell you how to implement QI in your services.

For Adult Social Care Services, the National Institute for Health and Care Excellence (NICE) have published a Quality Improvement resource for adult social care. It offers a downloadable resource for commissioners, aimed at helping discussions around quality improvement in the sector. It may well also be useful to providers. https://www.nice.org.uk/about/nice-communities/social-care/quality-improvement-resource

Mission Health, North Caroline, USA

Mission Health is the state's sixth largest health system provider. They already used evidence-based sepsis care bundles. Their problem was that processes for identifying patients with sepsis was fragmented and varied widely across the system, which had resulted in poor outcomes.

By using a comprehensive data-driven approach to support the early identification of sepsis and by standardising the management of potential sepsis, including the addition of evidence-based alerts into their system, Mission Health could see where the barriers to early recognition and treatment lay. This information was used to drive improvements.

Changing and improving their approach for early recognition and treatment of sepsis, they achieved substantial improvements outcomes. These included:

■ 1% relative reduction in mortality for patients with severe sepsis and septic shock.

■ 9% relative difference in mortality for patients that received the evidence-based protocols compared to those who did not – the evidence-based protocols substantially reduce mortality.

■ 4% relative reduction in emergency department length of stay for patients with severe sepsis and septic shock.

■ 4% relative reduction in critical care length of stay for patients with severe sepsis and septic shock admitted from the emergency department.

Their health system continues to use this plan to improve sepsis outcomes. They are working on plans to move the early identification screening tools to the outpatient setting, including urgent care centres and primary care settings.

Mount Sinai, New York

The Mount Sinai Health System is an integrated healthcare system providing medical care to local and global communities. The system includes the Icahn School of Medicine at Mount Sinai and eight hospital campuses in the New York metropolitan area.

Mount Sinai's 'Lose the Tube' project focused on improving the outcomes associated with the use of urinary catheters. The hospital had realised that catheters were being given to patients who didn't need them, and that they were being left in too long. This presented a significant risk of patients developing urinary tract infections, as well as being undignified and reducing both independence and mobility.

The Quality Improvement project was aimed at decreasing the number of catheter-associated urinary tract infections in the hospital. Over five months, a new system of nursing documentation and protocols were introduced, that ensured patients in need of catheters were appropriately cared for and that patients were not given catheters unnecessarily or for too long.

The project successfully reduced the infection rate from 2.67 per month to 0.2 month. Something as simple as more regular and systematic checks was able to dramatically reduce infection for Mount Sinai.

Part 4 –
Conclusion

To finish

I said at the outset that this book was never intended to be a 'How to Guide'. It is not a Haynes Manual of health and social care. Every service is unique. There will be similarities, but it is having a distinct response to the needs and preferences of local communities and individuals that sets services apart.

It is not having current policies aligned to best practice that will make a service exceptional. They should be a given.

It is not having current care plans that reflect the assessed needs of individuals. They should be a given.

It is about leaders creating a culture where staff feel confident to question and share concerns; it is about a culture where people feel equal; it is about a culture that encourages innovation and learning.

Mainly it is about a positive attitude and keeping the best interests of those who use the service at the very heart of every decision and action.

How does one finish a book like this? I think the message I hope people take away is:

"Never doubt that a small group of thoughtful, committed citizens can change the world. Indeed, it's the only thing that ever has."
Margaret Mead

Where next? This book is intended as a trigger to help start a process of thinking and reflecting, perhaps in a slightly different way. Within the series are other titles that may help you progress from thinking as you walk the dog or have a bath, to action. The Towards Outstanding Reflective Journal is a practical guide for individuals that asks the questions that leaders and staff should be asking themselves.

The Learning Pack is a series of sessions that can be offered to groups of staff to help them reflect on issues raised within this book and consider how they can improve the care or treatment provided. The sessions can be applied to most service types and can be used for one off learning days or as a course.

Appendix One: Fundamental Standards of Care

The fundamental standards for health and social care providers became law in April 2015. They are not about excellence – they are, as the name suggests, the minimum expectations of providers of health and social care. They are the level below which a provider should not fall. If they are not met, then there is a likely breach of regulation.

The standards were introduced as part of the government's response to the Francis Inquiry's recommendations and are intended to help improve the quality of care and transparency of providers by ensuring that those responsible for poor care can be held to account.

The fundamental standards define the basic standards of safety and quality that should always be met and introduce criminal penalties for failing to meet some of them.

The standards are used as part of the Care Quality Commission's regulation and inspection of care providers.

The Commission will hold providers to account if they are not being met, including through the courts where appropriate. Registration of new providers or locations will also be dependent on compliance.

As part of the fundamental standards, a new duty of candour and fit and proper persons requirement for directors was introduced for NHS providers from October 2014 and extended to all providers from April 2015.

The fundamental standards are:

■ Care and treatment must be appropriate and reflect service users' needs and preferences
■ Service users must be treated with dignity and respect
■ Care and treatment must only be provided with consent

- Care and treatment must be provided in a safe way
- Service users must be protected from abuse
- Service users' nutritional and hydration needs must be met
- All premises and equipment used must be clean, secure, suitable and used properly
- Complaints must be appropriately investigated, and appropriate action taken in response
- Sufficient numbers of suitably qualified, competent, skilled and experienced staff must be deployed
- Persons employed must be of good character, have the necessary qualifications, skills and experience, and be able to perform the work for which they are employed
- Registered persons must be open and transparent with service users about their care and treatment (the duty of candour)

Appendix Two: Safeguarding

Safeguarding is included as an appendix rather than in the main text because there must be a commitment to good safeguarding practice; it comes before any aspirations to excellence. There is no scope for debate or discussion. Any shortfalls in good safeguarding practice will prevent a provider being awarded an 'Outstanding' rating for the safe domain. A provider who can't deliver good safeguarding practice is a way off excellence.

Safeguarding is a key priority for the Care Quality Commission and people who use services are at the heart of regulation. The Commission work to help safeguard children and adults reflects both our focus on human rights and the requirement within the Health and Social Care Act 2008 to have regard for the need to protect and promote the rights of people who use health and social care services.

Safeguarding means protecting people's health, well-being and human rights, and enabling them to live free from harm, abuse and neglect. It's fundamental to high-quality health and social care.

The Commission's role in safeguarding is to monitor, inspect and regulate services to make sure they meet the fundamental standards of quality and safety. The published guidance about their role says:

"For safeguarding, we will do this by:

■ Checking that care providers have effective systems and processes to help keep children and adults safe from abuse and neglect.

■ Using Intelligent Monitoring of information that we receive about safeguarding (intelligence, information and indicators) to assess risks to adults and children using services and to make sure the right people act at the right time to help keep them safe.

■ Acting promptly on safeguarding issues we discover during inspections, raising them with the provider and, if necessary, referring safeguarding alerts to the local authority – who have the local legal responsibility for safeguarding – and the police, where appropriate, to make sure action is taken to keep children and adults safe.

- Speaking with people using services, their carers and families as a key part of our inspections so we can understand what their experience of care is like and to identify any safeguarding issues. We also speak with staff and managers in care services to understand what they do to keep people safe.

- Holding providers to account by taking regulatory action to ensure that they rectify any shortfalls in their arrangements to safeguard children and adults, and that that they maintain improvements. Regulatory action includes carrying out comprehensive and follow-up inspections, requiring providers to produce action plans, taking enforcement action to remedy breaches of fundamental standards, and acting against unregistered providers.

- Publishing our findings about safeguarding in our inspection reports, and awarding services an overall rating within our key question 'Is the service safe?' which reflects our findings about the safety and quality of the care provided.

- Supporting the local authority's lead role in conducting inquiries or investigations regarding safeguarding children and adults. We do this by co-operating with them and sharing information where appropriate from our regulatory and monitoring activity. We assist the police in a similar way.

- Explaining our role in safeguarding to the public, providers and other partners so that there is clarity about what we are responsible for and how our role fits with those of partner organisations."

Other titles in the Towards Outstanding series

For more information, visit www.pavpub.com

Towards Outstanding
A Staff Training Resource for Health and Social Care

This resource is designed to facilitate and support the delivery of training for care services staff. Like other Towards Outstanding titles, it is built on the premise that reflection is a critical tool for driving improvement. Along with the core text Towards Outstanding: A Guide to Excellence in Health and Social Care (to which trainees require personal or shared access) and Towards Outstanding: A Self-Development Reflection Workbook (of which they should own a personal copy), it explains why reflection, assessment and continuous improvement are critical ingredients of exceptional care. With this foundation in place, a series of sessions spanning a wide range of topics allow staff to explore and collaborative plan the best way for their own organisation and team to move forward. Interactive and engaging, the wisdom and practical guidance contained in this resource can set any service on the road to an 'Outstanding' rating.

ISBN: 9781913414771

Towards Outstanding
A Self-Development Reflection Workbook

Reflection is a process by which professionals consider experiences to gain insights about their practice. It supports people to continually improve the way they work and the care they provide, it allows for mistakes to be accepted and analysed rather than repeated, and it is encouraged by professional bodies wishing to foster improvements in services and continuous professional development. Specifically designed for staff working across health and social care, this self-development workbook guides users to reflect on experiences, focus their thoughts, generate new ideas about what good practice looks like, and understand the impact of their actions on others. Expert CQC inspector Terri Salt stresses that through careful reflection everyone in service can make a difference – and that only when every member of staff seeks to do so can services move beyond the ordinary and start to become genuinely 'Outstanding'.

ISBN: 9781913414733

Towards Outstanding
Enabling Excellence in Care Home Provision

Outstanding residential care is personalised not packaged, and prevention is far better than dealing with the results of poor care. Yet driving improvement in service provision requires a process of continuous organisational learning to embed best practice. This unique resource provides all that is needed to create a framework for assessing a care home's strengths and weaknesses and taking the first steps on the road towards an 'Outstanding' rating. Drawing on decades of inspection experience, Terri Salt provides a suite of forms and templates that – with appropriate planning, discussion and collaboration – can serve as the basis for a full quality assessment as well as being built into a regular cycle of monitoring and continuous improvement. Using these tools, staff can learn to enjoy the experience of delivering the very best care to patients – and leaders can provide them with the tools and freedom required to do so.

ISBN: 9781913414818